ART THERAPY AND
CANCER CARE

FACING DEATH

Series editor: David Clark, Professor of Medical Sociology,
University of Lancaster

The subject of death in late modern culture has become a rich field of theoretical, clinical and policy interest. Widely regarded as a taboo until recent times, death now engages a growing interest among social scientists, practitioners and those responsible for the organization and delivery of human services. Indeed, how we die has become a powerful commentary on how we live, and the specialized care of dying people holds an important place within modern health and social care.

This series captures such developments. Among the contributors are leading experts in death studies, from sociology, anthropology, social psychology, ethics, nursing, medicine and pastoral care. A particular feature of the series is its attention to the developing field of palliative care, viewed from the perspectives of practitioners, planners and policy analysts; here several authors adopt a multidisciplinary approach, drawing on recent research, policy and organizational commentary, and reviews of evidence-based practice. Written in a clear, accessible style, the entire series will be essential reading for students of death, dying and bereavement, and for anyone with an involvement in palliative care research, service delivery or policy-making.

Current and forthcoming titles:

David Clark, Jo Hockley and Sam Ahmedzai (eds): *New Themes in Palliative Care*
David Clark and Jane E. Seymour: *Reflections on Palliative Care*
David Clark and Michael Wright: *Transitions in End of Life Care: Hospice and Related Developments in Eastern Europe and Central Asia*
Mark Cobb: *The Dying Soul: Spiritual Care at the End of Life*
Kirsten Costain Schou and Jenny Hewison: *Experiencing Cancer: Quality of Life in Treatment*
David Field, David Clark, Jessica Corner and Carol Davis (eds): *Researching Palliative Care*
Pam Firth, Gill Luff and David Oliviere: *Loss, Change and Bereavement in Palliative Care*
Anne Grinyer: *Cancer in Young Adults: Through Parents' Eyes*
Henk ten Have and David Clark (eds): *The Ethics of Palliative Care: European Perspectives*
Jenny Hockey, Jeanne Katz and Neil Small (eds): *Grief, Mourning and Death Ritual*
Jo Hockley and David Clark (eds): *Palliative Care for Older People in Care Homes*
David W. Kissane and Sidney Bloch: *Family Focused Grief Therapy*
Gordon Riches and Pam Dawson: *An Intimate Loneliness: Supporting Bereaved Parents and Siblings*
Lars Sandman: *A Good Death: On the Value of Death and Dying*
Jane E. Seymour: *Critical Moments: Death and Dying in Intensive Care*
Anne-Mei The: *Palliative Care and Communication: Experiences in the Clinic*
Tony Walter: *On Bereavement: The Culture of Grief*
Simon Woods: *Death's Dominion: Ethics at the End of Life*

ART THERAPY AND CANCER CARE

Edited by DIANE WALLER and CARYL SIBBETT

OPEN UNIVERSITY PRESS

Open University Press
McGraw-Hill Education
McGraw-Hill House
Shoppenhangers Road
Maidenhead
Berkshire
England
SL6 2QL

email: enquiries@openup.co.uk
world wide web: www.openup.co.uk

and Two Penn Plaza, New York, NY 10121-2289, USA

First published 2005

Copyright © The Editors and Contributors 2005

A catalogue record of this book is available from the British Library

ISBN-13: 978 0335 21620 8 (pb)   978 0335 21621 5 (hb)
ISBN-10: 0 335 21620 X (pb)   0 335 21621 8 (hb)

Library of Congress Cataloging-in-Publication Data
CIP data has been applied for

Typeset by RefineCatch Ltd, Bungay, Suffolk
Printed in Poland by OZGraf S.A.
www.polskabook.pl

Contents

List of figures		vii
Notes on the contributors		xi
Series editor's preface		xv
Acknowledgements		xvii
Foreword		xix
Introduction		xxiii

1   On death and dying   1
      Ken Evans

2   'Betwixt and between': crossing thresholds   12
      Caryl Sibbett

3   Body image and the construction of identity   38
      Ken Evans

4   Liminal embodiment: embodied and sensory experience in
      cancer care and art therapy   50
      Caryl Sibbett

5   Shoreline: the realities of working in cancer and palliative care   82
      Michèle Wood

6   A woman with breast cancer in art therapy   102
      Elizabeth Stone Matho

7   Art therapy as Perseus' shield for children with cancer   119
      Cinzia Favara-Scacco

8   The efficacy of a single session   128
      Jacqui Balloqui

9   Art therapy with a late adolescent cancer patient: reflections on
     adolescent development, separation and individuation, and
     identity form   137
     Kathryn Horn Coneway
10   The Healing Journey: a ten-week group focusing on long-term
     healing processes   149
     Elizabeth Goll Lerner
11   Musing with death in group art therapy with cancer patients   163
     Paola Luzzatto
12   Fear of annihilation: defensive strategies used within art
     therapy groups and organizations for cancer patients   172
     Barry Falk
13   Creating through loss: how art therapists sustain their practice
     in palliative care   185
     David Hardy
14   Art therapy in the hospice: rewards and frustrations   199
     Timothy Duesbury
15   A 'don't know' story: art therapy in an NHS medical oncology
     department   210
     Maureen Bocking
16   An art therapist's experience of having cancer: living and dying
     with the tiger   223
     Caryl Sibbett

Index   249

List of figures

All figures illustrating artwork are available on the following website: **www.openup.co.uk/arttherapyandcancercare.** They will be referenced in the text and are listed below with a brief description of each illustration.

Figure 2.1   Artwork: house, boy playing
Figure 4.1   Artwork: clay foot
Figure 4.2   Artwork: hands
Figure 4.4   Artwork: clay face and hair
Figure 6.1   Artwork: breast
Figure 6.2   Artwork: clay torso of a woman
Figure 6.3   Artwork: painting: 'A well-closed money pouch for hiding money'
Figure 6.4   Artwork: painting of inverted parabola: 'Balm of light that softens and heals'
Figure 6.5   Artwork: painting of circle within broken circle: 'Watery curves'
Figure 6.6   Artwork: painting: 'Getting rid of . . .' (cluster of dots)
Figure 6.7   Artwork: patch of paint disturbed by wavy lines: 'More structured red'
Figure 6.8   Artwork:
Figure 6.9   Artwork: tree-like drawing: 'Power'
Figure 6.10   Artwork: painting of goblet filled with pleasure
Figure 6.11   Artwork: painting, upward swirling shapes: 'Papa, I see life in colour'
Figure 6.12   Artwork: painting, round shape with diagonal upward strokes: 'Gestures upwards'
Figure 6.13   Artwork: drawing of cemetery: 'Confronting death'

Figure 6.14   Artwork: drawing of spiral
Figure 7.1   Art therapy allows the spontaneous release of anguishing experiences
Figure 7.2   Regressive painting activities allow preschoolers to express the most anxiety-provoking experiences
Figure 7.3   Creativity helps parents to have a lively dynamic interaction with their child
Figure 7.4   Medical play to clarify illness and offer control over threatening reality
Figure 7.5   A six-week-old baby has primary needs to take care of. Creativity offers ways to let him 'speak' them out
Figure 7.6   A six-week-old baby has many things to 'tell' us, mostly if he is in a hospital
Figure 7.7   Art therapy creative core offers infinite ways to avoid dismissing children's needs
Figure 7.8   There are many creative ways to mould a hospital room into a cosy environment
Figure 7.9   Art therapy helps parents overcome their sense of impotence and uselessness, allowing emotional closure
Figure 8.1   Artwork: drawing of tree and dog
Figure 8.2   Artwork: drawing of black flower
Figure 8.3   Artwork: drawing of stream with trees and animals
Figure 8.4   Artwork: setting sun over sea, wall and trees
Figure 8.5   Artwork: bowl of fruit on table, dog on lead, vase
Figure 9.1   Artwork: circular photo collage
Figure 9.2   Artwork: drawing of house, large head, trees
Figure 9.3   Artwork: drawing of head surrounded by sets of features
Figure 9.4   Artwork: mandala
Figure 9.5   Artwork: white pastel on black paper – hands reaching out
Figure 9.6   Artwork: white dot surrounded by circle of stick figures
Figure 9.7   Artwork: image of tree/divided path
Figure 9.8   Artwork: circular photo collage, completed
Figure 10.1   Artwork: three abstract figures: 'Acceptance'
Figure 10.2   Artwork: drawing of angel, flowers
Figure 10.3   Artwork: painting of rose bush surrounded by tears
Figure 10.4   Artwork: painting of willow tree
Figure 10.5   Artwork: painting of dogs
Figure 10.6   Artwork: painting: diamond shape, dark mass with threads and rainbow
Figure 13.1   Artwork: young man dressed in the fashion of the 1950s
Figure 13.2   Artwork: what happen's next?
Figure 13.3   Artwork: on reflection cannot be sure
Figure 16.1   Artwork: self-collage of tree
Figure 16.2   Artwork: torso of woman with wounded head: 'Limbo'

Figure 16.3   Artwork: figure of a woman in foetal position: 'Living Bone?'

Figure 16.4   Artwork: clay figure of a woman: 'Clay Female'

Notes on the contributors

Jacqui Balloqui is an integrative psychotherapist in private practice specializing in traumatic loss and bereavement. She is also a practising artist and art therapist, trained at Goldsmiths College, where she was awarded the Corinne Burton Scholarship enabling her to specialize in palliative care. She works part-time as an art therapist at St Margaret's Hospice, Taunton, and is involved in ongoing art therapy research. She has previously worked in mental health as an assertive outreach worker and extensively with children and young people as a community artist and youth worker, specializing in multicultural work and anti-discriminatory practice.

Maureen Bocking has worked as the Corinne Burton Art Therapist in the Medical Oncology Department at St Bartholomew's Hospital, London since 1998. She also runs weekly open groups for patients in daycare at the North London Hospice, Finchley. Maureen has had wide clinical experience of work with children and adults in a variety of settings, both residential and community-based, and in education. She has been a tutor on the postgraduate art therapy training scheme at the University of Hertfordshire for the past two years. Her ambition is to retire to the country and paint.

Timothy Duesbury graduated from Goldsmiths College art psychotherapy course in 2000. He was awarded the Corinne Burton Scholarship at the commencement of his studies and through its financial assistance was able to extend his first art therapy post for two years. Prior to Goldsmiths he gained an honours degree in arts therapies at the University of Derby, where he had a placement at London Lighthouse with HIV clients. He has also worked at a central London hospital involved in the care of children living with cancer. He now works in palliative care in a charity in London, in an NHS unit in Surrey and in a private hospital for neurological rehabilitation.

Ken Evans combines his academic and professional interests by working as a consultant and lecturer in social policy and social sciences, contributing to the Master's degree in group and intercultural therapy at Goldsmiths College and to the research programme in that area. After graduating in philosophy at London, he took a BSc in sociology and psychology at Bristol, followed by an MA in social theory and a DPhil at the University of Santa Tomas, Philippines. He is a Fellow of the Royal Anthropological Society and has conducted research in mental health, elderly care, education and training for social work. His current interests are in combining and integrating theoretical perspectives from all fields of human traditions and categories in the application of care.

Barry Falk is an artist and art therapist. While training at Goldsmiths College he was awarded the Corinne Burton Scholarship, enabling him to specialize in work with cancer patients and those with terminal illness. He has pioneered art therapy services in palliative care in Sussex and also established the first art therapy service within early onset dementia care in Brighton. He has participated in a control group study evaluating the effectiveness of art therapy with older people with dementia carried out in Brighton and Newhaven between 2000 and the present, and is currently engaged, with Professor Waller, in a research project which aims to extend our knowledge of the value of art therapy for clients with cancer.

Cinzia Favara-Scacco was born in Catania, Italy and attended art school prior to taking a degree in psychology at the University 'La Sapienza' in Rome. She then went on to take a Masters in art therapy at the Pratt Institute in New York. During her placement at the Mount Sinai Hospital in New York, she was able to work with sick children and decided subsequently to specialize in work with children who have cancer. She returned to work in Sicily. Eight years on she is a psychologist and art therapist at the Paediatric Haematology–Oncology Unit of the Catania Polyclinic. She is involved in developing projects which offer support not only to children with cancer but also to their parents.

Elizabeth Goll Lerner has 23 years' experience in the field of art therapy. She has worked in a variety of in-patient and outpatient settings with a wide range of psychiatric and medical illnesses. She is in private practice and is an adjunct professor at the George Washington University's (Washington DC) graduate programme in art therapy. Her special interests are in mind/body medicine, archetypal psychology, psychosynthesis and transformational process.

David Hardy qualified as an art therapist from Goldsmiths College in 1996. He received a Corinne Burton Scholarship and did his placement within a hospice. Since then he has worked at Sir Michael Sobell House, a hospice in Oxford, and at the North Gate Centre in Colchester. Before training in art therapy he had worked as a staff nurse, mainly in palliative care.

Kathryn Horn Coneway is a 2003 graduate of the George Washington University art therapy programme in Washington DC. She was the 2002 recipient of the American Art Therapy Association Anniversary Scholarship Award and was a co-editor of the newsletter for the GW art therapy programme. She works at a cancer centre in a large urban university hospital with outpatient oncology, and in-patient bone marrow transplant patients. Her clinical experience includes work with disturbed children and adolescents in a therapeutic school setting, and with adult and adolescent cancer patients. Kathryn is also an exhibiting artist and finds that her own creative work informs her understanding and ability to guide her clients' process. She has worked as a documentary photographer and is particularly interested in integrating photography with other artistic modalities in developing interventions.

Paola Luzzatto has a background in philosophy and comparative religion. She trained in art psychotherapy at Goldsmiths College and in psychodynamic psychotherapy at the Tavistock Institute, London. Paola has worked with adult psychiatric patients in South London for several years. She then moved to New York and worked for ten years with cancer patients at the Memorial Sloan-Kettering Cancer Center. She has written a number of articles on art therapy theory and techniques in professional journals in the UK, Italy and the USA where she also teaches on many university art psychotherapy training programmes. She received the 2004 Clinical Award from the American Art Therapy Association for her work with adult cancer patients.

Caryl Sibbett is Lecturer in the Graduate School of Education of Queen's University, Belfast and course director of the MSc in art therapy, which she helped to establish as the first art therapy training in Northern Ireland. She is a HPC registered art therapist and a BACP/UKRC registered counsellor. She works in both private practice and as a sessional art therapist in diverse organizations, such as cancer care, probation and prisons. Caryl is active within the Northern Ireland Group for Art as Therapy (NIGAT) and a former Chair. Her PhD research focuses on liminality in art therapy and the cancer experience, and on her personal experience of having cancer. Caryl has published papers in several medical or psychological journals and has presented papers extensively, both nationally and internationally.

Elizabeth Stone Matho is in private practice in Grenoble, France, with children and adults in art therapy and psychotherapy. She works with oncology patients at the Centre Hospitalier Universitaire de Grenoble. Formerly on the faculty of New York University, where she did her graduate studies, she has been involved in the training and supervision of art therapists in Italy,

Switzerland and the USA for nearly thirty years. She is also a graduate of the New York School of Psychotherapy and Psychoanalysis. She has lectured widely in Europe and the USA and is the author of numerous articles on art therapy.

Diane Waller is Professor of Art Psychotherapy at Goldsmiths College, University of London and a UKCP registered group analyst. She was visiting professor at Queen's University, Belfast, School of Psychology from 2000 to 2004 and currently holds that position at the Universities of Brighton and Ulster. Her research and publications have included the history and development of art therapy in the UK and Europe, action research on art therapy training in addiction services, art therapy with eating disordered clients and evaluative studies with older people with dementia. Her background in ethnography, intercultural therapy and the process model of sociology has led her to question many of the assumptions present in the 'caring' professions. She is a member of the Health Professions Council and was the first Chair of HPC's Education and Training Committee. Her other main interest is in the traditional arts of the Balkans.

Michèle Wood graduated with a degree in psychology and went on to train as an art therapist in 1987 and obtained her MA in art psychotherapy in 1999. She has worked with clients in hospice care, adult mental health, eating disorders, mainstream primary education and medical oncology, and with adults and children living with HIV and AIDS. Michèle is a founding member of The Creative Response, a special interest group within the British Association of Art Therapists, for art therapists working in supportive and palliative care, and remains an active member of their committee. She is also a member of the BAAT Equality Steering Committee. Michèle currently teaches part-time on the MA art therapy programme at the University of Hertfordshire and works as an art therapist at Marie Curie Foundation Hospice, Hampstead.

Series editor's preface

A number of striking changes seem to be taking place in the way we view cancer in the contemporary world. A disease once deeply stigmatised in the west has now been transformed by a new 'gaze' which has brought it from the backstage areas of human social relations into a much more central place within the contemporary culture of health and illness – witness the explorations of cancer in popular magazines, newspapers, television, literature and film. The metaphorical and narrative aspects of cancer experience are an important part of this process – and this potential for representation within the disease, for narrative and story, for visual and three-dimensional expression, seems to resonate for many patients and sometimes for professionals as well. One particular aspect of this is that a striking metaphor of much health care practice relating to cancer care has become that of 'the journey' – to encounter the disease is to enter on a path that may have many features – stages and phases; predictable and unpredictable elements; and perhaps most tellingly, the potential for personal growth and discovery. The growing interest in patients' stories, narratives, journals and diaries is one aspect of this. The potential for artwork and art-making to illuminate these processes is another.

In recent years, art therapists have been undertaking their work in a variety of settings where people with cancer can be found: in oncology units, in hospices, in palliative care services, in patients' own homes. In addition, some specialist voluntary organisations and non-profit foundations have been developed which place the use of art therapy very centrally within their concept of care. There is a sense in which art therapy has become acknowledged as part of the legitimate spectrum of activities that make up the modern portfolio of cancer care. Art therapists have become more numerous, training and supervision opportunities have expanded, and awareness of the role of art-making and interpretation within the cancer 'journey' has never been greater.

All of these factors make *Art Therapy in Cancer Care* a welcome addition to the Facing Death series. Here is a book that makes a substantial contribution to our understanding of the place of art therapy in the cancer care setting. Its contributors are in the main experienced practitioners who bring to their writing an acuity of observation, an attention to detail and a sense of engagement with day to day practice that make for compelling reading. In particular this is a book that is rich in reflective and reflexive thinking – making for intellectual stimulation and challenge as well as practice innovation.

Almost 20 books have now appeared in this series. It is telling that we have so far been without a contribution on art therapy. Several earlier volumes have touched on related themes. Mark Cobb's analysis of spiritual care at the end of life[1] makes for interesting parallel reading. Likewise the collection of writings edited by Pam Firth, Gill Luff and David Oliviere on loss, change and bereavement[2] explores related territory. The collection on grief, mourning and death ritual, edited by Jenny Hockey, Jeanne Katz and Neil Small[3] is also complementary to the present volume.

Diane Waller is a Professor of Art Psychotherapy at Goldsmiths College, University of London. Caryl Sibbet directs the MSc in art therapy at Queen's University, Belfast. Together they have written and edited a series of fascinating chapters that cover theoretical exploration, detailed case studies, and commentaries on the organisational and practical issues that shape the delivery of art therapy. They raise questions about the place of art therapy within the evolving policy context for cancer care and highlight the importance of evaluation and the development of an evidence base for this sort of work if it is to gain further recognition and appropriate funding. *Art Therapy in Cancer Care* is a rich and stimulating collection of writings. I commend it wholeheartedly to readers of the *Facing Death* series and to anyone interested in the modern care of persons with cancer.

David Clark

References

1 Cobb, M. (2001) *The Dying Soul: Spiritual Care at the End of Life*. Buckingham: Open University Press.
2 Firth, P Luff, G Oliviere, D eds (2004) Loss, *Change and Bereavement in Palliative Care*. Buckingham: Open University Press.
3 Hockey, J., Katz, J. and Small, N eds (2001) *Grief Mourning and Death Ritual The Dying Soul*. Buckingham: Open University Press.

Acknowledgements

The editors would like to thank all of the contributors for their chapters and for being so efficient in meeting deadlines. Also to the many clients who have allowed their experience and art work to be included. We also much appreciate the efforts on our behalf of Rachel Gear, Hannah Cooper and the team at Open University Press/McGraw Hill, who have supported and encouraged us throughout, and the input of David Clark as series editor. Above all we are sincerely grateful to Sir Michael Burton for writing the Foreword and for his enthusiasm and generosity to the field of art psychotherapy in cancer care. We extend also our warmest thanks to the Trustees of the Corinne Burton Trust for their confidence in our work.

We are sad that Professor Ben Pimlott, late Warden of Goldsmiths College, who died in 2004 of Leukaemia, cannot share in this celebration of the Trust's work – we greatly miss his support and commitment.

Foreword

'She suddenly realised the crocodile was her cancer . . .'[1]

This is one of the many striking sentences in this extraordinary book. When my wife Corinne, artist, book illustrator, wife and mother of four young daughters, died, aged only 42, of cancer, in June 1992, and a large number of her friends and family wished to commemorate her name, we knew that we wanted to find a cause which would do good and fill, if possible, a previously unmet need, but also one which was both connected to her beloved art and also reflected the courage and determination with which she had fought against her cancer. She had, in those last hard months, been totally focused and implacably determined not to give in. Her way was not only to live her life, and, particularly, her role as a mother, to the full, until the very last gasp, but also to step up the hours of calm and concentration spent on art, especially, towards the end, in the pernickety skills of china painting. Her art not only took her full attention at a time when she might otherwise have given in to depression, but also encouraged those same virtues of calm, composure and pertinacity with which she fought against her disease. She would indeed have agreed with one of Caryl Sibbett's patients that *'during art-making time disappears'*.[2]

But we had no real idea, when we came to realise that the cause which we were looking for, and which seemed so obviously right, was the support of art therapy for cancer sufferers, what art therapy actually was. As Mandy

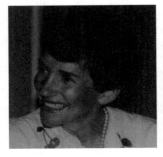

Corinne Burton, a talented artist and book illustrator, wife of Sir Michael Burton and mother of four daughters, Josephine, Isabel, Genevieve and Henrietta, died of cancer aged only 42 in June 1992. The Corinne Burton Memorial Trust, which supports art therapy in cancer care, was set up in 1992 by her family and many friends, to commemorate her.

Pratt says,[3] '*Art therapy is sometimes confused with diversionary creative activities*'. It is not simply the fact that art, like other recreations, can be therapeutic. This extraordinary book explains so much, but in 1992 we were only learners, and we did not know how much there was both to learn and admire. It was also early days for the particular field of art therapy in which it seemed so right for us to be involved – art therapy in cancer care, now the subject matter of this very book. There had been no tradition of art therapy being available for those suffering from potentially incurable diseases. As Professor Diane Waller herself says,[4] the psychotherapeutic profession has '*traditionally worked on a longer term basis*'. Cancer patients sadly cannot be guaranteed any '*longer term*'.

Only a small handful of pioneers were then working in the field: Camilla Connell, perhaps the doyenne of those practising in the area, at the Royal Marsden Hospital, inspiring author of the wonderful book '*Something Understood: Art Therapy in Cancer Care*',[5] Diane Waller herself, not then a professor but simply Head of Department at Goldsmiths College, London University,[6] and Mandy Pratt and Michele Wood,[7] who spearheaded the formation of the group Creative Response specifically for those art therapists who were becoming interested in specialising in palliative care, particularly in the cancer field. With their help and guidance we have been able to sponsor practising Corinne Burton Art Therapists – the most recent of these, Maureen Bocking, based at Barts and Royal London Hospitals, and enthusiastically supported by Dr Gallagher, Head of the Oncology Unit, is a contributor to this book – and Corinne Burton students. At Goldsmiths College itself we have funded a series of what has now amounted to 16 enthusiastic and talented art therapy students, many of whom, as can be seen from this book (to which four, Jacqui Balloqui, Timothy Duesbury, Barry Falk and David Hardy, have contributed), have gone on to make a valuable and original contribution to art therapy in cancer care.

So we were right at the cutting edge, and our learning process began quickly. What then have we learned of art therapy? So much of what there is to learn about art therapy is contained in this work. The book runs the gamut, from analysis of the philosophical justification for, and exposition of, the science of art therapy – accompanied by classical allusions from Charon to Perseus – through to an account of the problems, faced on a day-to-day basis by practising art therapists, not just the emotional problems, as patients to whom they have grown attached lose their battle,[8] but also the practical problems of working practices in hospitals and hospices, and working spaces (or the lack of them).[9]

Art therapy is described by Camilla Connell[10] by stressing '*how the symbolic component of art can facilitate the expression of strong and sometimes conflicting feelings which may be considered too difficult to put into words*'. She describes '*the facility of art therapy to mobilise previously untapped resources by accessing the unconscious*'. How does the art therapist set about his or her task, the task which Luzzatto describes[11] as the development of a *'personal imagery'* by the patients, on a *'creative journey'*? Jacqui Balloqui describes[12] *'the therapist's obligation to be constantly aware of personal thoughts, feelings and bodily sensations, as well as visual, verbal and bodily clues from the patient'.*

How do they do it? Timothy Duesbury[13] refers to the therapist's *'chronic niceness'*: which must be an awful strain – he himself recognises[14] *'the reward and the frustration of work in palliative care'.* The patients *'do not just bring with them cancer and death, but all aspects of their lives'*.[15] Significantly it is the patient who is encouraged first to paint or draw, or to use other artistic products such as clay or sand, and then to explain what he or she has produced – crocodile or otherwise. It is not the therapists who tell the patient what to draw, or what has been drawn, for they are not interpreters of dreams, like Moses, but rather mouthpieces for the patient, leaving it to the patient to describe what he or she feels or has expressed.[16] Maureen Bocking explains vividly how this occurs: *'I walk into people's personal spaces with my box of paper and art materials and our eyes meet.'*[17] She describes[18] how a young man who *'could not bear to see the sunshine outside the window, because he could not go out and live his normal life'* discovered that *'visualisation through art could set his mind free from the feeling of being trapped by illness, at least for a while'.*

But David Hardy explains how not only the patient's feelings are engaged, but the therapist's own emotions too, by reference to the concepts of *transference* and *reciprocity*;[19] while the academic analysis of the relationship between the patient and the therapist is fascinatingly explored by Caryl Sibbett.[20] We are also given an insight into the practicalities: the differences between working in a hospice and in a treatment centre,[21] and between working with individuals and with groups, where the process of death is the more obvious as the membership of the group changes or diminishes, and how the approach, and indeed the co-operation, of patients may depend upon such practical questions as the attitude of the nursing staff.[22]

The real achievement of art therapists in this field is to recognise their own limitations. They are dealing with a disease which they – indeed in most cases the doctors – cannot cure. Yet their role is a vital one in giving the patient an insight, and hopefully an additional will to fight. The cancer patient is in limbo.[23] The art therapist can help to provide a way out of limbo or at least a signpost. Luzzatto describes[24] how *'it is quite common that a patient draws a symbol of vulnerability and mortality, and in the same picture adds a symbol of strength and life. Here the power of art therapy is particularly effective: what is not possible in the verbal process is possible with symbolic imagery'.* Caryl Sibbett, whose patient so vividly depicted and described her cancer as a crocodile and *'it's never the same again, because you know the crocodile exists and you are always waiting for him to come and bite again'*,[25] describes her own unfortunate experience of having cancer as *'living and dying with the tiger'*.[26] The therapist is giving the patient the best chance to hang on in and win.

Corinne fought her own tiger on her own, and held it at bay for as long as she possibly could by positive thinking and positive doing. That is the help which art therapists can give, and perhaps the very fact that a famous passage by Dylan Thomas is drawn on not once but twice in the course of this book, both by a contributor[27] and, perhaps even more significantly, by a patient, who made a reference to it the title of one of her own last sketches.[28] means that it should be the inspiration for all art therapists in cancer care:

'*Rage, rage against the dying of the light.*
Do not go gentle into that good night.'

Sir Michael Burton
A Trustee of the Corinne Burton Memorial Trust

The Corinne Burton Memorial Trust is a registered charity (No. 1015586) and welcomes any donations: its address is c/o Citroen Wells, Devonshire House, 1 Devonshire Street, London W1N 1DR

Notes

1 Sibbett, Chap 2, p. 17.
2 Sibbett, Chap 2.
3 Quoted by Falk at Chap 12, p. 175.
4 Introduction at p. xxiv.
5 Whose publication in 1998 the Corinne Burton Memorial Trust was fortunately able to help support.
6 Author of many books, including *Art Therapies and Progressive Illness: Nameless Dread*, 2002.
7 Editors of *Art Therapy in Palliative Care: The Creative Response*, 1998.
8 Esp. Evans, Chap 1.
9 See e.g. Falk, Chap 12 and Duesbury, Chap 14.
10 Quoted by Hardy, Chap 13, pp. 185–6.
11 Chap 11, pp. 165–70 and as described by Hardy, Chap 13, pp. 187–8.
12 Chap 8, p. 134.
13 Chap 14, p. 202.
14 Chap 14, p. 208.
15 Duesbury, Chap 14, p. 208.
16 See e.g. Horn Coneway, Chap 9, p. 145 and Hardy, Chap 13, p. 193.
17 Chap 15, p. 212.
18 Chap 15, p. 214.
19 Chap 13, p. 187; see also Balloqui at Chap 8, pp. 129, 135.
20 Chaps 2, 4, 16.
21 Falk, Chap 12.
22 Falk, Chap 12, p. 177.
23 Sibbett, Chap 2, pp. 16–8.
24 Chap 11, p. 170.
25 Chap 2, pp. 17–8.
26 Chap 16, title.
27 Evans, Chap 3, p. 39.
28 Cited by Luzzatto, Chap 11, p. 169.

Introduction

Diane Waller and Caryl Sibbett

For many years, the province of the art therapist was mental health services. Art therapists pioneered work with so-called chronically mentally ill patients in large psychiatric hospitals. With the move to close these hospitals and establish more day-based and acute services, and with the welcome increase of training possibilities, research and professional development, art therapists have taken their experience of working with extreme emotional distress into a new area, that of working with people who are suffering from serious and even incurable illness such as HIV/AIDS, cancer, Parkinson's, Alzheimer's, Huntington's Chorea, motor neurone disease and brain injury. Art therapists have had to come to terms with the fact that many of their clients are almost certainly likely to deteriorate and to die, so they have needed to face death as a central aspect of their work. With cancer patients, there is of course possibility of cure or remission, but often the person exists in a kind of limbo, as Caryl Sibbett so poignantly describes, and it is difficult to stay with one's client in this space.

It does seem that art therapy can be helpful for people with cancer, whatever their status – recently diagnosed, during treatment, in remission, facing death – but unfortunately there has been a hard struggle to establish services. All the more reason, then, why the work of the Corinne Burton Trust is so inspiring. The Trust, formed after the tragic early death of Corinne Burton, an artist who had herself benefited from art therapy in the days before she died, has already had a significant influence on the development of art therapy services in hospitals and hospices. It has sponsored art therapy posts in the UK and, very importantly, sponsored at least one full-time art therapy trainee each year from Goldsmiths College by paying fees in total and providing the equivalent in fees for two years' service development, post-graduation. It seemed essential, then, to mark the ten years of the Trust's existence by preparing a book which would celebrate the efforts of many of the graduates and to put these efforts in the context of theory and practice by pioneers in this field. At the same time, we do not wish to overlook the excellent contribution to cancer care that has been made by the Arts for Health movement, notably by Michael Petrone – himself a sufferer who has, by the example of his own artwork and writing, and by his generous sharing of experience, helped hundreds of cancer sufferers and care staff to engage in creative activity. Our thanks are also due to Professor Betty Bednarski, who was very enthusiastic about our idea for the book and kindly sent us *Illness and Healing: Images of Cancer* by Robert Pope, and *The Art of Robert Pope* by Jock Murray, Professor of Medical Humanities in Halifax, Nova Scotia. An exhibition of Pope's work was sponsored by the Foundation of the same name, which we feel has much in common with the Corinne Burton Trust. Although there are obviously differences in Arts for Health and art therapy, practitioners of both are convinced of the healing potential of all the arts. For the purposes of this book, we will mainly focus on visual art therapy while acknowledging that much work is being done by the other arts and arts therapies (music, drama, dance movement, poetry for example).

This book, then, is conceived around three main issues and these will run throughout the text: first, a broadly theoretical perspective on art therapy and cancer care – this is not presented as a single chapter but many of the contributors have introduced the literature that they have found helpful and which relates to the particular aspect of art therapy and cancer which preoccupies them. The fact of death and dying, the effects of cancer on identity, on body image and gender disruption will be discussed from several perspectives.

A second aspect of the book will focus on examples from experienced practitioners from the UK, Italy, France and the USA. These discuss various client groups – children, adolescents, adults. Practice is informed by theory, and we will see that the contributors to this book often refer to each other's already published work, demonstrating that there is a strong network of practitioners working in palliative care, both across the UK and abroad. There are chapters by the graduates who held the Corinne Burton Scholarship or who have been sponsored by this Trust, and who have gone on to set up art therapy services. Their case studies and discussion of the realities of establishing services, and of working as usually the solo art therapist in a team, show that they are really pioneers in this field. We learn how they sustain their work and themselves in emotionally demanding circumstances. We also learn how institutional dynamics, and whether or not the treatment is supported at a high level, can affect the outcome for patients.

A third aspect is the personal reflections of art therapists who have themselves experienced cancer, showing how they have sought to understand their reactions as both professionals and patients. They draw on theory from philosophy, psychology, the arts and anthropology to sustain themselves, but they also discover, sometimes unexpectedly, other support systems. They describe how this personal experience has affected their practice and given them a greater understanding of the need to be flexible in providing services.

A combination of approaches can be found in the book, reflecting the training, background and personal experience of the therapist or writer. Readers may observe some differences in style and approach from the contributors who are working in the USA, where more structured and 'directive' methods have tended to be favoured over the psychodynamic, 'non-directive' approaches of the UK. Narrative research methods have been found to be extremely important in both countries, and are relevant to art therapists, as patients can tell their story both in words and images. Both editors were fortunate enough to attend the British Medical Association Conference, Narrative Research in Health and Illness (September 2004) and were moved by the many presentations which featured cancer experience. Insights from anthropology and sociology, as well as from psychoanalytic theory and aesthetics, inform several contributions. Some chapters focus on the actual hands-on work with clients, discussing the context in which they work and the importance of institutional support, whereas others are philosophical in nature but raise and discuss many of the same questions that we all have to consider when we enter this field.

As an introduction to the book and to place it within the context of the Facing Death series, Ken Evans shares his thoughts on death and dying and thinks about his early encounters with death. He leads us into thinking about good and bad death and dying, describing a good death as one where engagement with the dying is maintained until the final moments and possibly beyond this time, and to considerations about what it means to be human, to be a person. Following on, and developing the profound ideas from Evans' paper, Caryl Sibbett explores the significance of rites of passage, particularly the liminal phase, in relation to the cancer journey and art therapy in cancer care. She considers the relevance to such rites of passage of symbolic expression and experiences of 'flow', communitas and the ludic. Her chapter also examines the relevance to art therapy of time and timelessness, space, and Foucault's concept of the hererotopia. As if continuing a dialogue, Ken Evans' second chapter discusses the social construction of identity and its maintenance as a continual process throughout our lives. Psychological theories provide a base line for other explanations about identity, especially the highly detailed descriptions that underpin the current wide-ranging psychotherapeutic theories of 'self'. These issues are explored as a context to discussion about body image, given that our bodies become the means through which we express institutional contradictions. Evans begins to bring in a theme which we will see emerging in later chapters, that of the powerlessness experienced by cancer sufferers as they hand themselves over to institutions, and indeed the powerlessness felt by therapists in the face of negative institutional dynamics and the fact of the imminent death of their patient.

The important role of the senses in relation to the cancer journey is discussed in Caryl Sibbett's second chapter about body and embodiment. She discusses aspects of art therapy and the cancer experience related to various senses – touch, movement, kinaesthetic. Issues relevant to body image are explored, including disfigurement and scarring. Scars can be experienced ambiguously as negative, and/or as a mark of survival or of the 'warrior'. Orbach's concept of the true and false body is introduced and linked with Winnicott's true and false self. Gender issues are discussed, together with the role of art therapy in helping patients to express and manage potential gender disruption – as with deprivation of gender identity in the form of hair, breast, ovaries, testicles, prostate.

Michèle Wood, another long-standing pioneer of the profession in the UK, looks at where art therapists are employed and how they are located within their organizations, with some links to the British National Institute for Clinical Excellence guidelines. In her aptly titled chapter, 'Shoreline: the reality of working in cancer and palliative care', she explores essential aspects of an art therapist's practice: confidentiality, dilemmas around the storage, retention and disposal of clients' artwork, and the ethics of using the artwork for teaching and publication are discussed. Wood asks how the reality of cancer and the sense of impending death can impinge on therapeutic boundaries. This chapter, which contains a helpful literature review, leads us into the area of clinical practice with specific client groups.

We begin with Elizabeth Stone Matho's moving account of individual art therapy with a woman with breast cancer, in which her practice is informed by a psychodynamic model. Elizabeth was trained in the USA but has spent much of her recent working life in Italy, France and Switzerland and her approach reflects this interesting multicultural dimension. This is a very erudite demonstration of the best of art therapy, with a clear interaction between the client, the therapist and the images. We become intimately involved with the client's story through her remarkable clay models and the dialogue between her and the art therapist.

The chapter by Cinzia Favara-Scacco, an Italian colleague with experience of work in England and the USA, again brings us close up to the cancer patient, this time a child. Favara-Scacco's chapter introduces the painful prospect of childhood cancer and how the art therapist may structure the sessions to enable the child and his parents to remain close together, through that desperately painful phase of the child's dying, right up to his actual death. Jacqui Balloqui, a recent Corinne Burton graduate, describes how effective a single session of art therapy can be. This concept has also been discussed by Wood (see Chapter 5) and is a difficult one to grasp in a psychotherapeutic profession which has traditionally worked on a longer term basis. Kathryn Horn, working in the USA, presents a case study of a young woman. She describes the way that creativity can aid the process of individuation and the role of the art therapist as a witness and guide in creative therapy. The case study involves the young woman's active treatment and the period immediately following it, and how the developmental tasks of late adolescence were disrupted by the diagnosis. The chapter will show how art therapy allowed her better to anticipate difficulties and to communicate her needs to others. A different aspect of group art therapy is provided by Elizabeth Goll Lerner, also from the USA. This chapter describes a group that allows patients the opportunity to explore their relationships to their illness from a physical, emotional, psychological and spiritual perspective. Participants are invited to find a voice that relates to their essential experiences and their authentic self. Questions are asked, such as: How do people react to serious illness at different life stages? How does this change over time, and how do the groups affect the participants? Paola Luzzatto, a long-standing Italian pioneer in art therapy with cancer patients, presents 'Musing with death' in which she discusses three different types of group art therapy at the Memorial Sloan-Kettering Cancer Center in New York. Luzzatto was trained in Britain and worked for many years pioneering art therapy services for people with eating disorders and addiction, before moving to the United States where she has developed services with cancer patients. Luzzatto encourages her patients to make use of their dreams within the art therapy groups and reflects on the different art therapy techniques which can be used to their best advantage.

Barry Falk continues the group work theme, but in his chapter considers two groups set up in different British institutions in the South of England. These are outpatient groups, proving to be an important place for dealing with emotions that arise following diagnosis and treatment. Falk asks how one assesses whether clients will best benefit from group work or individual work. He also looks at the impact of institutional dynamics on the progress of the clients.

The theme of sustaining practice within palliative care, and the effects of this work on the therapist, is raised and developed by both David Hardy and Timothy Duesbury, both (like Barry Falk) graduates of the Corinne Burton scheme. David Hardy discusses the effects on the therapist of working with terminally ill clients within a hospice setting. Issues such as the culture of illness, fears of the client which transmit to the therapist, transference and counter-transference and the role of supervision are considered in depth. Timothy Duesbury looks at the difficulty of working with a psychodynamic model of art therapy in a hospice where this model was not formerly used. He looks at the difficulties of introducing such an approach to the team who had been used to art activity sessions. The chapter points out the necessity for art therapists to ensure that they liaise regularly with the rest of the team, and the importance of multidisciplinary working – otherwise art therapists may become embroiled in battles which might be a reflection of the clients' own battles against their illness, and thus find themselves exhausted and isolated.

The concluding chapters concern the art therapists' own stories as well as those of their patients. Maureen Bocking, a Corinne Burton art therapist in a large London teaching hospital, entitles her chapter 'A don't know story', and explores why she was drawn to this area of work and what she brings to the art therapy setting. This reflective chapter introduces us to the need to be adaptable and flexible as art therapists, yet to maintain the necessary professional boundaries to ensure effective practice. She tells us about two patients, 'Jill' and 'James' and gives us her reflections on their sessions, referring to Patrick Casement's important book, *On Learning from the Patient*. The book ends with Caryl Sibbett's third chapter, which concerns her own story as an art therapist. It examines two main aspects: her own experience of having cancer from diagnosis to treatment, including discussion of a medical error applied to herself and finding out that others shared this experience; and the issue of self-care – one's need, as an art therapist working with cancer, for self-care. This chapter powerfully brings together many of the themes addressed directly or indirectly by others throughout the book, including the danger of isolation, the need to recognize transference, counter-transference and projection, the significance of body image and the difficulty of maintaining relationships. The metaphor of Charon, the ferryman who sailed people across the Styx to death, is aptly used to ask what this recurring experience is like for therapists, how they survive it, and how it impacts on them.

This, we feel, is an apt conclusion to the journey of art therapists, their colleagues and their patients to a better understanding of how the art therapy process may benefit their quality of living and help them, where necessary, to face death. For the future we would like to recommend that there is increased attention to the emotional and spiritual needs of the cancer patient. There are many signs that these are now much more widely acknowledged among health and social care staff. However, we feel that the opportunities to engage in the arts therapies are as yet minimal, despite the numerous reports from patients that it has helped them. Most art therapists are employed on a sessional basis, which means that it is difficult for them to become part of the multi-professional team. They can become as isolated as the cancer patient, bearing much of the pain that is an inevitable outcome of the therapeutic relationship. It is also difficult for these colleagues to carry out the necessary research which will provide a sounder evidence base for art therapy with cancer patients. Although there are some embryo studies in place (including one by Diane Waller in cooperation with Barry Falk based in East Sussex), we cannot yet point to a range of studies which would confirm, in a form more acceptable to the employers of health professionals, the findings of the contributors to the book. We do, however, have the testimonies from a considerable number of cancer patients about how the art therapy process has helped them, which is obviously of central importance. Research projects may build on this evidence and develop it further in the interests of better service provision. The model of narrative research, which we mentioned earlier on, seems to us a very suitable one and ensures that the patient's voice is given a central position. We feel that generally there is still insufficient attention paid to the psychological needs of patients with any serious illness. There are major advances in medical treatment and it is important that this is not carried out apart from the psychological or psychosocial services, or we will remain in a divided 'mind and body' state.

Note

Illness and Healing: Images of Cancer by Robert Pope and *Reflections: The Art of Robert Pope* by Jock Murray are published by the Robert Pope Foundation, PO Box 425, Hantsport, Nova Scotia, Canada BOP 1PO.

1 On death and dying

Ken Evans

My own first encounter with death occurred while I was still a boy: the death of my father and a sister within weeks of each other. First, the sudden death of my eldest sister, who was 21, killed in a motorbike crash, hit by a truck while travelling at a hundred miles an hour. I had tried to visualize it, the energy and the impact, and had hoped that it had happened with such speed that there had been no time for her to know it. And then, shortly after the funeral, the slow painful death of my father, and my visits to the hospital every evening watching him haemorrhaging in the final stages of tuberculosis of his lungs, coughing up mouthfuls of blood, his emaciated body retching with each painful cough, and the white bed linen soaked in thick concentrated gore, he knowing that I was there but unable to speak. I could only think of it in terms of him fighting, fighting for his life, fighting death itself, and me watching helplessly and uselessly as he was dying. Up until this moment, death had been something at a distance; my only thoughts about death had been of fictionalized war heroes, of submariners and fighter pilots that I had read about, and who had sacrificed themselves for their country. It took me a long time after this to realize that the only way that we can cope with death is to fictionalize it, to deconstruct and reconstruct it, and to change it in one of a million ways in order to transcend it, to conquer it, to nail it, not to deny it, but neither to be totally destroyed by it.

Thinking back to this time, I can hardly remember any grieving, or the pain of coming to terms with the fact that I would not be seeing father and sister any more. But I can remember dreams and guilt that they had died without our settling our small disagreements. That bit is still painful and I try not to return to those memories, partly believing that to some extent I have let them go – that is, to the extent that we can ever let go of such memories.

The following brief discussion is about dying, or, more correctly, it is about one aspect of it. It is about the social acts of engagement and disengagement that occur during the last moments of people's lives. And it is also about some of the wider issues which are embedded in those final moments. I am not an expert on the subject, or even a specialist, and I am not even sure if there is such, but I have witnessed many deaths, of friends and family and as part of my work with elderly dementia sufferers, and, despite what the textbooks say about grieving, every dying performance is particular and different. My particular interest in this chapter is concerned with how couples deal with the final moments of their ultimate separation and the possibility of love after death.

For the patient, in extreme medical circumstances, after the feared diagnoses, and the options, and the preparations, and the treatment, and sometimes the extensive surgery, all that we are left with privately is the diminished sense of who we are and who we have been.

Whatever it is that interrupts our lives, at first it is a set of feelings that tells us that we are not well, and challenges us to imagine what our illness might or might not be, or the possibility that it is something that will kill us. In the brief rational moments we tell ourselves that it is just a pain, sometimes not even that – rather more a discomfort that comes and goes and so there is no need to alarm anyone. No need to share our inner thoughts with those we love or give any indication that there is anything to worry about. After all, it could be something that we have amplified through some mysterious act of our imagination. Such a thought, rather than being even slightly heroic, is built into our idea of what it is to love someone. In illness, as in death, the first inclination is to deny it as a first line of defence against despair. We don't intend it to be a game – after all our life is at stake – but it bears a remarkable resemblance to the very first game of all: the game of beep-o, which both excites us and puts us in touch with other persons and, perhaps for the first time in our lives, allows us to experience a sense of engagement, with others and also with ourselves.

At some point in our meandering thoughts we relent, we acknowledge that something is wrong, and share our fears with others. We do this incrementally, as if we had an itinerary, visiting the various separate groups which form the structure of our life. Those on the periphery, perhaps our work colleagues, provide a means to a kind of ventilation. To merely mention the fact that we are ill provides an opportunity to test responses, to try out the role of being seriously ill. In this we are testing others and ourselves, and measuring our own shock against theirs. This is the beginning of the contradictions that are woven into the fabric of terminal illness. To be ill and to expect to recover is normal and ordinary; we speak of being ill, of catching something, of having certain symptoms we can shed. But we do not have serious illnesses as some kind of possession; in fact they seem to possess us. They invade us, and claim us, for it seems that we are no longer the host, but the supplicant. Modern medicine places us in the perverse position of having to transfer the focus of our attention away from ourselves as subject, towards our condition as object. And this is amplified through our medical treatment, which becomes a regime, a ritual through which we reify the clinical description of the diagnosis. Up to this point we are initiates, feeling our way around the complexities of a frighteningly modern institution, for we have entered the social space of the condemned. The connection is not made by those who operate this place because, unlike the leper colonies and the gulags of former times, we are all functioning as guards, sharing in the rituals of modern-day palliative care, which unintentionally isolates the dying from the living.

The social and psychological demands on kith and kin are distinctively heavier and different. We find that some of our closer friends claim some limited ownership of us through their support; this is a legitimate kind of ownership expressed in terms of group identity, of belonging, and in this sense we belong more to those closest to us, hence it is our loved ones who must most share and carry the burden of our illness. And so we find ourselves at the centre of a strange event, a point of discovery. Our status as persons has changed; we are alienated from the normal and the healthy, and now defined by the name of our illness. We enter a new world of categories, where we become initiated into statistical probabilities for our survival, with a special kind of folklore about heroes and warriors who have fought the battle, and nearly won, or have lost and forfeited their lives. There seem to be so many people involved in this process, but we rapidly discern the limits of their involvement; however close they might be they cannot know how it feels to be in your body. By some strange alchemy there is a growing sense of becoming alienated from our own flesh, as we attempt to maintain engagement with our nearest and dearest. We wish to remain like them, and enter into a tacit pact to facilitate, to cooperate, to be disciplined, to diligently embrace our medical regime.

The pressures on our closest relationships, spouses, partners, or parents, amplify the ambiguities that are the essence of all close human relationships. The complex interactions that weave the good and the bad experiences together through the push and pull of everyday living create a shared life story, which manifests itself through many narratives. These are the stories we tell ourselves when we reminisce, and through which we confirm or deny key aspects of our feelings about each other. But throughout the course of our time together they also reflect the temperature of our love at any one time. This is part of the dynamic of living and loving another person, and included in this dynamic is the status of external relationships, how we as individuals, and as a 'pair', currently relate to other family members, friends and colleagues. The intrusion of 'the illness', to use George Simmel's[1] model of relationships, is to shift the dyadic to the triadic; the twosome becomes a threesome, a catastrophic ménage a trois, in which the 'illness' too frequently becomes the dominant partner. Besides the physical and domestic upheaval, and the resetting of lifestyles, the new psychological and emotional demands create both pressures and vacuums. The shared narratives are reinterpreted, producing cycles of fusion and fission, sucking the energy from whatever it is that holds two people together in some bearable balance of affection. In many cases the psychological processes mimic the physical course of the disease, eroding the substantial strands that hold the various parts of our selves together. And in the end, at the finish of that inevitable process, is the discovery by surviving partners of the extent of their own damage.

During the final stages even the physical laws of the universe seem to change. Time and space distort, so that some days pass instantly and other moments stretch into an eternity. Our sense of place and moment takes on surreal qualities – of being simultaneously unique and universal; there is time to ponder our shared human condition, and the urgency to fill the precious moment. The 'illness', the condition itself, becomes the master of all events; even the smallest interlude is slotted into place, into a pattern defined by the medical regime, governed by the illness and administered through the collective activities of the palliative care team. At some imperceptible point the importance and centrality of the illness shifts, or rather the *modus operandi* of existence switches from one opposition to another, from between that of illness and health to between that of life and death. While both of these two oppositions have existed and run side by side during the whole course of the illness, and while in essence the consequences of both are the same, our psychology opts for hope against despair. It is a symbolic choice, and even if we acknowledge the inevitability of death to ourselves, we might feel the obligation, for one reason or another, to deny it. Of course the whole of human communication is symbolic, but at this extreme moment of our life the sharing of a loved one's death evokes unfamiliar thoughts and beliefs. Our mind works in pictures, not words, and we grapple to express the inexpressible. We are with them, trying against the odds to hold on, to let go, and to carry some of the pain, to seek relief and release. At some point in our disorganized thoughts we feel the disengagement, as if losing the grip of someone drowning.

To be near someone who is dying almost inevitably causes us at some point to reflect on our own mortality, and this 'empathy' can occasionally alarm us; our feelings about the dying and death fluctuate between ourselves and the dying person. In our modern society we are not prepared for death, of others or ourselves. It is a matter we generally prefer not to consider or discuss, and it is for that reason that it is recognized by many as the final taboo, the one human activity we are unable to control or negotiate. Consequently in our society we hand over the activities that surround death and dying to groups of specialists, the medical teams, social workers, morticians. And perhaps it is this arrangement that underwrites and substantiates the pain accompanying disengagement. In some other societies the experience of death and dying includes preparation for separation without disengagement. But in modern societies, where commercial and materialistic values predominate, death is final. We cannot turn back the clock either personally or culturally, and we cannot reclaim what is already lost. But there is no doubt that there is a heavy psychological and emotional cost to living in Max Weber's 'disenchanted world'.[2]

From my own professional experience working in social care of the elderly, many with terminal illnesses, I have witnessed many deaths. Some of these people I had known personally and been able to establish a relationship with, but also there were many others, who now seem to me to have been merely passing through, as if my workplaces were clearing centres for the dying. And when I compare this experience with other experiences of and about death, in other places where I have worked with the dying, for example in rural villages in the Philippines, it seems self-evident to me now, although we rarely state it, that death and dying is primarily a social act. It is certainly culturally bound; it transcends the merely physiological processes, and this act of dying, this performance, to some extent can be good or bad. For, despite what we may wish, the pain for all those involved in this final social act is not evenly distributed socially or culturally, but is bundled up in clusters of unarticulated memories, and carried more or less, in one way or another, by surviving loved ones until the moments of their own departure. Even after we accept the cultural differences, and (perhaps) the benefits of dying in a collectivist culture, and the different ontologies and meaning systems, and also the vast economic differences that underpin our attitudes to death, this is no reason why we, in our individualist culture, should tolerate bad deaths.

The idea that death and dying could be either good or bad might seem to belong to the realms of philosophy, because in an everyday sense death is separation, and painful at every level of experience. But when commenting on someone's life we distinguish between a good and bad life, a bad life perhaps blighted by relationships. In the same way, some deaths are clearly worse than others, depending on the causes and the circumstances, but if we restrict our attention to just one category, that of terminally ill hospital patients, cases where many variables are the same, there are still significant differences between those who die well and those who have bad deaths. In this sense, in our culture there are very few 'good deaths'. It is not easy to monitor such events, but a 'good death' would clearly not invoke the terrible raging of Dylan Thomas's famous poem[3] but would rather maintain the momentum of a gentle journey and a fond farewell. And as death and dying continues to affect kith and kin for some time after the event, a good death is where engagement with the dying is maintained until the final moments, and possibly beyond this time.

In thinking about death and dying, we are confronted by a kind of information overload. So many sources of our knowledge carry fragments about death and, if Freud is correct, then our fear of death is instinctive, hard-wired into the architecture of our minds. But instincts alone cannot explain human behaviour, even when relating to something as powerful as death. Our culture and individual personality factors combined with the unique family relationships change the universal performance of dying into what becomes the personal and individual event, which is ambiguously shareable and unshareable. And it is this veiled ambiguity of our emotions about death and dying, between the unique and the generalizable, expressed in the poem by John Donne that begins 'No man is an island',[4] which adds to our confusion when discussing deathly matters. On the one hand it is natural, part of the universal cycle of life for which there are no exemptions, while on the other it is the unique flow of feelings about the death of our particular loved ones which are acutely private, incommunicable, and ultimately beyond the reach of all other persons. And it is our relationship with the deceased person, which for our own protection we try to place beyond the reach of others and which in this sense maintains the connection between the living and the dead, which could be described as a kind of engagement.

By engagement, I mean a shared awareness of self with and of another person, which includes recognition, communication, intuition and empathy. To some extent the ebb and flow of affection in personal relationships involves a series of disengagements and re-engagements, which does not suddenly stop when someone dies but in fact continues to alternate after their death as if they were still alive. I have also noticed that surviving partners frequently use the present tense when referring to their deceased loved one, and that their conversations sometimes indicate that there is an ongoing sense of togetherness, and a sense of a continuing relationship. During the last thirty years of various interpretations of John Bowlby's work on separation,[5] a theoretical dichotomy of opposing views has arisen which is sometimes applied to bereavement counselling. The basic opposition is between 'letting go' and 'holding on', and because Bowlby stands within a Freudian framework, letting go carries positive values, while holding on is considered neurotic.

But it could be argued that, in the cultural eclecticism of the present day, this should not matter because there are a wide range of beliefs that permit individuals the freedom to deal with their personal matters as they choose. We should be able to grieve in the way that best suits us, but in actual fact this is not always possible, for whatever our individual beliefs and value systems, which would cause us to act in a particular way, most dying occurs within the institutional framework of society, which in physical terms means in hospitals. And although there is some 'flexibility' between the means of wider society and the needs of individual persons in how the dying of individuals might be managed, it is the institutional values which predominate.

In institutional terms a good death is one which minimizes both suffering and the pain of the patient.

And it is these same institutional values, which support life and which are dedicated to extending life so efficiently and effectively, that inform the systems of care, with equal efficiency, to discharge the remains once life has ended. From the point of view of the health services, after a person has died their responsibilities have finished; it is in Durkheim's[6] terms a simple matter of division of labour, part of the modern social agenda. In traditional societies, the governance of care within the family is seamless from beginning to end, but in modern societies, which other sociologists tell us are based on contract values, all services are delivered at a price, except perhaps for the one exception in the entire system – that of the social and emotional aspects of death and dying. The state institutions, which control so many aspects of our lives, have no dominion here, except for regulating the disposal of human remains and the taxation of their estates. Beyond this there is a social void, and also a psychological one that strikes at the very centre of modern social values, and that goes to the heart of the matter, which is our present-day understanding of what it means to be a person.

One might imagine that our sense of identity would be central to our general understanding of our world, and that who and what we are would be fundamental to everything we do, for not to have some idea of ourselves is surely the critical test of sanity, indeed of existence and being. Yet strangely, for the majority of people and for our institutions this is a matter of little real concern. Perhaps for most of us it is taken for granted that we simply 'are', and that any speculation about 'being' and associated issues is best left to philosophers and other specialists. It might also be an assumption that such matters are safe in their hands, and that they are able to define for us what it is to be human and to be a person. If that is the case then we are mistaken, for definitions that value who and what we are, as persons, have been steadily diminishing over the last two centuries and now, at the start of the twenty-first century, have almost completely been eliminated.

The causes and reasons for this are complex, but for anyone interested in these issues, the difficult problem is in negotiating the gap between theorizing, with all of its convolutions, and the practical requirements of assisting ordinary people when these fundamental questions might be raised. A brief answer might be that the world has changed, and that our species, at one time central to the whole cosmos, has been relocated as one species among many, at one end of the evolutionary spectrum. But it is far more complicated even than that, and the consequences are more serious than simply changing cosmologies, because who and what we are affects how we treat one another, and ultimately how we feel and think about ourselves, and about others, even after they have died. And this in turn sets the agenda for all the myriad interactions that combine to underpin social life.

This is not a matter of concern at the mundane level, for in ordinary everyday conversations we continually test ideas about ourselves and seek reassurance. But in extraordinary circumstances, for example when someone is dying, the questioning might dig deeper and activate different levels of discourse. It is at these points that ordinary language fails, and that we discover the poverty of our current vocabulary and terminology to express our deeper feelings about ourselves and our mortality. And if language shapes our thinking, as some psychological theories suggest, then it is necessary to examine the forces and influences that have reshaped human consciousness to understand why a void at this level of human interaction has become the tolerated norm.

Whenever issues concerning changes in consciousness are discussed, a small number of key points of reference are identified, including the Enlightenment, Darwin's theory of evolution, Marx's false consciousness, Freud's personality theories, perhaps Weber's ominous warning of disenchantment,[7] and more recently the bundle of new sciences which include genetics and neurology. Their influence is set against a cultural and intellectual historical background, beginning at the end of the nineteenth century, with its response to burgeoning mass society, giving rise to massive and massing processes including mass production, mass consumption, mass media, mass destruction, mass murder in the form of genocide, and so on. Consequently the scale of human history has expanded to gargantuan levels, diminishing by comparison the meaning of individual people's lives. In all of this it has been impossible for individuals to try to make sense of the impact of these processes on personal relationships, or to understand how changes in personal values and manners have impacted on ordinary everyday relations. To try for an explanation at a very general level we only have to look around us, for examples of what might be described as objectification of human relations, which are freely evident even in the most casual of human interactions. In fact, even at such minimal levels of personal exchanges as purchasing a newspaper from a street vendor, where once there was a cheery 'Thank you' there is now at best a grunt.

Or we can read the signs of consciousness, not in behaviours but in bodily appearances which, perhaps more than anything else, have come to define a sense of 'being' in the present time. Concern with appearances, as one strand of materialism, is bound up with an inversion in values relating to the human person. Whereas in the past it was viewed as shallow to be concerned with external physical appearances compared with interior qualities, now the external and the visual is the paradigm. The older values, rooted in classical philosophy, having survived more or less for two and a half millennia, have finally been overturned and replaced by an international and institutionalized fascination with bodies. This concentration on the physical body is expressed most powerfully through various forms of consumption, becoming, as Marx warned, the central component of capitalism and the primary means through which all commodities are absorbed, the body finally itself becoming commoditized as 'object'. While this is also self-evident in an everyday sense, in the display of bodies in their various forms – as clothes hanger, as object for adaptation, to be reshaped, worshipped, decorated, pierced, exchanged, and sold – it is through changing images of bodies in cultural artefacts that we glimpse this relentless exteriorization. Even the briefest review of how artists have represented bodies over the last hundred years will show both its objectification and fragmentation.

But whatever the symbolic components of a new materialistic consciousness as expressed through the arts, nothing can compare with the brave new scientific reductionism of the new sciences. With their roots in the scientific thinking of the Enlightenment, and driven by neo-Darwinism, this combination of 'sciences' draws together several strands of ideas including evolutionary psychology, neuro and cognitive sciences, and a genetics-based techno-biology. This potently seductive mixture rides high on its technological steed, cracks the genetic code and provides colourful pictures of brains in action. It also fertilizes barren women, clones sheep, grows human cells from aborted foetuses, and defines consciousness in terms of 'a bundle of neurons'. This blend of ideas is disseminated through high-profile media stories, and constitutes a new wave of super-science, marking out the territory for the final phase of human evolution.

The effect of this omni-directional cultural onslaught is to diminish any hold we might have on the belief that there is anything special or unique in being human. The discourses provided by psychology and sociology, which have attempted to explain human processes, are surprisingly blunt instruments for the purposes of opening up the human mind. And even in the friendly territory of psychotherapy, perhaps, one might think, the one remaining place where we might expect to find a residuum for the 'human person', we find instead complex theorizing about selves, and constructs completely bereft of any organic qualities. Whatever the fears for personal survival in an increasingly hostile world, it feels as if all avenues of escape from this cultural wasteland have already been cut off. Slowly but surely progress is demolishing the human soul. Only the laments of a few poets and music makers alert us to the fact that we are the manufacturers of our own extinction, not only in a physical sense, but also metaphysically and spiritually.

To the average person who has perhaps only the vaguest notion of current debates about what it means to be human and to be a person, there is little consolation. And whether a person is trying to come to terms with his or her own terminal illness or that of a loved one, the consequence of this void is despair, and it is this despair that makes for a bad death. If we are at all concerned about this then we urgently need to review our understanding of both life and death, and consider how we might recover some of the wisdom from the past about the art of dying, the *ars moriendi*. In traditional societies the line between life and death is less distinct, symbolized by personal actions such as not cutting one's hair or fingernails during grieving, and so blurring the lines between the material world and the spiritual, between the living and the dead. In these societies even food is served to them, as the newly deceased temporarily inhabit the middle ground between those who have breath and those without breath. The effect of these rituals is to strengthen attachments between surviving members of families and friends and the deceased person, and to provide a communication channel through which they can express their feelings, both positive and negative. The rituals that surround death have the effect, among other things, of bridging the space between the personal and the public, and as such 'normalize' the changing status of the dying and those who mourn. In modern societies these rituals have almost disappeared. My own experience of working in other more traditional cultures suggests to me that their acceptance of death as a natural organic process, as elementary as the changing seasons, protects them from despair and maintains their continuing affections for 'those who have gone ahead'.

Both individually and institutionally we are ill prepared for death. At its very least it is an embarrassment; at its most profound it is the basis for all that is tragic. We assume in our modernity that we as human beings have come of age, and that we have triumphed over nature – not that we would put it that way, for to suggest that there is a war between humans and nature is to locate the debate in the primitive mythopoetic world, which we also wish to be rid of. In our Brave New World we can already read our life-chances in our DNA, and we can construct replacement organs, make the infertile fertile, clone ourselves, reconstruct our appearances, and hold back the years. And such is the power of our new beliefs in conquering death that the storage of frozen bodies in the USA has already become a problem. There are plans to construct vast cryopreservation vaults, in which bodies can be stored until the time when life can be regenerated. In the twenty-first century not only have we become alienated from life, but we have also become alienated from death.

And while we cannot turn back the clocks, we can re-examine how the idea of a 'good death' has varied over time and between cultures, how we can educate and prepare ourselves, how we might discover the essential new rituals for our final rites of passage and how the social and healthcare professionals can assist more in this process.

Notes

1   Georg Simmel, German sociologist and associate of Weber, identified the 'dyad', a group of two members, as the basic element of social exchange, whereas the 'triad' is a three-person group. For further reading on this, refer to Simmel, G.

(1949) The sociology of sociability, *American Journal of Sociology*, 55 (3): 254–61.

2   Max Weber's famous phrase – 'disenchantment of world' – referred to the process of increasing rationalization in modern society, partly as a consequence of bureaucracy. It means, literally, a world without spontaneity.

3   Thomas's famous poem, 'Do Not Go Gentle Into That Good Night', angrily advises that we should 'Rage, rage against the dying of the light' and not meet death calmly and with acceptance.

4   John Donne was a seventeenth-century English poet and an Anglican priest. His prose poem that begins 'No man is an island' is in fact a Meditation (No. 17), and is about the inherent unity of all humankind, especially when it concerns death and dying.

5   Bowlby contributed to our understanding of 'our sense of loss' by examining processes of attachment. See *Attachment and Loss*, Vol. 1: *Attachment*. Harmondsworth: Penguin.

6   Durkheim saw the division of labour in society as fragmenting human experience, as parcelling it into meaningless events. 'The division of labour in society' (1893) was his doctoral thesis, and became a controversial book: Durkheim, E. (1997) *The Division of Labour in Society*. New York, London: Free Press, Macmillan.

7   Weber, *op. cit.*

2 'Betwixt and between': crossing thresholds

Caryl Sibbett

Introduction

This chapter will explore from an anthropological perspective the relevance of the liminal, transitional or threshold phase of rites of passage to art therapy and cancer experiences. It will focus particularly on the relevance of ritual and four characteristics of liminality: *limbo, power / powerlessness, playing* and *communion* (communitas). Liminal space and time experience, 'flow' experience and the use of symbolic objects will also be discussed. Chapter 4 will explore the relevance of a fifth characteristic, *embodied experience*.

Chapters 2, 4 and 16 will draw on a research study into liminality in my own cancer experience and that of other participants. Participants' voices, verbal and pictorial, will be included at times to explore whether rites of passage, ritual and liminality are relevant metaphors to conceptualize art therapy and practice with clients dealing with the potentially liminal nature of the cancer experience, itself perhaps a rites of passage experience. Chapter 16 explores liminality in my own cancer, art-making and professional experience, so any case examples in Chapters 2 and 4 will mostly be from other participants.

Motivation and methodology

The three chapters I have authored draw on research undertaken for my PhD using 'arts-based autoethnography' (Slattery 2001). Autoethnography is 'an autobiographical genre of writing and research connecting the personal to the cultural', where autoethnographers focus 'outward on social and cultural aspects of their personal experience; then, they look inward, exposing a vulnerable self' (Ellis and Bochner 2000: 739). Therefore the methodology features 'auto/biography' (Stanley 1992).

I was in my final dissertation year of a Masters degree when I received a diagnosis of leiomyosarcoma, a rare soft tissue cancer. In trying to understand my own experience I discovered the term 'liminal', originating from the Latin for threshold and meaning 'the border realm between life and death' (Bolen 1998: 15). This seemed congruent with my experience as I wavered on the margin between life and death. Liminality was emerging as a metaphor for my experience and, being curious, I explored the concept in depth.

Beginning a literature review I was excited to discover an article by Little *et al.* (1998) that specifically emphasized liminality as 'a major category of the experience of cancer illness'. Little *et al.* (1998: 1490) assert their belief that 'liminality is a fundamental category of the experience of serious illness that needs separate recognition and examination in any account of serious illness . . .'. I subsequently selected this topic as the focus of my PhD because I wanted to explore the source authors on liminality to see which, if any, of its characteristics were relevant. I therefore embarked on a systematic investigation of the relationship between key aspects of liminality and art therapy and my cancer experience and that of those clients who participated in the research. This involved an exploration of the relevance of ritual space and activity in art therapy. These issues will be explored in this chapter and developed further in Chapters 4 and 16.

In the auto/biographical research my own experience was the main focus yet, true to autoethnography, this widened to include data gathered from participating clients. The overall sampling approach taken was non-probabilistic or purposive theoretical sampling, relevant in ethnographic research (Brewer 2000: 79). Methodological triangulation or 'crystalliza-tion' (Richardson 2000: 934) was used, featuring multi-modal data collection sources and methods including interviews, focus groups, art reviews and questionnaires using a design congruent with that recommended in medical research and audit (Bhattacharya 2004). Concept mapping was used to understand the relationships between complex qualitative concepts and themes and was valuable as an analogous pictorial social research approach (Trochim 2000). I checked the congruence of my emerging findings with the experience of other healthcare practitioners and researchers.

I will now explore the relevance of liminality to the cancer and art therapy experiences by first summarizing the classic anthropological model of rites of passage, then discussing the relevance of ritual and then focusing on four characteristics of liminality.

Rites of passage

One way of conceiving cancer experiences and art therapy is from an anthropological perspective, paralleling such experience with a rites of passage transition and associated ritual. Classic anthropology theory proposes that transitions can give rise to rites of passage characterized by three phases (Van Gennep 1960):

- *Separation* – from an earlier status in social structure and a change in space and the 'quality of *time*' to being 'out of time' (Turner 1982: 24).
- *Liminality* – 'ambiguity' (Turner 1982: 24), 'neither here nor there; . . . betwixt and between' (Turner 1995: 95) transition experience.
- *Incorporation* – or reincorporation; the passage is 'consummated' and the person is in a 'relatively stable' position (Turner 1982: 24).

Writing of the 'cancer experience', Bronson (1994) describes how, at a conference on cancer, Achterberg compared cancer to 'a rite of passage' with its three phases of 'a separation and wrenching away from life as usual' (like diagnosis), a 'transition time . . . like the solitary journey of cancer treatment', and 're-entry' into society as a changed person. Froggatt (1997) suggests that the hospice culture offers what might be described as a 'rites of passage' model that facilitates the transitions of the liminal dying or bereaved. Little *et al.* (1998) emphasize that liminality is 'a major category of the experience of cancer illness'.

Rites of passage, ritual and liminality are important aspects of therapy where therapists can act as 'ritual elders' facilitating transformation (Moore 1991, 2001). Kenny (1996) recounts how Ruud (1995) described music therapy as modern 'rites de passage' and associated liminality with improvization. Ritual, rites of passage and liminality are important in drama therapy (Mitchell 1999: 12–13) and performance studies (Schechner 2003). Schechner (2003: 58) suggests that in 'ritual and aesthetic performances, the thin space of the limen is expanded into a wide space both actually and conceptually. What is usually just a "go between" becomes the site of the action . . . It is enlarged in time and space yet retains its peculiar quality of passageway or temporariness'.

Ritual

Writing of rites of passage, Turner (1988: 25) explains that rituals '*separated* specific members of a group from everyday life, *placed them in a limbo* that was not any place they were in before and not yet any place they would be in, then *returned* them, changed in some way, to mundane life'. The term ritual refers to the systematic use of rites or behaviour that may be private or social and that 'may involve sacred or secular symbols' (Cohen 2002).

Achterberg *et al.* (1994: 3) assert that rituals 'give significance to life passages'. It is possible to conceive of aspects of both people's cancer experiences and, perhaps particularly, art therapy experiences in terms of rituals.

In medicine, Wall (1996) suggests that the term 'ritual' can have a value as a 'vehicle for the transmission of meaning' in surgery where, as a 'rite of passage', it helps move patients from 'illness' to 'health'. Kleinman (1989: 130) proposes that medical record-keeping is 'a profound, ritual act of transformation through which illness is made over into disease, person becomes patient . . .'. Dyer (2002), a professor of psychiatry who had cancer, recounts how 'the ritual of blood counts and treatments' was part of his cancer experience. Ritual and image-making can help individuals navigate through illness (Achterberg *et al.* 1994). Rituals are important in psychotherapy and play a role in transition and continuity (Van der Hart 1996). Kirmayer (2003: 249) notes that Frank (1973) includes 'ritual time and place' as one of the five universal elements that occur in systems of symbolic healing. Achterberg *et al.* (1994: xv) propose that 'an image or a symbol that effects healing – is most fundamentally evoked through some form of ritual. A healing ritual forms the "container" for using the imagination for healing.'

Rituals are 'an important aspect of all art therapy groups' (Skaife and Huet 1998: 12). Examples of 'rituals of art therapy' include 'time for making images followed by discussion, often in a circular group; the display of work, shifting focus from one group image to another or holding the group image in view', so art therapy 'becomes a ceremony of redefinition' (Barber and Campbell 1999: 30).

Liminality

Rites of passage are fundamentally characterized by the liminal phase (Mahdi *et al.* 1996), which is the most important as it is the core of where transition occurs (Lertzman 2002). Turner outlined key characteristics of liminality experienced by 'threshold people' (1995: 95) including:

1 *Limbo* – 'ambiguity', 'social limbo', being 'out of time' (Turner 1982: 24), 'neither here nor there; . . . betwixt and between' (Turner 1995: 95).
2 *Power/powerless* – 'submissiveness and silence' (Turner 1995: 103), structural inferiority and outsiderhood (Turner 1975: 231), reduced status, 'passive' (Turner 1995: 95).
3 *Playing* – 'playful experience' (Turner 1988: 124–5), 'ludic (or playful) events' and use of 'multivocal symbols' (Turner 1982: 27); experience of 'flow' (Turner 1982: 55–8), potentially transforming, possibility (Turner 1986: 42, 1990: 11–12).
4 *Communitas* – 'intense comradeship', 'communion' (Turner 1995: 95–6).

5 *Embodied experience* – experiencing physiological 'ordeals' (Turner 1995: 103), 'pain and suffering' (Turner 1995: 107), stigma, 'effacement' (Turner 1982: 26), 'polluting' (Turner 1967: 97), 'sexlessness' (Turner 1995: 102), androgyny (Turner 1967: 98), involving 'performance' and 'expression' such as in 'acts' and 'works of art' (Turner 1982: 12–15).

Limbo

The first characteristic of liminality to be explored in its relevance to cancer experiences and art therapy is *limbo*. Turner (1988: 25) discusses how during rites of passage people can find themselves '*in a limbo* that was not any place they were in before and not yet any place they would be in'. He describes this as a state of 'ambiguity', 'social limbo', and being 'out of time' (Turner 1982: 24), 'neither here nor there; . . . betwixt and between' (Turner 1995: 95). People do not necessarily move through the three phases of rites of passage but can get held in liminality (Turner 1974).

Halvorson-Boyd and Hunter (1995: 1), two healthcare professionals writing of their own cancer experiences, assert: 'We live in limbo: after cancer, we know that we are on uncertain ground.' They describe the cancer experience as 'entering the unknown' (Halvorson-Boyd and Hunter 1995: 2) and add: 'We are in limbo . . . We enter limbo when we are diagnosed, but in our shock and terror we don't notice' (Halvorson-Boyd and Hunter 1995: 15). Kleinman (1989: 181) describes how some patients' narratives describe 'chronicity' as 'like being in limbo emotionally and interpersonally' with 'an intuition that illness involves rites of passage between different social worlds'.

Little *et al.* (1998: 1490) propose that liminality in serious and chronic illness like cancer is experienced in two stages: 'An immediate phase of *acute liminality*, and an enduring phase of *sustained liminality* which may last for the rest of the patient's life.' The liminality of having cancer can bring a 'disorientation . . . and a sense of uncertainty' and people can fluctuate between states of 'acute' and 'sustained liminality' (Little *et al.* 1998: 1492–3). Acute liminality features heightened fear and reduced control, as experienced during diagnosis, waiting for scan results, feeling new pain or finding a lump. Sustained liminality features times of less fear and reassertion of some control. However, as Halvorson-Boyd and Hunter (1995: 2) suggest: 'Limbo is the borderland where we will live for the rest of our lives.' Kleinman (1989: 181) asserts that: 'Social movement for the chronically ill is back and forth through rituals of separation, transition, and reincorporation, as exacerbation leads to remission and then circles back to worsening, and so on.'

Muzzin *et al.* (1994) comment that the cancer experience has been characterized as a 'living–dying' experience and they add that a person never really 'gets over' cancer, but rather cancer is a 'sword of Damocles' that continues to hang over individuals and their families for the rest of their lives. Riskó *et al.* (1998) also refer to the 'Damocles sword syndrome' that can be experienced by cancer patients. Self (1999), a psychiatric senior house officer, comments on her personal experience of having osteosarcoma: 'I was fascinated to hear the term "Damocles syndrome" used to describe the psychosocial stresses experienced by survivors of childhood cancer. No story could more accurately describe the legacy of overcoming the original diagnosis.' Dyer (2002), a physician with cancer, suggests that 'recovery from cancer was much like recovery from alcoholism; once you had it, you were always in recovery (or remission), never really cured'.

The art therapy clients who participated in this study reported this limbo experience in various ways. One said a particularly difficult aspect was 'the limbo of waiting for the treatment or tests and of waiting to go back to work and drive again' and on another occasion reported: 'Limbo is a very important element and the worst aspect. Waiting at the start then now for the treatment to begin.' Another client reported as difficult the 'limbo of waiting for the treatment or tests', while another said that 'waiting is the worst'. The experience in waiting rooms can be a liminal experience for carers as well as patients (Cohn 2001).

Limbo in art therapy could link to how it acknowledges the importance of 'staying with the uncertainty or not knowing what it "means" or "says" which is central to the therapeutic process' (Case and Dalley 1997: 65). This is about 'cultivating the ability to wait', which Claxton (1998: 174) regards as similar to Keats' 'negative capability' (Rollins 1958: 193). Limbo also relates to the liminal space–time that art therapy offers, as discussed below.

Metaphor is useful when conceptualizing cancer because patients use multiple, sometimes contradictory and often embodied metaphors when describing their experience (Gibbs and Franks 2002). Metaphors such as cancer 'eating' can appear in narratives and the word cancer is itself a metaphor, as Hippocrates likened the veins radiating from lumps in the breast to crabs (Skott 2002). Lakoff and Johnson (1980: 5) suggest that metaphor works by 'understanding and experiencing one kind of thing in terms of another'.

One client, a woman in her fifties diagnosed with breast cancer, created a visual and verbal metaphor for her cancer and limbo experience. In an early group session she chose clay for the first time. As she worked I observed an animal-like shape began to form. She later reported being surprised to see a crocodile begin to emerge, then becoming absorbed in making it. She reported experiencing emotion as she suddenly realized the crocodile was her cancer. On looking at the clay crocodile she said: 'He's mean.' She related her story in metaphorical terms. 'Before getting cancer I was sitting by the water in the sun, OK and relaxed. Then suddenly out of the water sprang a crocodile who bit me! It's never the same again because you know the crocodile exists and you are always waiting for him to come and bite again.'

Liminal space

Turner (1982: 25) notes that in rites of passage the change in social status is often 'accompanied by a parallel passage in space . . . the literal crossing of a threshold which separates two distinct areas'. 'Threshold', 'liminal' or 'ritual space' is important in self-discovery and transformation (Bly 1993: 194–9). Perhaps one way of conceiving liminal space is to use Foucault's (1986) concept of the '*heterotopia*', a real place set apart from other places. Perhaps some of the spatial locations in cancer experiences might be described as heterotopic and I suggest that heterotopia could be a metaphor for the art therapy space and indeed the artwork spaces within therapy.

Foucault (1986: 24–25) proposes that heterotopias probably occur in every culture although they take varied forms. One category features 'crisis heterotopias' which are 'privileged or sacred or forbidden places' for those in crisis, but he suggests these are being replaced in our society by 'heterotopias of deviation' meant for people regarded as different to the norm. The latter might link to the aspect of stigma potentially associated with liminality (Turner 1967: 97) and cancer (Muzzin *et al.* 1994; Colyer 1996; Flanagan and Holmes 2000) and indeed with seeking psychological help (Pandey and Thomas 2001). Perhaps, as discussed further in Chapter 4, art therapy can provide a constructive heterotopic crisis space that can reduce stigma.

Foucault (1986: 25) suggests that the heterotopia is 'capable of juxtaposing in a single real place several spaces, several sites that are in themselves incompatible' and can take the form of 'contradictory sites'. Perhaps in art therapy contradictory artworks, or symbol meanings within artworks, can coexist. In art therapy artwork enables symbolic expression of 'seemingly contradictory ideas and feelings simultaneously', thus accommodating potentially ambivalent feelings about cancer (Miller 1996: 133).

Foucault (1986: 24) uses the metaphor of a 'mirror' for a heterotopia. He suggests that in the mirror 'I discover my absence from the place where I am since I see myself over there' and 'I come back toward myself; I begin again to direct my eyes toward myself and to reconstitute myself there where I am.' Simon (1992: 199) asserts that: 'Art as therapy is a mirror that the patient makes to find his own self reflected.' Perhaps art therapy and the artwork offer heterotopic spaces and mirrors for discovery and reconstitution of the self that could be termed a form of 'reauthoring' (White and Epston 1990) or 'narrative reconstruction' (Williams 1984).

One client, diagnosed with a type of facial cancer, reported having difficulties at home in looking at the reflection in the mirror. The client said: 'You know. Because every time I looked in the mirror that was not me. You know, who the hell is this person looking back at me?' In the art, a series of images was created of a shape whose meanings unfolded to represent a self-image. The client began to speak of 'my face' and related how cancer had impacted on self-image. The art became a type of mirror and the client reported that art therapy had promoted greater acceptance of self-image and added: 'I'm much better now; I can look in the mirror and see I am sort of back. It's been a hell of a long time.' Perhaps the heterotopic mirror function of the art provided a 'site of alternate ordering' (Foucault 1986: 24) and in the *self-made* mirror of the art the client had been able to see the self reflected (Simon 1992: 199) and engage in self 'gaze' and, as Foucault (1986: 24) says, 'begin again to direct my eyes toward myself and to reconstitute myself there where I am'.

Liminal time

Turner (1995: 96) asserts that liminal experience is a 'moment in and out of time'. Foucault (1986: 26) suggests that heterotopias are linked to 'slices in time' and the 'heterotopia begins to function at full capacity when men arrive at a sort of absolute break with their traditional time'. In cancer experiences 'acute liminality' can involve a 'discontinuity of subjective time' (Little *et al.* 1998: 1492) and a sense of timelessness (Dreifuss-Kattan 1994: 126). Yet paradoxically survivors can be 'acutely aware of time', divide their lives into 'the time before and after cancer' and regard time as 'precious' (Halvorson-Boyd and Hunter 1995: 152–3).

Turner (1982: 55–9) suggests that in liminality there can be an experience of 'flow' (Csikszentmihalyi 2002) or timeless absorption in the moment. 'Flow' will be discussed further in the section on Playing. Bolen (1998: 86–7) proposes that two types of time are relevant in cancer experiences: *kairos*, experienced as 'non-linear', a 'losing track of'; and *kronos*, a measured and linear form of time. During life-threatening illness like cancer, art activities can give an experience of 'kairos' or non-linear 'soul satisfying and soul nourishing' time (Murray 2000). Kairos is 'the right or opportune moment' and 'reigns where creative purposes are to be achieved' (Aldridge 2000: 3). Bartunek and Necochea (2000) note that White (1987: 13) clarifies that the term kairos originates in archery and weaving. In archery it relates to an 'opening' or 'opportunity', specifically 'a long tunnel-like aperture through which the archer's arrow has to pass'. Interestingly, Turner (1982: 41) asserts that liminality can have positive and active qualities especially when the transition or threshold is 'protracted and becomes a "tunnel", when the "liminal" becomes the "cunicular" '. However, in CT and MRI scans the *spatial* experience of a tunnel can be claustrophobic for some patients. In weaving, kairos relates to ' "the critical time" when the weaver must draw the yarn through a gap that momentarily opens in the warp of the cloth being woven' (White 1987: 13). Overall White summarizes that it means 'a passing instant when an opening appears' which must be moved through to achieve success.

Perhaps art therapy can enable experiences of flow and kairos by creating an opening or opportunity for 'ritual and aesthetic performances' in which Schechner (2003: 58) suggests the limen is 'expanded into a wide space both actually and conceptually' and 'becomes the site of the action'.

All clients reported often being absorbed in art-making and losing track of time. One client reported that during art-making 'time disappears'. Another client reported: 'When I was working I was able to just move into the art. When I went home I felt really uplifted. I was able to get a really good night's sleep.' On a research questionnaire in response to the question 'How is/was the art therapy experience for you?' another client's response included: 'No perception/awareness of time while doing art.'

Hartocollis (1983) and Sabbadini (1989) propose that varieties of time and timelessness experience feature in psychoanalysis. Similarly Schubert (2001) comments that analysis has to handle an apparent contradiction in that it creates and uses both a timeless perspective, as in regression and rhythmic recurrence of sessions, and a linear time perspective, in its time-limited nature and development towards set goals. He suggests this parallels the timeless nature of the unconscious versus the linear time of conscious reality.

Perhaps in relation to time *and* space, Foucault (1986: 26) asserts that heterotopias have 'a system of opening and closing that both isolates them and makes them penetrable'. They are 'not freely accessible' but either entry is 'compulsory . . . or else the individual has to submit to rites and purifications. To get in one must have permission.' Perhaps this parallels medical systems and art therapy which both have ritual-like procedures of assessment, entry and time boundaries. Toombs (1990) cautions that in temporal experience of illness there can be a disparity between the patient's experience of 'flux of subjective time' and the physician's approach based on objective time. As an art therapist I needed to be aware that clients can use therapy to escape from 'our fear of losses, separations, endings' and to 'escape from it into timelessness' or an 'addiction to the experience of time-lessness' (Molnos 1995: 19–20). Dreifuss-Kattan (1994: 125–8) suggests that artworks become 'transitional objects between . . . past time and present time', allowing for 'a temporary defense against timelessness in its traumatic, fragmenting aspect', and helping patients face mortality and experience the duality of 'end' *and* 'endlessness'.

Bakhtin (2000: 84) uses the term *chronotope*, meaning 'time space', to refer to 'the intrinsic connectedness of temporal and spatial relationships that are artistically expressed in literature'. Perhaps Bakhtin's (2000) concept of the 'chronotope' could be applied to the artwork that embodies clients' expression of 'time space'. He proposes that in 'the literary artistic chronotope, spatial and temporal indicators are fused into one carefully thought-out, concrete whole. Time, as it were, thickens, takes on flesh, becomes artistically visible; likewise space becomes charged and responsive to the movements of time, plot and history' (Bakhtin 2000: 84). Embodiment will also be discussed later and in Chapter 4.

Power/powerlessness

A second characteristic of liminality to be explored in its relevance to cancer experiences and art therapy *is power/powerlessness*. Turner (1975: 231) suggests that liminality is associated with structural inferiority and outsiderhood, submission to 'authority' (Turner 1995: 103), being 'passive' (Turner 1995: 95), 'submissiveness and silence' (Turner 1995: 103) and also with 'ritual powers' (Turner 1995: 100).

A cancer diagnosis can begin 'a series of frightening events over which the patient has little control' (Cunningham *et al.* 1991: 71). Lack of control over one's body and uncertainty about the possibility of recurrence are distressing (Moch 1990). Little *et al.* (1998: 1485) describe how an 'initial acute phase of liminality is marked by disorientation, a sense of loss and of loss of control, and a sense of uncertainty'. Sometimes then an 'adaptive, enduring phase of suspended liminality supervenes, in which each patient constructs and reconstructs meaning for their experience by means of narrative'. In acute liminality 'patients resign themselves to the system and surrender control, recognising that the label "cancer" demands these surrenders, and that it accords the system special duties and powers. Some patients were relieved to hand over control; others resisted' (Little *et al.* 1998: 1487). The issue of power in healthcare is complex (Canter 2001) and perhaps patients' degree of trust in the fiduciary relationship with a doctor and/or art therapist can depend on whether they perceive the practitioner's power as 'legitimate', 'expert' and 'referent' (French and Raven 1959) or not.

One lymphoma patient valued how art as therapy allowed self-expression and self-control, since doctors controlled her body (Lynn 1995). Medical art therapy can promote 'personal empowerment' (Malchiodi 1999: 14; 1996) and artwork is a 'vehicle' to discover and activate 'deeper resources' (Connell 1998: 90). Art enables a dialogue with our destructive and creative forces, enabling patients to activate change and find solutions from within, rather than relying on external treatment (Adamson 1984: 8). It can promote the expression of emotion and reduce feelings of helplessness and hopelessness (Hiltebrand 1999).

Turner (1982: 26) describes how liminal persons undergo a 'leveling' process which can feature symbols of effacement such as being 'stripped of names and clothing', 'eating or not eating specific foods', 'wearing of uniform clothing, sometimes irrespective of sex'. Some clients told me of difficulties encountered with restrictive hospital food and of self-chosen diets outside hospital selected to try to promote health. Males and females also spoke of the embarrassment of wearing the hospital gowns during examinations or scans and of feeling 'exposed' and 'vulnerable'. I needed to be aware that art therapy plastic aprons might stimulate emotion by reminding clients of gowns. Therefore when appropriate I encouraged clients who wished to bring their own aprons. Promoting client choice was important with regard to art materials and therapy decisions in general and this was facilitated through the therapy contract and regular contract reviews.

All clients commented on issues relating to power. One client, a man in his thirties diagnosed with a brain tumour, reported experiencing 'helplessness and no control over it and over what the doctor will decide. I can try to convince him to do chemo but it's his decision.' Another client, diagnosed with a type of facial cancer, reported: 'It's like I am trying to get rid of this anger and this cancer, maybe weakening it or diluting it. This is coming out of me onto these [the artworks]. I feel I lost control and I need to get that back', and she reported that art therapy gave her a sense of greater control. Many clients reported an increased sense of empowerment through the art therapy. One, diagnosed with ovarian cancer, reported: 'You helped me be in control of things and the media in the drawing helped me find control.' Another client discussed how creating rectangles had helped her in 'trying to show a sort of order, regularity'. Another said art therapy 'gave me something positive and powerful during my week'. Another reported: 'I feel more empowered about my situation.'

Yet *losing* control to the art materials during spontaneous art-making might also help a person come to terms with lack of control. One male client reported: 'Art – not conscious control as it does what it wants, I follow, yet a progressive sense of mastery over the art materials – it's a paradox.' As an embodied image, it 'engages the artist/client in its making; it is as if the picture seems to lead, becoming something rather different than originally intended' (Schaverien 2000: 59).

The next section on playing also discusses the relationship between various types of play and power or powerlessness.

Playing

A third characteristic of liminality to be explored in its relevance to cancer experiences and art therapy is *playing*. Liminality is associated with 'varieties of playful experience' (Turner 1988: 124–5). Indeed, Wilson (1980) reconfigures the classic three-phase rites of passage model and parallels separation with 'preparation', liminality with 'play' and incorporation with 'a game' where people develop new thoughts and behaviours. Turner discusses the relevance to rites of passage of Caillois' (1962) theory of play.

A surrealist and anthropologist, Caillois outlined types of play ranging from play bound by conventions (*ludus*) to spontaneous improvization (*paidia*). Turner (1988: 125) notes that *paidia* stems from the Greek word for 'child' (Caillois 1962: 27) and it is defined as 'free improvization' (Caillois 1962: 13) and 'spontaneous manifestations of the play instinct' (Caillois 1962: 28). *Ludus* involves a 'tendency to bind it with arbitrary, imperative, and purposely tedious conventions' (Caillois 1962: 13) and 'calculation and contrivance' (Caillois 1962: 31).

Therapy has been conceived of as a form of playing; in fact Winnicott (1996: 57) makes 'a plea to every therapist to allow for the patient's capacity to play'. The presence of the art therapist is important because 'it would seem that play lacks something when it is reduced to a mere solitary exercise' (Caillois 1962: 39) and such players 'need an attentive and sympathetic audience' (Caillois 1962: 40). One client reported valuing how art therapy gave her 'permission to play . . . freedom of expression'. Another reported it was valuable to 'be given "permission" to play', and another said: 'It was lovely to be allowed to "play" again.'

Permission is both internal and external, thus relating to Rogers' (1996: 353–9) summary of 'inner' and 'external' conditions fostering creativity. I endeavoured to provide the external conditions: first, 'psychological safety', established by regarding both client and artwork as of unconditional worth, being non-judgemental and empathic; second, 'psychological freedom . . . of *symbolic* expression'. These could foster inner conditions in the client: first, 'openness to experience' and a 'tolerance of ambiguity'; second, an 'internal locus of evaluation'; third, 'the ability to toy with elements and concepts', i.e. 'the ability to play spontaneously with ideas, colors, shapes, relationships . . .'.

The aspect of needing to find external and inner permission to play was evident in my experience with another client, a man in his seventies diagnosed with prostate cancer. In his first group session after I had explained the nature of art therapy and that it did not require skill, he declined to make art but said he would observe. However, noticing that he was curiously watching the others making art, I encouraged him again to try the materials. He did so but soon stopped, telling me that he was no good at art. I asked him what made him think that and he replied: 'I was told at school I was no good at art, that I'd got no imagination.' This imposed self-concept had stayed with him.

I had noticed that when he had begun to make the art he seemed initially absorbed until he sat back and looked at it and seemed to judge it. I shared my observation and assumption with him and asked him how he had felt when actually making the art. He replied: 'It felt good', so I encouraged him to try again, suspending the judgement. He chose a pencil first and drew the outline of a house with a door and smoking chimney, a path and smaller building. He then chose soft pastels, coloured the house and path and added items in the garden that he described as grass, a wheelbarrow, two trees and a swing.

Several factors prompted me to ask him a particular question. These included the way he had engaged with art-making, the absence of any humans in the art yet symbols indicating habitation, and the fact that this could be our first yet last session due to his terminal condition. I asked him: 'I wonder who uses the wheelbarrow and who swings on the swing?' He immediately replied: 'The wee boy who lives in the house plays on the swing.' Later he called me over and excitedly showed me that he had drawn a figure in a space beside the path. He said to me: 'Look! The wee boy has come out to play.' I replied: 'You have made a space for the wee boy to come out to play.' He looked at me with an emotional expression and we both acknowledged that he was talking about the 'wee boy' in the picture and also the child in him who was now playing. I found this an emotional and powerful moment in our therapy. (See Figure 2.1, on website.)

This gentleman went on to have a number of sessions before he died and in what turned out to be his last session he drew a number of flags of his own design. He told me they were 'flying in celebration' but he did not know what of.

Types of play and their relationship to power or powerlessness

My professional and personal experience indicated that cancer experiences feature diverse types of play and each seemed to be in a relationship with power or powerlessness. These included play associated with Caillois' (1962) types of play: role play (*Mimicry*), chance or fate (*Alea*), competition (*Agôn*), vertigo (*Ilinx*).

Mimicry

This type involves play that is like 'wearing a mask, or *playing a part*' (Caillois 1962: 20). This could relate to various forms of disguising such as masking emotions to protect others and denial, which may be adaptive as a normal reaction allowing adjustment or maladaptive if problematic. One client told me that a male figure in her artwork was saying 'Please help me' and when I asked what help he wanted the client replied he was saying 'Please help me . . . stop hiding . . . It's like help me you haven't done me right.' The client explained that he had been coloured pink as a positive colour because that was how she herself portrayed to her family, yet she reported: 'I really wanted to do it black because that was how I was feeling.' A suppressed voice was perhaps given a means of expression.

Alea

This type of play relates to chance or fate. The player is 'entirely passive . . . All he need do is await, in hope and trembling, the cast of the die . . . *alea* is a negation of the will, a surrender to destiny' (Caillois 1962: 17–18). Superstitious thinking could be evoked which could be conceived as negative or positive. Halvorson-Boyd and Hunter (1995: 3), both cancer patients and healthcare professionals, describe how, when writing about their illness, 'We had to face the irrational fear that talking about survival would jinx our own cures.' I personally can identify with that. Caillois (1962: 46–7) suggests that a 'corruption' of *alea* can involve 'superstition' and talismans. However, Schaverien (1992, 1994) suggests that in art therapy the artwork can have a positive function as a 'talisman'. McNiff (1998: 69) also comments that physical objects made in art therapy become 'props, talismans'.

Ritual art-making can have associations with power, play and the auspicious. Ritual threshold art symbols called *kolams* (Kavuri 1998; Nagarajan 1997), *muggu* or, when coloured, *rangoli* (Kilambi 1985; Reddy 1998), are made by Hindu women in the 'liminal space of the threshold' of houses (Kavuri 1998). A 'kolam' has associations with play and warding off bad luck and is created in a 'ritual performance' at a 'contingent moment' or threshold time, such as morning, and kolams are associated with the woman's sense of 'agency' (Kavuri 1998).

Clients reported feeling at times that their future seemed dependent on 'fate' or 'survival probability' figures. Some reported heightened superstitious behaviour and having 'lucky' objects or, like Halvorson-Boyd and Hunter (1995: 3), avoiding talking about being 'clear' or cured in case 'something bad' happened. At times I personally felt powerless, like a piece of meat being played with by something. In artwork clients often reported aspects, colours or specific symbols seeming to evoke hopes of future good fortune or fears of bad fortune. Some clients found spontaneously or deliberately created aspects of the art to be like a talisman or 'guardian angel'. One client created an image of a creature that she said was a companion that she evoked when frightened.

Agôn

This play is 'competitive', 'like a combat' (Caillois 1962: 14). Metaphors for cancer include 'invading', 'fight', 'war' and 'enemy' (Sontag 1978: 63–5; Skott 2002) and betrayal by one's body (Spiegel 1993: 16–17). Cancer can be conceived as the enemy within. Artwork is valuable in addressing how cancer can represent 'a bad internal object' (Dreifuss-Kattan 1994: 125). Bronson (1994) describes a 'cancer experience' conference where Bolen observed that many cancer patients 'bore the marks of a warrior, the scars . . .'. In the cancer experience, 'Putting up a good fight is socially endorsed' (Little *et al.* 1998: 1491).

One client drew images of a figure that had multiple meanings. It was the thing being fought such as 'a cancer cell being squashed until he's not there', yet also the 'fighter', the part of her fighting the cancer. In cancer group art therapy, themes of dealing with possibly ambivalent feelings of treatment being paradoxically both 'healer' and 'hurter' can be processed (Minar 1999).

In studying Ndembu rites of passage Turner (1967: 59–92) found that many rituals featured the symbolic colours red, black and white, with white being linked to life, purity and health, black to impurity and death, and red to blood and power. Bly (1993: 200) suggests that Europeans have similar meanings for these colours. These three colours are the first to be named in many languages (Berlin and Kay 1969). Red can represent ambiguity as in 'betwixt and between' situations and 'conceptual boundary crossings' (Jacobson-Widding 2001: 2247). Owoc (2002), citing Taçon (1999: 122), asserts that 'colour plays an important role in the recording of change', in that new identities are 'given substance' and 'particular events are highlighted or defined through the deliberate use of colour and coloured materials'. She adds that colour is often 'intimately involved' in the 'communication of change, time, and identity'.

In my art and that of my clients, specific colours generally had multiple meanings that could be influenced by personal and cultural factors. Sometimes white was referred to as positive, black as negative and red as linking to blood, but not always. One client reported a 'fight' going on in the art between the lighter colours and the darker ones representing cancer and said 'I don't like using the dark colours.' One picture was of coloured shapes, some black, all outlined in black. She spoke of the lighter colours moving to fight the darker shapes: 'I feel that is trying to push that out . . . The yellow and the peach triangles are very positive. Movement . . . they are washing over the darkness.' However, reflecting on the same picture she commented positively on the black outlines: 'Although I've outlined it in black I think it's more like a fence to try and keep it in. The cancer, I suppose, to keep it in one place so it won't travel to anywhere else.' Another client reported a gradual move from darker to lighter colours in her art to be positive and reported it was good 'bringing out colours that I thought were buried'. However, another client reported having 'no sense that black is bad and white is good'.

It is important to point out that Turner (1982: 27) emphasizes that liminality involves the use of 'multivocal symbols', i.e. 'symbol-vehicles – sensorily perceptible forms', such as 'trees, images, paintings . . . that are each susceptible not of a single meaning but of many meanings'. This parallels Jung's (1981: para. 199) concept of the 'shimmering symbol', whose meaning in art therapy is not fixed, but living (McNiff 1992: 105). Symbols carry a sense of 'and–and–and', this being 'the essence of art as therapy and the therapist must beware of defining symbols as fixed signs' (Simon 1997: 116). Modell (1997) suggests that metaphorical expression enables a fluid experience along two spectra of *fixed* to *open* as well as *personal* to *collective* meanings. Thus I believe art therapy can promote a both/and perspective rather than an either/or perspective.

Ilinx

Such play is 'based on the pursuit of vertigo and . . . an attempt to moment-arily destroy the stability of perception and inflict a kind of voluptuous panic upon an otherwise lucid mind' and is etymologically linked to whirlpool (Caillois 1962: 23–4). It can be an embodied experience. The existential experience of one's own mortality is perhaps relevant here. Writing of limi-nality in cancer experiences, Little *et al.* (1998: 1491) note the awareness of one's 'boundedness' and quote Jaspers (1986: 112), who wrote: 'The move-ment of fright, expressed as vertigo and shuddering, becomes, in anxiety, the turning point where I become conscious that I can be annihilated.'

Symbolic objects

Turner (1982: 32) suggests that ritual objects can be played with but liminal play is not 'leisure', rather it is 'in earnest', associated with 'work' and involves 'performing symbolic actions and manipulating symbolic objects' or ritual objects to bring about change. Art therapy is not just a diversion or pastime (Schaverien 1992: 2). McNiff (1998: 69) argues that the physical objects made in art therapy 'have especially potent powers for stimulating ritual, performance, and creative movement. They become props, talismans, and ritual objects.' Artwork can act as a 'transitional object' (Winnicott 1996: 1) in therapy and act as a defence against anxiety, particularly at times of transition (Arthern and Madill 1999: 1). Young (1994) asserts that Winnicott (1996) believed that the transitional object 'is the rite of passage for entering the realms of symbolism and culture'. Arthern and Madill (2002: 384) suggest that clients can use transitional objects within 'ritualised sequences of behaviour'. They propose a five-phase spiral theory of how transitional objects enable clients to move through a holding process (Arthern and Madill 2002: 379) in which the:

1 client cannot hold a positive sense of self;
2 therapist holds for the client;
3 transitional object holds;
4 client holds the transitional object and can evoke the therapist's holding capacity;
5 client holds without a transitional object.

Artwork can function as a 'container' (Bion 1959: 308–15), a 'talisman' (Schaverien 1992) and be the focus of transference. Schaverien (1994: 82) argues that art therapy is different from psychotherapy in that the artwork can become a 'scapegoat' and then 'disposal' can occur through its destruc-tion or leaving with the art therapist. She adds that the act is 'empowered through ritual, and so becomes an "enactment" . . .'. Moon (2001: 39) describes this as 'a positive enactment of ritual transference and disposal'.

Thus artwork, as transitional object, container and scapegoat, has a potential to enable people both to develop their capacity to hold positive as well as difficult aspects and to dispose of particular aspects. In clients' and my own artwork these functions were important in working on self/body image, and feelings such as anger.

Flow

Writing of play, Turner (1982: 55–9) suggests there is a relationship between the liminal and Csikszentmihalyi's (2002; Csikszentmihalyi and Csikszent-mihalyi 1988) concept of 'flow', a holistic sensation experienced when one is totally involved in an activity. Csikszentmihalyi (2002: 49–70) describes characteristics of flow: a merging of action and awareness; a loss of self-consciousness yet paradoxically a resulting stronger sense of self; a centring of attention; a loss of ego as kinaesthetic awareness is heightened, a trans-formation of time experience; a challenge yet achievability as there is a developing 'capacity to manipulate symbolic information' (Csikszentmihalyi 2002: 50); and autotelic experience, i.e. worth doing for its own sake (Csik-szentmihalyi 2002: 67). He also suggests that 'the *possibility*, rather than the *actuality*, of control' (Csikszentmihalyi 2002: 60) is experienced and this contributes to feeling empowered through playing.

This links to the 'reverie' art-making offers (Milner 1977: 163; Simon 1992: 88), to Maslow's (1971: 63) 'absorption' component of 'peak experi-ence', to Winnicott's (1996) 'relaxed state' which generates 'creative playing', and possibly to meditative experience such as 'jhana' or 'total immersion' in an object the mind is centred on (Gunaratana 1988).

All clients reported experiencing various aspects of flow during art-making, particularly absorption or reverie. A client reported it helpful: 'Being able to relax, clear my mind and be totally absorbed with one thing.' Another client stated: 'Becoming involved in my project that I forgot about *all* my worries while I was doing it.' Another said: 'You do get into it. I noticed it here and I noticed it at home when I'm doing it. You just go into it. It has been helpful because it's "me time". I can just feel myself calming down and letting go.' She added that art therapy had helped her to 'really express that movement and freedom, you really do get into it. I can move this and hopefully achieve something.' Another client reported often feeling in a 'daydream state when making the art'. Another reported: 'Absorbed my mind completely. Involvement and absorption in creating.'

Communitas

A fourth characteristic of liminality to be explored briefly in its relevance to cancer experiences and art therapy is *communitas*. Turner (1982: 58) notes that whilst 'flow' is experienced within an individual, 'communitas' is experienced between individuals. A form of social 'anti-structure', it is a 'liberation of human capacities of cognition, affect, volition, creativity, etc., from the normative constraints incumbent upon occupying a sequence of social statuses' (Turner 1982: 44). In this form of shared experience, social interaction, communion or connection, 'fellow liminars' treat each other as equals irrespective of previous status differences (Turner 1967: 7).

Montgomery (2002: 34–5) comments that groups with specific goals like 'coming to terms with a diagnosis of cancer' have a 'homogeneous popula-tion with a shared and clearly stated aim'. Social support in cancer groups can be life-enhancing and empowering (Spiegel *et al.* 1989). Montgomery (2002: 38) cites research suggesting that 'group cohesion' is linked to effi-cacy of group therapy (Tschuschke and Dies 1994). Sharing, witnessing and active participation can help individuals build a bridge from 'alienation' towards social experience (Winnicott 1996). Art therapy group-studio chemistry can be based on 'the process of individual people performing the intimate and isolating rituals of painting within a communal environment' (McNiff 1995: 182). McNiff adds: 'It is this process of making art together and then bearing witness to the arrivals in a sacred way that establishes the healing imagination of the environment.'

As noted by Barber and Campbell (1999: 30), art therapy rituals can be paralleled with Myerhoff's (1982: 105) concept of 'definitional ceremonies', in which White (2000) notes that 'socially marginal people, disdained, ignored groups' can engage in 'collective self definitions', as can individuals with 'spoiled identities' (Goffman 1963). Sadly, Myerhoff herself died of cancer. White (2000) summarizes that in the 'tellings and retellings' of defi-nitional ceremonies people's lives are 're-membered', thus enabling people to revise 'the membership of their association of life', contributing to the 'production of multi-voiced identities'. In art therapy groups, the therapist, group and artworks perhaps provide a 'reflecting team' or 'outsider-witness group' (White 2000) in which such definitional ceremonies occur. However, perhaps ritual is a better term than ceremony. Turner (1982: 80–1) explains that 'Ceremony *indicates*, ritual *transforms*, and transformation occurs most radically in the ritual "pupation" of liminal seclusion – at least in life-crisis rituals.' He adds that 'living ritual' can be 'likened to artwork'. Perhaps in art therapy what might be called *redefinitional rituals* can occur.

Clients reported the communitas aspect in a number of ways. One client, a woman in her fifties diagnosed with breast cancer, reported that group art therapy was valuable in developing 'bonding with others who know what you have been through'. Another reported the 'positive support of therapist and other members of the group' as valuable. In a focus group and inter-views all participants reported that knowing I had experienced cancer too had positively affected their sharing and the relationship. I disclose my situ-ation briefly as appropriate if there is a possibility that clients might discover this aspect, for instance if I encountered them unexpectedly whilst attending hospital (which has happened) or if I became ill. Although common feelings can be experienced, each patient has a unique experience of cancer and this can be affected by many variables including the type and phase of cancer and prognosis. Care is needed when creating art therapy groups to ensure the group make-up is appropriate and to try to avoid cross-traumatization.

Conclusion

In this chapter, I have discussed liminality and four of its characteristics – *limbo, power, playing* and *communitas* – and their relevance to cancer experiences and art therapy. Chapter 4 will explore a fifth characteristic: embodied experience, and Chapter 16 will explore liminality in my *own* experience as a cancer patient, art-maker and art therapist.

I have suggested that Turner's model of liminality illuminates both the art therapy and cancer experience and so has particular relevance for art therapy with cancer patients. It is probable that liminality and its characteristics are valuable lenses through which to explore the lived experience of other life-threatening illnesses and other liminal experiences. Turner's model suggests that at times of transition and anxiety people are stimulated to engage in ritual and symbolic expressions and performances associated with rites of passage. The model throws light on some factors that prompt humans to make art at transitional times potentially for individual and evolutionary functions.

Perhaps art therapy can provide an opening for symbolic and metaphorical expression of liminal cancer experience. Amidst limbo it can offer therapeutic liminal or heterotopic space and therapeutic time and timelessness experience, and foster capabilities for staying with uncertainty. Amidst diminished power it can offer empowerment and constructive lack of control. Amidst hiding, chance-driven, competitive and frightening forms of play it offers improvizational play with symbolic objects and colours, thus stimulating flow experience and promoting empowerment and a both/and rather than an either/or perspective. Amidst alienation it provides opportunities for creative communion and comradeship. In general it offers a potential for *redefinitional rituals*. This is facilitated by an attentive therapist and 'reflecting team' that includes the artworks and, in groups, group members.

The use of multivocal symbols allows previously suppressed voices to be expressed and join the dominant voices, thus enabling a process of 'social inclusion' (McLeod 1999) to previously unshared material. Such experience could also develop a person's capacity for crossing thresholds and thus deal with the 'oscillating trajectory' between acute and sustained liminality (Little *et al.* 1998: 1493) and the 'shifting perspectives' dynamic of cancer experience (Paterson 2001; Thorne *et al.* 2002: 449). One client reported: 'The journey is brighter . . . but you also know that there's still going to be times when you go back to being bewildered, stunned, frightened, you know, and it's just a passage.' Perhaps art therapy accommodates, and can potentially promote better tolerance of, the unique, ambiguous and shifting meanings inherent in cancer experiences.

References

Achterberg, J., Dossey, B. and Kolkmeier, L. (1994) *Rituals of Healing: Using Imagery for Health and Wellness*. New York: Bantam Doubleday Dell.

Adamson, E. (1984) *Art As Healing*. London: Coventure.

Aldridge, D. (2000) Music therapy: performances and narratives, *Musictherapy World 'Research News 1'*, November, http://www.musictherapyworld.de/modules/archive/stuff/papers/TalkPSYCH3.pdf (accessed 7 August 2004).

Arthern, J. and Madill, A. (1999) How do transitional objects work? The therapist's view, *British Journal of Medical Psychology*, 72(Pt.1): 1–21.

Arthern, J. and Madill, A. (2002) How do transitional objects work? The client's view, *Psychotherapy Research*, 12(3): 369–88.

Bakhtin, M.M. (2000) *The Dialogic Imagination* (edited by Michael Holquist, translated by Michael Holquist and Caryl Emerson). Austin, TX: University of Texas Press.

Barber, V. and Campbell, J. (1999) Living colour in art therapy: visual and verbal narrative of black and white, in J. Campbell, M. Liebmann, F. Brooks, J. Jones and C. Ward (eds) *Art Therapy, Race and Culture*. London: Jessica Kingsley.

Bartunek, J.M. and Necochea, R.A. (2000) Old insights and new times: Kairos, Inca cosmology, and their contributions to contemporary management inquiry, *Journal of Management Inquiry*, 9(2): 103–12.

Berlin, B. and Kay, P. (1969) *Basic Color Terms: Their Universality and Evolution*. Berkeley, CA: University of California Press.

Bhattacharya, R. (2004) *Designing a Questionnaire for Medical Research and Audit*. The Royal College of Surgeons of Edinburgh, Surgical Knowledge and Skills Web Site. Lectures and Tutorials: Assessment and Monitoring, http://www.edu.rcsed.ac.uk/lectures/lt25.htm (accessed 7 August 2004).

Bion, W.R. (1959) Attacks on linking, *International Journal of Psychoanalysis*, XL: 308–15.

Bly, R. (1993) *Iron John*. Longmead: Element Books.

Bolen, J.S. (1998) *Close to the Bone: Life-threatening Illness and the Search for Meaning*. New York: Touchstone/Simon & Schuster.

Brewer, J.D. (2000) *Ethnography*. Buckingham: Open University Press.

Bronson, M. (1994) Reinterpreting the cancer experience, *Breast Cancer Action, Newsletter*, 25, August. Report of the conference 'Cancer as a Turning Point: From Surviving to Thriving', http://www.bcaction.org/Pages/SearchablePages/1994Newsletters/Newsletter025L.html (accessed 5 August 2004).

Caillois, R. (1962) *Man, Play and Games*. London: Thames and Hudson.

Canter, R. (2001) Patients and medical power, *British Medical Journal*, 25 August, 323: 414, http://bmj.bmjjournals.com/cgi/content/full/323/7310/414 (accessed 2 August 2004).

Case, C. and Dalley, T. (1997) *The Handbook of Art Therapy*. London: Routledge.

Claxton, G. (1998) *Hare Brain, Tortoise Mind. Why Intelligence Increases When You Think Less*. London: Fourth Estate.

Cohen, M. (2002) Death ritual: anthropological perspectives, in P.A. Pecorino (ed.) *Perspectives on Death and Dying*. Online Textbook. Department of Social Sciences, Queensborough Community College, City University, NY, http://www2.sunysuffolk.edu/pecorip/SCCCWEB/ETEXTS/DeathandDying_TEXT/table_of_contents.htm (accessed 2 August 2004).

Cohn, E.S. (2001) From waiting to relating: parents' experiences in the waiting room of an occupational therapy clinic, *American Journal of Occupational Therapy*, 55(2): 167–74.

Colyer, H. (1996) Women's experience of living with cancer, *Journal of Advanced Nursing*, 23(3): 496–501.

Connell, C. (1998) *Something Understood. Art Therapy in Cancer Care*. London: Wrexham.

Csikszentmihalyi, M. (2002) *Flow*. London: Rider.

Csikszentmihalyi, M. and Csikszentmihalyi, I.S. (eds) (1988) *Optimal Experience: Psychological Studies of Flow in Consciousness*. New York: Cambridge University Press.

Cunningham, A. *et al.* (1991) A relationship between perceived self-efficacy and quality of life in cancer patients, *Patient Education and Counseling*, 17: 71–8.

Dreifuss-Kattan, E. (1994) *Cancer Stories: Creativity and Self-Repair*. Hillsdale, NJ: The Analytic Press.

Dyer, A.R. (2002) *A Helicopter Named Icarus: Essays on Health, Healing, Medicine and Spirituality*. Unpublished online book. Department of Psychiatry and Behavioral Sciences, James H. Quillen College of Medicine, East Tennessee State University, http://faculty.etsu.edu/dyer/books/icarus/ (accessed 3 August 2004).

Ellis, C. and Bochner, P.A. (2000) Autoethnography, personal narrative, reflexivity: researcher as subject, in N.K. Denzin and Y.S. Lincoln (eds) *Handbook of Qualitative Research*. Thousand Oaks, CA: Sage Publications.

Flanagan J. and Holmes, S. (2000) Social perceptions of cancer and their impacts: implications for nursing practice arising from the literature, *Journal of Advanced Nursing*, 32(3): 740–9.

Foucault, M. (1986) Of other spaces, *Diacritics 16*, Spring, 22–7, http://www-unix.oit.umass.edu/~bweber/courses/foucaultspaces.html (accessed 7 August 2004).

Frank, J.D. (1973) *Persuasion and Healing: A Comparative Study of Psychotherapy*. Baltimore, MD: Johns Hopkins University Press.

French J.R.P. and Raven, B. (1959) The bases of social power, in D. Cartwright (ed.) *Studies in Social Power*. Ann Arbor, MI: Institute for Social Research.

Froggatt, K. (1997) Rites of passage and the hospice culture, *Mortality*, 2(2): 123–36.

Gibbs, R.W. and Franks, H. (2002) Embodied metaphor in women's narratives about their experiences with cancer, *Health Communication*, 14(2): 139–65.

Goffman, E. (1963) *Stigma: Notes on the Management of Spoiled Identity*. New York: Simon & Schuster.

Gunaratana, H. (1988) *The Jhanas in Theravada Buddhist Meditation*, The Wheel Publication No. 351/353. Kandy, Sri Lanka: Buddhist Publication Society, http://www.accesstoinsight.org/lib/bps/wheels/wheel351.html (accessed 8 August 2004).

Halvorson-Boyd, G. and Hunter, L.K. (1995) *Dancing in Limbo: Making Sense of Life After Cancer.* San Francisco, CA: Jossey-Bass.

Hartocollis, P. (1983) *Time and Timelessness or the Varieties of Temporal Experience (A Psychoanalytic Inquiry).* New York: International Universities Press.

Hiltebrand, E.U. (1999) Coping with cancer through image manipulation, in C.A. Malchiodi (ed.) *Medical Art Therapy with Adults.* London: Jessica Kingsley.

Jacobson-Widding, A. (2001) Color classification and symbolism, in N.J. Smelser and P.B. Baltes (eds) *International Encyclopedia of the Social and Behavioral Sciences.*

Jaspers, K. (1986) *Karl Jaspers: Basic Philosophical Writings.* New Jersey, NJ: Humanities Press.

Jung, C.G. (1981) *Alchemical Studies. Collected Works 13.* London: Routledge & Kegan Paul.

Kavuri, S. (1998) Ritual domestic threshold drawings of South India: a visual trope of the socialized Hindu feminine, *Iconomania: Studies in Visual Culture,* Electronic Journal, http://www.humnet.ucla.edu/humnet/arthist/icono/kavuri/kolam.htm (accessed 12 August 2004).

Kenny, C.B. (1996) The dilemma of uniqueness: an essay on consciousness and qualities, *Nordic Journal of Music Therapy,* 5(2): 87–96, http://www.hisf.no/njmt/kenny.html (accessed 5 August 2004).

Kilambi, J.S. (1985) Toward an understanding of the muggu: threshold drawings in Hyderabad, *Res: Anthropology and Aesthetics,* Autumn, 10: 71–102.

Kirmayer, L.J. (2003) Asklepian dreams: the ethos of the wounded-healer in the clinical encounter, *Transcultural Psychiatry,* 40(2): 248–77.

Kleinman, A. (1989) *The Illness Narratives: Suffering, Healing, and the Human Condition.* New York: Basic Books.

Lakoff, G. and Johnson, M. (1980) *Metaphors We Live By.* Chicago, IL: University of Chicago Press.

Lertzman, D.A. (2002) Rediscovering rites of passage: education, transformation, and the transition to sustainability, *Conservation Ecology,* 5(2): 30, http://www.consecol.org/vol5/iss2/art30 (accessed 13 August 2004).

Little, M., Jordens, C.F., Paul, K., Montgomery, K. and Philipson, B. (1998) Liminality: a major category of the experience of cancer illness, *Social Science & Medicine,* 47(10): 1492–3.

Lynn, D. (1995) Healing through art, *Art Therapy: Journal of the American Art Therapy Association,* 12(1): 70–1.

McLeod, J. (1999) Counselling as a social process, *Counselling,* 10: 217–22.

McNiff, S. (1992) *Art as Medicine – Creating a Therapy of the Imagination.* London, Boston, MA: Shambala Publications.

McNiff, S. (1995) Keeping the studio, *Art Therapy: Journal of the American Art Therapy Association,* 12: 179–83.

McNiff, S. (1998) *Art-Based Research.* London: Jessica Kingsley.

Mahdi, L.C., Christopher, N.G. and Meade, M. (eds) (1996) *Crossroads: The Quest for Contemporary Rites of Passage.* La Salla, IL: Open Court Publishing Company.

Malchiodi, C.A. (1996) Art as empowerment for women with breast cancer, in S. Hogan (ed.) *Feminist Art Therapy: Visions of Difference.* London: Routledge.

Malchiodi, C.A. (ed.) (1999) *Medical Art Therapy with Adults*. London: Jessica Kingsley.

Maslow, A.H. (1971) *The Farther Reaches of Human Nature*. New York: The Viking Press.

Miller, B. (1996) Art therapy with the elderly and the terminally ill, in T. Dalley (ed.) *Art as Therapy: An Introduction to the Use of Art as a Therapeutic Technique*. London: Routledge.

Milner, M. (1977) *On Not Being Able To Paint*. Oxford: Heinemann Educational Books.

Minar, V. M. (1999) Art therapy and cancer: images of the hurter and the healer, in C.A. Malchiodi (ed.) *Medical Art Therapy with Adults*. London: Jessica Kingsley.

Mitchell, S. (1999) Reflections on dramatherapy as initiation through ritual theatre, in A. Cattanach (ed.) *Process in the Arts Therapies*. London: Jessica Kingsley.

Moch, S. (1990) Health within the experience of breast cancer, *Journal of Advanced Nursing*, 15(12): 1426–35.

Modell, A.H. (1997) The synergy of memory, affects and metaphor, *The Journal of Analytical Psychology*, 42(1): 105–17.

Molnos, A. (1995) *A Question of Time: On Brief Dynamic Therapy*. London: Karnac Books.

Montgomery, C. (2002) Role of dynamic group therapy in psychiatry, *Advances in Psychiatric Treatment*, 8: 34–41, http://apt.rcpsych.org/cgi/reprint/8/1/34 (accessed 8 August 2004).

Moon, C. (2001) Prayer, sacraments, grace, in M. Farrelly-Hansen (ed.) *Spirituality and Art Therapy: Living the Connection*. London: Jessica Kingsley.

Moore, R.L. (1991) Ritual, sacred space, and healing, the psychoanalyst as ritual elder, in N. Schwartz-Salant and M. Stein (eds) *Liminality and Transitional Phenomena*. Wilmette, IL: Chiron Publications.

Moore, R.L. (2001) *The Archetype of Initiation: Sacred Space, Ritual Process, and Personal Transformation*. Philadelphia, PA: Xlibris Corporation.

Murray, T.J. (2000) Personal time: the patient's experience, *Annals of Internal Medicine*, 132(1): 58–62, http://www.annals.org/issues/v132n1/full/200001040-00010.html (accessed 2 August 2004).

Muzzin, L.J. *et al.* (1994) The experience of cancer, *Social Science & Medicine*, 38(9): 1201–8.

Myerhoff, B. (1982) Life history among the elderly: performance, visibility and re-membering, in J. Ruby (ed.) *A Crack in the Mirror: Reflexive Perspectives in Anthropology*. Philadelphia, PA: University of Pennsylvania Press.

Nagarajan, V.R. (1997) Inviting the goddess into the household: women's kolams in Tamil Nadu, *Whole Earth*, Summer, http://www.findarticles.com/p/articles/mi_mOGER/is_n90/as_19777421/print (accessed 23 February 2005).

Owoc, M.A. (2002) *Munselling the Mound: The Use of Soil Colour as Metaphor in British Bronze Age Funerary Ritual*. Mercyhurst Archaeological Institute, Erie, Pennsylvania. Research project, http://mai.mercyhurst.edu/PDFs/MAO_Munsell.pdf (accessed 13 August 2004).

Pandey, M. and Thomas, B.C. (2001) Rehabilitation of cancer patients, *Postgraduate Medicine*, 47(1): 62–5.

Paterson, B.L. (2001) The shifting perspectives model of chronic illness, *Image: Journal of Nursing Scholarship*, 33(1): 21–6.

Reddy, P.C. (1998) Muggu – A Folk Art Form of Indian Women, *FOSSILS News*, No. 18–20, Newsletter of Folklore Society of South Indian Languages.

Richardson, L. (2000) Writing: a method of inquiry, in N. Denzin and Y. Lincoln (eds) *Handbook of Qualitative Research*. Thousand Oaks, CA: Sage Publications.

Riskó, Á., Deák, B., Molnár, Z., Schneider, T., Várady, E. and Rosta, A. (1998) Individual, psychoanalytically oriented psychotherapy during oncological treatment with adolescents suffering from malignant lymphoma. Online article based on lecture given at 4th International Congress of Psycho-oncology, Hamburg, Germany, 3–6 September, Oncopsychology Unit, National Institute of Oncology, Budapest, Hungary, Website, http://www.psycho-oncology.net/en1.html (accessed 23 February 2005).

Rogers, C.R. (1996) *On Becoming A Person*. London: Constable.

Rollins, H.E. (ed.) (1958) Letter to George and Tom Keats, 21 December 1817, in *The Letters of J. Keats: 1814–1821*. Cambridge: Cambridge University Press.

Ruud, E. (1995) Improvisation as a liminal experience: jazz and music therapy as modern 'rites de passage', in C.B. Kenny (ed.) *Listening, Playing, Creating: Essays on the Power of Sound*. New York: State University of New York Press.

Sabbadini, A. (1989) Boundaries of timelessness. Some thoughts about the temporal dimension of the psychoanalytic space, *International Journal of Psychoanalysis*, 70 (Pt.2): 305–13.

Schaverien, J. (1992) *The Revealing Image: Analytical Art Psychotherapy in Theory and Practice*. London: Routledge.

Schaverien, J. (1994) The scapegoat and the talisman: transference in art therapy, in T. Dalley *et al.* (eds) *Images of Art Therapy*. London: Routledge.

Schaverien, J. (2000) The triangular relationship and the aesthetic countertransference in analytical art psychotherapy, in A. Gilroy and G. McNeilly (eds) *The Changing Shape of Art Therapy: New Developments in Theory and Practice*. London: Jessica Kingsley.

Schechner, R. (2003) *Performance Studies: An Introduction*. London: Routledge.

Schubert, J. (2001) Between eternity and transience: on the significance of time in psychoanalysis, *Scandanavian Psychoanalytic Review*, 24: 93–100, http://www.spaf.a.se/spr/pages/back_issues/vol24_nr2/Schubert.pdf (accessed 10 August 2004).

Self, M. (1999) The sharp edge of Damocles, *Student BMJ*, March, 7: 85, http://www.studentbmj.com/back_issues/0399/data/0399pv1.htm (accessed 27 July 2004).

Simon, R.M. (1992) *The Symbolism of Style: Art as Therapy*. London: Routledge.

Simon, R.M. (1997) *Symbolic Images in Art As Therapy*. London: Routledge.

Skaife, S. and Huet, V. (1998) Introduction, in S. Skaife and V. Huet (eds) *Art Psychotherapy in Groups: Between Picture and Words*. London: Routledge.

Skott, C. (2002) Expressive metaphors in cancer narratives, *Cancer Nursing*, 25(3): 230–5.

Slattery, P. (2001) The educational researcher as artist working within, *Qualitative Inquiry*, 7(3): 370–98, http://www.coe.tamu.edu/~pslattery/documents/QualitativeInquiry.pdf (accessed 2 August 2004).

Sontag, S. (1978) *Illness as Metaphor*. New York: Farrar, Straus & Giroux.

Spiegel, D. (1993) *Living Beyond Limits. New Hope and Help for Facing Life-Threatening Illness*. New York: Times Books.

Spiegel, D., Bloom, J., Kraemer, H. and Gottheil, E. (1989) Effect of psychosocial treatment on survival of patients with metastatic breast cancer, *The Lancet*, 2(8668): 888–91.

Stanley, L. (1992) *The Auto/Biographical I*. Manchester: Manchester University Press.

Taçon, P. (1999) All things bright and beautiful: the role and meaning of colour in human development, *Cambridge Archaeological Journal*, 9(1): 120–3.

Thorne, S. *et al.* (2002) Chronic illness experience: insights from a metastudy, *Qualitative Health Research*, 12(4): 437–52.

Toombs, S.K. (1990) The temporality of illness: four levels of experience, *Theoretical Medicine*, 11(3): 227–41.

Trochim, W.M. (2000) Concept mapping, in *The Research Methods Knowledge Base*, 2nd edition, http://www.socialresearchmethods.net/kb/conmap.htm (accessed 3 August 2004).

Tschuschke, V. and Dies, R.R. (1994) Intensive analysis of therapeutic factors and outcome in long-term inpatient groups, *International Journal of Group Psychotherapy*, 44: 185–208.

Turner, V.W. (1967) *The Forest of Symbols: Aspects of Ndembu Ritual*. Ithaca, NY: Cornell University Press.

Turner, V.W. (1974) Liminal to liminoid in play, flow and ritual: an essay in comparative symbology, *Rice University Studies*, 60(3): 53–92.

Turner, V.W. (1975) *Dramas, Fields, and Metaphors: Symbolic Action in Human Society*. Ithaca, NY: Cornell University Press.

Turner, V.W. (1982) *From Ritual to Theatre: The Human Seriousness of Play*. New York: Performing Arts Journal Publications.

Turner, V.W. (1986) Dewey, Dilthey, and drama: an essay in the anthropology of experience, in V. Turner and E. Bruner (eds) *The Anthropology of Experience*. Champaign, IL: University of Illinois Press.

Turner, V.W. (1988) *The Anthropology of Performance*. New York: Performing Arts Journal Publications.

Turner, V.W. (1990) Are there universals of performance in myth, ritual, and drama?, in R. Schechner and W. Appel (eds) *By Means of Performance*. Cambridge: Cambridge University Press.

Turner, V.W. (1995) *The Ritual Process: Structure and Anti-Structure*. New York: Aldine de Gruyter.

Van der Hart, O. (1996) *Rituals in Psychotherapy: Transition and Continuity*. New York: Irvington Publishers.

Van Gennep, A. (1960) *The Rites of Passage*. London: Routledge & Kegan Paul.

Wall, L.L. (1996) Ritual meaning in surgery, *Obstetrics and Gynecology*, 88(4, Pt.1): 633–7.

White, E.C. (1987) *Kaironomia: On the Will-to-Invent*. Ithaca, NY: Cornell University Press.

White, M. (2000) Reflecting teamwork as definitional ceremony revisited, Dulwich Centre Website. Chapter 4 in White, M. (2000) *Reflections on Narrative Practice: Essays and Interviews*. Adelaide: Dulwich Centre Publications, http://www.dulwichcentre.com.au/reflectingarticle2.html (accessed 7 August 2004).

White, M. and Epston, D. (1990) *Narrative Means to Therapeutic Ends*. New York: W.W. Norton.

Williams, G. (1984) The genesis of chronic illness: narrative reconstruction, *Sociology of Health & Illness*, 6(2): 175–200.

Wilson, B. (1980) Social space and symbolic interaction, in A. Buttimer and D. Seamon (eds) *The Human Experience of Space and Place*. London: Croom Helm.

Winnicott, D.W. (1996) *Playing and Reality*. London: Routledge.

Young, R.M. (1994) Potential space: transitional phenomena, in *Mental Space*, online book. *The Human Nature Review*, http://human-nature.com/rmyoung/papers/paper55.html (accessed 5 August 2004).

3 | Body image and the construction of identity

Ken Evans

Illness

Modern attitudes to illness are well informed; alongside all of the other everyday warnings we are warned to be vigilant, to look for lumps and bumps and seek treatment without delay. It is part of our general assumptions that from time to time we become ill, and expect to recover. Modern medicine genuinely is able to cure most routine illnesses. But when we are smitten by a life-threatening illness, we already know the reputation of our opponent, and most of us know about our chances of survival. And because we also have some idea of biology and knowledge about our immune system, and can visualize, and can transport the pictures from the media into our own bodies, we are overwhelmed by our own helplessness to do anything about it. On discovering something that might be 'life-threatening', we immediately respond with desperation and panic. At this point it is easy to relinquish some of our independence, and we hand over ourselves, bit by bit, to the medical institutions. Erving Goffman (1963)[1] describes this process brilliantly, in terms of our sensations and feelings of utter powerlessness when faced by the immense and immovable power of social institutions, especially when we are ill. But institutional influences are not only experienced externally, for our institutionalized understanding of who and what we are penetrates deep into our psyche, to such an extent that in cases of AIDS and cancer some patients express feelings of claustrophobia, of being trapped inside a diseased body, or disgust at the physical disorder that is their disease. Whatever we were before this discovery begins, we crumble, and we assume a new identity – that of AIDS victim or cancer patient.

Cancer, AIDS and other degenerative diseases are not like other illnesses;

they don't come and go. They come, they stay, and they take over, and they erode us cell by cell. But through the power of our imaginations, we augment our suffering further; relentlessly eating ourselves away from within. The sheer terror of this is beyond anything fiction could impose. The symbolic pincer-like destructive power of cancer appositely describes the closing claws of the external institutions, and the internal instruments of our own minds. The internal contradictions exacerbated by the urge to self-destruction, and the longing to survive, become part of a new understanding of who we have become. We are no longer even approximations of the images of other bodies, which still surround us. We are no longer like other people, no longer persons in the same sense, or selves; we have now become negatives of the normal world. The caring institutions, by proxy and without our permission, have indirectly reconstructed for us our new social identity.

From the time when we guess that our treatment is failing we are thrust into an even more excruciating ambiguous condition, like an unwelcome guest, too embarrassed to leave, but wishing away the time of our departure. Our loved ones join in our fight, not for our physical survival but for the maintenance of just a little bit of 'dignity', a desperate claim for a good death. For them, as our survivors, all of the pain is theirs. In our spiritless world, our diseased bodies are trash, to be disposed of efficiently and effectively, yet we still go through the rituals demanded by our institutions. Instead of black plastic refuse sacks, we are trundled away in mass-produced environmentally friendly boxes, to be burnt or buried. But it need not be like this. There are other ways of dealing with terminal illness, which require resistance to, and even rebellion against the operating social institutions that exist to administer our care. Such rebellion requires us to resist institutional definitions of who we are. Surely it is within everybody's capacity to redefine selfhood and what it means to be a person, and not just a body. It is also possible to resist the power of commercialization, and also to reinterpret the ancient ideas of spirit. This resistance to conformity is more than just natural anger – the kind of anger expressed by Dylan Thomas in his poem, 'Do not go gentle into that good night', and even more than a 'romantic' reaction against an oppressive material culture. In fact, as Marx predicted, such rebellion is the only rational response to the contradictions within the present-day capitalistic/materialistic paradigm, but not quite in the way he expected.

Identity

Identity is socially constructed and is maintained as a continual process throughout our lives. This process begins before we are born, through the expectations of our parents and other members of our families, and proceeds via our primary socialization as children, through adulthood and even into old age. We deceive ourselves if we claim that identity is an inherent and unchangeable cluster of characteristics that constitute our individuality, although a common-sense view encourages us to do just that. In fact, common assumptions about identity have absorbed a mish-mash of ideas drawn from a variety of explanations and theories that support an egocentric view of self. To be otherwise is regarded as aberrant, perhaps to be even psychologically unwell, because current attitudes about mental health draw on a misunderstanding and theoretical confusion about personhood.

Psychological theories provide a baseline for other explanations about identity, especially the highly detailed and convoluted descriptions that underpin the current wide-ranging psychotherapeutic theories of 'self'. These psychotherapy theories themselves constitute a strange intellectual territory, many of them evolving directly or indirectly from Freudian ideas, creating a self-supporting paradigm of what it means to be a person. For this reason these theories of 'self' acquire an untouchable quality, which sustains and authenticates them. As such they form the canon of psychotherapy and, in their most extreme forms, these theories and some variations assume a doctrinal and dogmatic quality. Even some of the alternative views are constrained by the requirements of artificial academic demands, by an insistence that they should be in essence linked in some way to a general Freudian ethos. The consequences are that the whole set of activities that constitute the realm of psychotherapy are intellectually incestuous and introverted. Mainstream psychotherapy tends to operate in a social and political vacuum, enabling it to resist external criticism. This is one of the reasons it can claim a kind of monopoly when defining 'self'.

From a sociological viewpoint, identity is a social construct, the outcome of social interactions within a particular social milieu. And although there are some theoretical tendencies to reify these processes, mainstream sociology, alongside anthropology, considers each person as very much a child of their time and place. This is not to claim heuristic superiority of sociology over psychology, for both disciplines offer explanatory models that are capable of reductionism, but because psychology has been claimed by medical sciences as underpinning its own understanding of the human person it is important to identify the nature of its influence.

Explanations of the nature of self and the human person are problematic, and cannot be the preserve of any single perspective, because it is not an objective entity and is subject to dynamic influences ultimately beyond the complete control of any individually identifiable agencies. But perhaps the biggest difficulty of all is that in constructing models of being we are attempting to assemble more than is necessary for the explanation of everyday actions and activities. Our overviews of ourselves have become monsters, heavy-handed caricatures that crush or demolish that incredible lightness of being, which through intuition we reach for in our explanations, but fail to touch. Eventually we retreat from the 'scientific' to the aesthetic in our bid to maintain contact with the sublime, and we shift from the material to the invisible, and from the obvious external and physical descriptions, to descriptors which deny measurement and control.

In pre-scientific times, and still in other cultures, this intangible essence is active as the fundamental motivator, as an inner dynamic that is both the energy that drives all our actions and the core itself, by definition – that spiritual element we call the soul. But we moderns are uncomfortable with this; it is no longer a reasonable part of our working paradigm. Because at some point in time that viewpoint and the vast theological edifice constructed around it, and which permitted the grossest ecclesiastical totalitarianism to dominate human existence, finally gave way to a more open understanding of the nature of humanity. But in that process of rationalization the severity of our intellectual surgery pared away all that was tinged with the superstitious, in favour of what is demonstrable and responsive to hard scientific examination.

The consequences of this paradigmatic change include everything we choose to call modern; in fact the definition of modernity specifically requires the disenchantment defined by Weber and other social commentators who were writing in the shadow of increasing late nineteenth-century bureaucratization. In Marxist terms, we have replaced one form of false consciousness with another, and it is debatable which is the more oppressive. From this perspective we can view both the massive power of the universal church and centralizing tendencies of capitalistic technology as variants of mass control. Both developed systems of privilege and control, both were and are undemocratic, and both hijacked and monopolized key elements of our understanding of ourselves, and used them through the controlling social institutions to define for us and to operate as the parameters of our shared reality.

Selfhood

The construction of social identity requires analysis at several different levels, but very briefly the process entails the examination of structures within structures, through which the prototypical images of selfhood are communicated. This diffusion flows in all directions, but the structures through which centralizing powers choose to exert their influence define current social norms. This process has the appearance of being untidy in Western countries, because there is no apparent direct link between the institutions, and none with any obvious monopolistic totalitarian single elite. Instead the centralizing tendencies are ideological, expressed through the bureaucratic, commercial and political channels that shape and define all social institutions. Every society shapes its individuals through its institutions, which most of us regard as benign. Indeed, how could we think otherwise? 'Normality' is derived from the status quo, and through our participation we reinforce the norms and values that frequently oppress and control us. Our resistance to these controls is not viewed as a serious threat to the system; indeed, it may even be viewed positively as justification for the necessity of the intransigence and rigidity of the regulating methods.

Individualism

One of the amazing contradictions of advanced capitalism is the myth of individualism. This myth is the essential element on which the notions of personal freedom and choice are dependent, and which underwrites and justifies the whole system of competition and consumption in modern Western societies. But advanced capitalism can only exist in mass society, where commodities and services are mass-produced. On the one hand we are encouraged and cajoled to express our individuality, whilst at the same time we are seduced to follow current fashions and become like everyone else, in our lifestyles, modes of consumption, appearances and in what we wear. But current fashions include much more than clothes, for every aspect of consumption is manipulated to maximize profits, including the ready-made off-the-shelf *items* that we acquire one way or another, and that we assemble to construct a personal identity. The more we spend, the more choice we believe we have 'to be'. While in fact the reverse is true, for the higher our consumption, the more embedded are the central values of greed and acquisition that punctuate every point of social interaction, binding us more and more into the systems of consumption. Acquisition and desire become the central theme running through our notions of what it is to be a person. All institutions eventually adjust and adapt to accommodate this world view; families, education, entertainment, food, healthcare, and so on. In all areas of life, we are tricked into thinking that in consuming increasingly standardized products we achieve individuality, whilst at the same time we are conforming to current tastes and fashions and looking increasingly like everyone else.

This pattern of behaving is discernible in our most intimate relationships, such is our desire to conform, and we consume and are consumed by sameness. Selves are structured according to over-simplified formulae; personhood is categorized by typologies. It is hardly surprising that any idea of soul or spirit could not continue to exist in such an explicitly conformist and consumerist environment, for without a heavy-handed church (ecclesiastical) authority capable of monopolizing such an idea, and besides any other reason (philosophical, psychological, theological, anthropological, etc.), there is no profit in it for anyone. But contradictions create stresses that are not easily absorbed by the systems that contain them. Sometimes these stresses are released through social action, such as industrial strikes, or disagreements between cultures, and when the system adjusts to close off such forms of ventilation the internal stresses distort reality, at both social and individual levels. At personal levels such institutionalized contradictions cause madness and disease.

The term 'madness' is broader than any of its modern equivalents and notional insanity; it includes deviance, ecstasy and the outer limits of so-called normal behaviour. One form of current madness, which is a direct consequence of our attempts to deal with these institutional contradictions and our confusion about identity, is expressed through body image. If the above discussion about externalization of self is true, then it would be reasonable to assume that our bodies have become the ultimate focus of our sense of self, and that we are how we look. It is in this way that almost all consumption, in one form or another, is dedicated to this idealized body image; it also means that our bodies become the means through which we express the institutional contradictions. But on top of these contradictions is the added burden of chasing the impossible vision of physical perfection, presented to us through all media. As a result, chasing the impossible enslaves us further; we wish to look like our idols, and also to be ourselves, which we imagine is something different. We also pay homage (lip-service) to the 'true' values of what lies deep within ourselves, whilst exhausting ourselves with the external surface, which is only skin deep.

Our modern faith in materiality should have logically eliminated any ambiguity of feelings about our bodies; we should have transcended Descarte's dualism,[2] but actually now the body has become the main expression of institutional contradictions. While on the one hand we worship it, on the other it is the main focus of our despair and contempt. Eating disorders such as anorexia nervosa and obesity are social diseases as much as psychological and body disorders and together with all of the other eating disorders they are just one example of the confusion we feel about our bodies; they are also strong supporting evidence for the above thesis. Current beliefs about body shape, underpinned by the commercial machinery of the fashion industry, also serve to support the view for many that our body is all that we are. Bodies and body images surround us as constant reminders of what we are.

Visible bodies

'Visuality' is one of the epithets attached to the twentieth century, and it is through the development of photography and television that visual media have become the predominant channels of communication. Everything that can be translated through pictures is reconstructed to fit within the frame of reference of 'advertisers'. Unwittingly, graphic designers have become the new 'lackeys' of commercialism and capitalism, and their frame of reference has become ours. The hegemony of the advertising world is complete; all images, even those at one time considered sacred, are now recycled for the purpose of profit. The message is that through the purchase of products we can achieve a kind of hypothetical beauty. We know that the fashion models are not ordinary or average; we also know that we are not like them, and we might even know that we do not wish to become like them, but nevertheless their images represent the 'ideal' and the 'desirable' sustained by all of the social institutions. The pervasive message is that well-being and success, and even life itself, are rooted in these images, and because they are displayed continuously and ubiquitously they are no longer processed as new information – in effect they have become the screen-savers of our minds.

The primacy of the body has become the dominant belief about 'self' in modern Western societies. The point of departure from what we might describe as a religious world view to the scientific, with its concomitant shift in consciousness and meaning, occurred in the seventeenth century. Up until that time humans were distinguished from all other creatures through possessing dual natures, of body and soul. The interplay between these two dimensions dominated all institutions, and defined the whole trajectory of European history before the beginning of the scientific ages now labelled the Enlightenment. We should not casually dismiss the powerful symbolism of the term Enlightenment, for as well as realizing Plato's directive which challenged us to face the light and perceive reality – literally to come out of the cave, demolishing the darkness of superstition, and generally freeing up the democratic social processes – it offered us the supreme and most coveted prize of personal freedom.

Freedom

This freedom in its entire variety – political, religious, of thought, of speech, of being and of everything else – also included the idea of freedom as dynamic and continuous, so that human history and evolution are represented as a momentous historical struggle with the forces of nature, overcoming, taming, reshaping and controlling it. It is within this process that the internal contradictions emerged. Somehow, somewhere along the line in this process, the struggle for freedom, to escape the various forms of control, became inverted. Freedom and control became dual aspects, two sides of the same coin. And it is against the background of this struggle with nature that we locate the ultimate freedom of choice of becoming whoever we wish to be (for individually we now have the means to substantially change our appearance). And whilst this has already partly been achieved socially, through the elementary democratizing processes of modernizing society, we are caught in the double bind of the need to resist modern society's external controls, whilst exercising our freedoms. When this is expressed physically at an individual level, through one form or another of body modification, the objectification of self is so persuasive that the psychological causes and consequences are neither recognized nor acknowledged.

Body modification

The roots of our desires to change ourselves run deep and most likely are hard-wired, alongside other aspects of consciousness, into the structures of our brains. Archaeological and other evidence indicates that humans, for a variety of reasons, have always needed to experiment with impersonation, to become momentarily someone or something else. This imperative lies at the heart of all drama and disguise, and reinforces our understanding about the essential fluidity of human personality. Costume, dress, hairstyle and cosmetics are universal, in all cultures, throughout all stages of history. And although, as Shakespeare claims, 'Apparel oft proclaims the man', the things we wear as such are external props for the construction of identity; they are essentially different from our bodies. We use them to change our general appearance, but really they are external, because they can be removed. Body modification is different, and its variety and forms are evident in most societies, which is why it is not regarded as problematic.

Some aspects of body modification are regarded as commonplace. For example, male facial shaving, and even circumcision, which is considerably more permanent than the daily use of a razor, is understood as normal and essential in particular cultures. Piercing of the ears and other body areas have been practised since the early beginning of human cultural development, and are justified by their ritualistic purposes. The important point here is that meaning and justification are culturally contextualized; what is 'normal' in a given culture at any one time might easily become aberrant and even pathological in another. All human activities and meaning are socially constructed; through socializing processes, meanings attached to body modification are internalized and consequently impact on us psychologically and physically. All body modification, however diminutive, is never a matter of surface change, but an expression of dissatisfaction about who we believe we are.

The desire to change our bodies contains a wish to become somebody or something else, and is an expression of power, both over others and also over ourselves. Psychological theories concerning anorexia and bulimia focus on 'the need to control' as one of the many features of these conditions. Such eating disorders are also about consumption and consuming, and could justifiably be described as a pre-eminently capitalistic body problem. Their victims consume images of desirable bodies instead of nutritional food, and the bulimic cycle of ingesting and expelling is generally accompanied by similar behaviours relating to personal relationships and the acquisition of possessions. These two conditions are seen as pathological because if untreated they become life-threatening, but they are also enigmatic because sufferers combine mixed feelings of love and hate about their own bodies, and it is this ambivalence about bodies that has become one of the major themes of modern Western culture.

The expansion and affordability of plastic surgery, sex-change surgery, pigment modification, bodybuilding and body moulding are externalized indicators of deep-seated feelings about bodies. Besides the psychological fetishism associated with these, there is commodity fetishism, which in effect means that we are able to purchase modified parts of ourselves, thus turning our bodies into financial statements. This is the ultimate expression of capitalistic power, because the power to consume is an expression of wealth. To understand this it is necessary to invoke Marx's theory of 'commodification',[3] which lies at the heart of his theory of alienation. Quite obviously, although he was unable to predict the emergence of plastic surgery consumerism, it might be seen as an inevitable development within the whole process of mass-production and mass consumption, and as such it has become the exemplary definition of commodification and alienation. And it is not only for wealthy celebrities but increasingly for ordinary people, for cosmetic plastic surgery has already become commonplace in modern Western societies, and is now within the means of average consumers. Advertisements abound in daily newspapers for what are described as 'nip and tuck' treatments, 'nose jobs' and 'boob jobs', and these light-hearted descriptions further attest to its availability and its product image.

The main point of this analysis has been to explore some of the main influences that have shaped current attitudes about bodies, drawing some inferences about the psychological consequences of materialism, disenchantment and the internal contradictions bound up with the central tenets of consumer society. Some of these contradictions have always existed in one form or another: for example, in pre-enlightenment times debate about the interaction of spiritual and material elements was one of the main driving forces of Western philosophy. And even though there is no resolution to this question there was, for our predecessors, a gentle acceptance of the inexplicable. By comparison, present-day contradictions are more brutal, for the physical dimension has become the only dimension. Now there is no escaping the conclusion that we do not live *inside* our bodies because we *are* our bodies, and nothing more. One dire consequence of this paradigmatic shift is how we respond to illness, disease and death, especially in cases when that body is attacked by enemy cells, as in cancer, for example. For dualists, who held that there was a distinction between themselves (that is, their inner core of being that was their soul) and their bodies, disease constituted an enemy. The disease attacked their bodies but it never became part of them, because their soul was untouchable, and the disease was to be fought as an impostor. But for materialists for whom the body is all, when they become ill they themselves become 'a diseased body' and, if persistent, the disease becomes the main focus, around which their identity is reconstructed. Both world views, that of the dualist and that of the materialist, hold their own contradictions and their own consistencies. While for dualists disease was an affliction to be suffered but was incapable of changing their sense of self, incapable of afflicting their essential inner core, for materialists, for whom the body is all, they themselves actually become the disease.

Independence

The interplay of social influences that shape identity is initially external; during the earliest stages of social development socialization is predominantly conformist. In its broadest sense, to become civilized is to learn to follow the rules. Most children in most cultures find some aspects of this oppressive, but at some stage in our development we gain the feeling that we ourselves play a part in becoming who we are. This sense of self is particularly strong in Western societies, and is a consequence of the interplay of beliefs and ideas that are deeply embedded in our (European) individualist cultures. These ideas are also bound up with our notions of freedom and individuality, and we sustain our beliefs in these ideas as the basis of our claims to our human dignity, and to our human rights. At some stage in our lives we achieve a special kind of freedom, which we call 'independence', which allows choice within the parameters set by society. In fact, independence is the source of our individuality, and the focus of selfhood that sets us apart from society; once it is achieved we guard against the intrusion of social institutions to snatch it away, and we defend it at all costs.

The fear of losing our independence has become a major feature of modern living, and in various ways this fear is the primary motivation for our daily activities, because our independence has many interconnected strands. To let go of one strand can paralyse us with fear, because the warnings of loss are as ubiquitous as those of bodies. In fact those warnings of the threat of loss coincide with, and are built into, the very images of the bodies that we admire so much, sometimes metaphorically, sometimes actually. Threats to health and home, for example, are printed in bold type on cigarette packets, on every mortgage letter and in our employment contracts. But our greatest fear of loss of independence is through illness. For when we become ill we lose the power to defend ourselves, and the very institutions that should provide some protection have the power to swallow us up, and to take from us the last vestiges of what we treasure most – our independence. This process is well documented elsewhere, so there is no need to labour the point here, but because current attitudes locate illness in the body, it is important to examine the effects of this at the personal level.

Rebellion

At the heart of our current social and intellectual paradigm are the beliefs, ideas and theories of modern science and technology, and it is here that the seeds of resistance, and of a possibility of an alternative understanding, are sprouting up. The relationship between modern science and the many technologies that fuel modern commercialism is a complex one. Somewhere within this relationship there is the scientific quest to construct a theory of everything, including explanations of human consciousness. After successfully decoding the human genome, offering scientists the means ultimately to understand every living cell of our bodies, human consciousness has become the final scientific frontier. But the human mind is resistant to investigation, and the new neuro-sciences with their advanced scanning techniques are no further foreward in explaining mind and its immateriality. Until fairly recently scientists had avoided the study of consciousness because they had viewed it as impossible, and consequently their solution was to deny its existence. But now that it is once more a subject for scientific interest, they cannot deny it and they cannot explain it; it is inconsistent with their material explanations, but they cannot trash it as the scientific paradigm has trashed the concept of the soul.

Bodies, souls and identity

Our ideas and beliefs about spirituality are locked into the old religious paradigms, which for most of us are intolerable, but the pervasiveness of commercialism, consumerism and corporate control is equally repugnant. Our options for rational discourse about spirituality, logically consistent with the rest of our understanding about the world we inhabit, and authenticity of self are diminishing, but this should not push us into seeking irrational and easy solutions, such as so-called New Age experiments with spirituality, or uncritical acceptance of the claims of proselytisers of new religions. We should also resist the so-called experts, such as philosophers and theologians whose views have failed to connect with the needs of the common man. Yet for many people today there is a yearning, an expression of dissatisfaction with the simply materialistic definitions that are the prime movers of present-day institutions. We need to listen to our own inner voices, and to other ordinary persons who communicate their pain, their confusion and their expressions of hope. And we need also to search for the ways in which a sense of a spiritual dimension manifests itself in ordinary everyday events and experience, and we should not be embarrassed to respond to our emotions and intuitions. But we cannot simply return to the past, and in some way revert to previous world views. The only truly authentic way to make sense of what might be considered as spiritual, is individually and personally to construct for ourselves explanations and models which inform the basis of our relationships with all others, both friends and strangers. For if spirituality is about anything it must be principally about membership and belonging to a particular class of animal, whose primary qualification is consciousness and self-awareness. Whatever our ethnic and other differences, we humans all share this faculty, and it is from this that we derive whatever sense of spirituality we possess. While physically and materially we vary, the attractiveness of the concept of souls is that each one of us is fully equal; souls then are perfectly democratic and egalitarian. It is only our bodies, bound by time and space, which distinguish and identify us as unique and individual persons. But the concept of soul, which has been one of the central concepts of Western philosophy for nearly three thousand years, has gradually been diminishing since the seventeenth century; one of the unintentional consequences of modern science has been to reduce us to mere flesh and bones. And it is this fear that we might not be much else that feeds current anxieties about the future, especially in matters relating to cloning and body modification. We cannot return to the past but we can learn from it and seek inspiration and understanding about this strange sense we have that we are more than simply our bodies, and that our sense of self is not entirely physical.

Notes

1   Goffman also touches on the effects of institutionalization on identity in *Asylums*, his book on mental patients and other inmates of institutions.
2   Descarte's dualism refers to his theory that humans consist of two substances: a physical, material substance and a non-physical substance that provides the motivation of the material substance.
3   Marx's concept of commodification refers to the tendency in advanced capitalism to convert everything into a commodity which has only a financial value, and which also includes human values, actions and sentiments.

Reference

Goffman, E. (1963) *Stigma. Notes on the Management of Spoiled Identity.* New York: Simon & Schuster.

4 | Liminal embodiment: embodied and sensory experience in cancer care and art therapy

Caryl Sibbett

Introduction

One way of conceiving of cancer experiences and art therapy, as noted in Chapter 2, is from an anthropological perspective, paralleling their characteristics with those of the liminal or threshold state (Turner 1995) of a rites of passage transition (Van Gennep 1960). In that chapter I discussed the relevance of liminality and four of its characteristics – *limbo, power/ powerlessness, playing* and *communitas* – to art therapy and cancer experiences. This chapter will explore the relevance to these topics of a fifth characteristic of liminality: *embodied experience*. This acknowledges the body's 'central place in our personal and social life' (Synnott 2001: 2). The chapter will draw on research undertaken for a PhD as a form of 'arts-based autoethnography' (Slattery 2001) and 'auto/biography' (Stanley 1992).[1]

The importance of embodiment in cancer and art therapy experience was an important finding in this study and I will attempt to clarify what I mean by embodiment. I mean that when exploring the lived experience of liminality in cancer and art therapy it is important to pay attention to the bodily aspects involved. It is also important to acknowledge that such bodily experience is influenced by factors such as gender and culture. Cancer experiences can give rise to bodily sensations, perceptions and changes that have physical and practical consequences and also stimulate emotions and often symbolic meanings for the patient. Art therapy can enable expression and processing of these and, in itself, also feature bodily sensations and perceptions and related emotions and symbolic meanings for both the client and art therapist.

Embodied experience

Turner (1982: 12–14) notes that Dilthey (1976) links 'experience' with the phenomenological concept of '*Erlebnis*', which relates to our 'lived experience' engaging in 'embodied action' (Burch 1990). This is congruent with the embodiment paradigm (Merleau-Ponty 1962) and 'corporeal turn' (Sheets-Johnstone 1990; Ruthrof 1998), which emphasizes that the 'body is also, and primarily, the self. We are all embodied' (Synnott 2001: 1). Thus it is important to acknowledge the significance of the body in cancer experiences (Picard 1997; Waskul and van der Riet 2002; Thomas-MacLean 2004) and art therapy (Simon 1992; Lark 2001).

Turner (1982: 12–15) believes that experience 'presses out' to an 'expression' that completes it and takes the form of 'ideas', 'acts' and 'works of art'. Expression involves 'performance' and generation of 'myths, symbols, rituals, philosophical systems, and works of art' (Turner 1982: 52, 1995: 128). This is congruent with art therapy in which experiences are expressed particularly through symbols, rituals and potential embodiment into artwork.

Cancer is an embodied experience but paradoxically, whilst we are a 'psychosomatic unity', we can become 'alienated' from our bodies, which can be perceived as turning against us and untrustworthy (Macquarrie 1973: 92–96). There are suggestions that cancer can be caused by negative emotions (Sontag 1978: 51) and some patients can feel responsible for it (Rix 2000), thus letting down or being betrayed by their body. In liminality the 'self' can be 'split up the middle' and become both 'subject and object, something that one both is and that one sees and, furthermore, acts upon as though it were another' (Turner 1988: 25). Perhaps art therapy can help address such a splitting as Borgmann (2002) cites Baron (1989: 148), who states that it promotes the 'intimate connection between the mind and body, psyche and soma, (which) becomes apparent when exploring the imagery and artwork of an individual with cancer'. The mind–body interrelationship that is difficult to experience can be 'glimpsed in artwork' as the physicality and symbolic aspects of art enable 'wordless layers of experience to be rendered in concrete form' (Wood 1998: 34–5).

Embodied liminality

Turner (1995: 107) proposes that liminality is an 'embodied' state and this features various dimensions that might be summarized as relating to realities and/or perceptions of:

1 *Physicality* – experience of 'pain and suffering'; 'physiological processes' such as 'death and birth' (Turner 1995: 107); 'ordeals . . . often of a grossly physiological character' (Turner 1995: 103); engagement of '*all* the senses' (Turner 1982: 81).

2 *Structural inferiority and power* – experience of 'humiliations, often of a grossly physiological character' (Turner 1995: 103); 'effacement' (Turner 1982: 26); stigma and perceptions of being 'polluting' (Turner 1967: 97); outsiderhood (Turner 1975: 231); 'marginality and structural inferiority' (Turner 1995: 128). Yet, perhaps in compensation for structural inferiority, liminars can experience 'ritual powers' (Turner 1995: 100); 'a special kind of freedom, a "sacred power" '; 'close connection with the non-social or asocial powers of life and death'; and regard 'cosmological systems' as important (Turner 1982: 26–7).

3 *Sexual embodiment* – 'sexlessness'; 'sexual continence' or 'discontinuance of sexual relations'; 'the absence of marked sexual polarity' (Turner 1995: 102–4).

4 *Expression* – 'performance' and 'expression' such as in 'ideas', 'acts' and 'works of art' (Turner 1982: 12–15); generation of 'myths, symbols, rituals, philosophical systems, and works of art' (Turner 1982: 52, 1995: 128).

The rest of this chapter will explore these dimensions of embodied liminality by means of discussing how the last – *expression*, as relevant to art therapy, relates to each of the first three – *physicality, structural inferiority and power, sexual embodiment*, in the context of cancer experiences. Research examples from art therapy practice will be cited.

Physicality

The first dimension of liminal embodied experience that I will explore is *physicality*. This includes various aspects such as experience of 'pain and suffering', 'ordeals' and engagement of 'all the senses' (Turner 1982, 1995).

'Pain and suffering'

Pain reflects our embodied nature since it is an experience of an embodied mind (Kleinman 1994: 8). 'Total pain' presents as 'a complex of physical, emotional, social, and spiritual elements' (Saunders 1996) and exploring this concept, Clark (1999: 727–8) cites Morris (1991: 3), who argues that pain 'emerges only at the intersection of bodies, minds and cultures'. This perhaps indicates the liminal or interstitial nature of pain.

Change in embodied experience, such as suffering, loss of trust, or control over one's body, is a key distressing aspect of the illness experience (Morse *et al.* 1995). Between 33 and 50 per cent of cancer patients, higher in palliative care, experience pain that can be caused by tumour involvement, diagnostic and therapeutic procedures and treatment side effects (McGuire 2004). In my study, these causes featured in most clients' reports of pain and suffering. All clients reported heightened vigilance about their body sensations.

Art therapy enables symbolic expression of pain (Miller 1996: 133) and it has been claimed that it can help its management (Thomas 1995; UMCCC 2004). One client, a man in his fifties diagnosed with advanced terminal liver cancer, reported that claywork helped his pain management. At the start of a session he was eager to use clay for the first time in his life. He began shaping it and a foot about 13 centimetres long began to appear, with carefully sculpted toes (Figure 4.1, on website). He spent approximately fifteen minutes smoothing it and I had an impression that he was massaging it. Later I shared that I had observed him moving his hands over it for some time. He responded: 'I realized it was my foot and it felt like I was massaging it.' He added that he often experienced pain in his feet and he said 'massaging this (clay) foot helped ease the pain in my feet'.

'Ordeals'

Most clients also reported experiencing bodily ordeals of some kind including surgery, reconstruction, nausea, diarrhoea, insomnia, 'sweats', body weight change, appetite change, burned skin or damage from radiotherapy, hair-loss, numbness, vertigo and infection. A client spoke of experiencing repeated attempts at needle entry until 'I shouted at them to stop and get me someone who can do this quickly'. Fatigue, however, was the most commonly disclosed experience.

Fatigue is the most frequently reported cancer-related symptom (Glaus *et al.* 1996; Richardson and Ream 1996), reported by more than 75 per cent of cancer patients (Portenoy and Itri 1999). Such clinical fatigue is significantly different from and more negative than fatigue within the general population (Glaus 1993; Portenoy and Itri 1999). Differences include that it appears more rapidly, lasts longer, impairs self-esteem and significantly increases physical impairment, tiredness, weakness, social limitation, distress and need for rest (Glaus *et al.* 1996; Magnusson *et al.* 1999; Holley 2000). Potter (2004) found that, with advanced cancer, fatigue brought interconnected physical, psychological, social and spiritual consequences and adjustment and hope could be fostered through sensitive communication about fatigue and its meaning. It has been claimed that art-making can 'reveal our energy levels, our feeling states, and our self-concepts' (Rogers 1993: 69).

Most clients reported such fatigue and also that art-making affected energy levels, sometimes reporting it to be 'stimulating' or 'energizing' and other times 'very relaxing' or 'soothing' and occasionally 'draining'. One client reported: 'It was relaxing, social, therapeutic and creative.' Another client, a lady in her forties diagnosed with breast cancer, noted a theme appearing in a number of artworks where clay figures seemed to be 'tired' or 'leaning as if exhausted' and she related this to her fatigue.

Another client, a man in his thirties diagnosed with a malignant brain tumour, reported that some pastel pictures gave him a 'a profound sense of being energized which could last beyond the making and could be re-engaged with afterwards', and of being 'energized in the core of my body'. However, he reported one gave him the sense of being 'tired' or 'drained' after creating it. On one occasion he reported having a semi-dream state immediately after a session in which he experienced 'blue energy' in his body. He reported experiencing it as 'darker blue than the light blue with white energy that seemed to be in me and come out of me – in the abdominal area – as if consciousness was not in my head but had gone into my body, the core of my body'. He also described it as 'a sense of self extending beyond the bodily self' and as 'blue healing energy or light' which he then intended to visualize to help him, and he also used this colour in his art which he reported as beneficial.

Multi-sensory experience

In liminality, Turner (1982: 81) notes that all senses can be involved, including 'kinaesthetic' experience, and he links this with the social drama aspect of ritual. All senses are affected in cancer experiences. For instance, chemo-therapy can evoke changes in touch, taste, smell and sight (McDaniel et al. 1995; Comeau et al. 2001). The multi-sensory nature of art-making lends itself to expression of these aspects of cancer experiences.

Art-making is a 'visceral experience' that can reveal 'kinesthetic messages' (Rogers 1993: 69) and offer 'kinesthetic release' (Hill 2002). Haptics and touch senses are important in art-making, with 'hands' playing a prime role, and these 'skin senses' or 'somaesthesia' link with the kinaesthetic senses of body position and movement (Prytherch and McLundie 2002). Lowenfeld suggested that there are two art orientations: visual, looking *at* art from the outside as an observer; and haptic, experiencing more in sensory and kinaesthetic terms and feeling involved *in* art (Lowenfeld and Brittain 1987).

All clients reported multi-sensory aspects of cancer and its treatment such as changes in sensations relating to sight, taste, smell, touch, movement, warmth/coldness, sound, wetness/dryness, heaviness and other body sensa-tions. All clients also reported that the multi-sensory aspect of the art-making and using 'different media' was important in expressing and processing the bodily experiences relating to cancer. Examples reported similarly included sight, touch, movement, sound, warmth/coldness, wetness/dryness, smell and other inner and outer body sensations.

One client reported: 'It is also a physical expression because you are touching the work and that feels really very good too.' Another said that he found the 'multi-sensory', 'tactile', 'kinaesthetic' aspects very important as was 'my body's role in the making and experiencing of art'. He described how he would 'sense where the pastel felt right to go in a picture' by moving his hand over the page and he related how, between sessions, he 'honed this sense and now I apply it beyond the art, such as to the room in general and to what feels right in a space'.

Sometimes changes in sensory or skin experience could be regarded as somewhat embarrassing and this will be discussed in the next section.

Structural inferiority and power

The second dimension of liminal embodied experience that I will explore is *structural inferiority* and *power*. This includes various aspects such as body/self-image and stigma, embodied boundary, cultural inscribed embodiment, and ritual power (Turner 1967, 1982, 1995).

Turner (1995: 128) emphasizes that such experiences of 'liminality, marginality, and structural inferiority are conditions in which are frequently generated myths, symbols, rituals, philosophical systems, and works of art', which are *expressions* that can be 'reclassifications of reality' and our 'relationship to society, nature, and culture'. Perhaps in this way art therapy can offer a constructive liminal or heterotopic (Foucault 1986) or chronotopic 'time space' (Bakhtin 2000: 84) where negative self-concepts and cultural stereotypes can be reclassified.

Body/self image, stigma

Body image is influenced by cultural factors including gender, age, ethnicity, social class, the media (Grogan 1999) and health conditions (Cash and Pruzinsky 2004). Synnott (2001: 1–2) asserts that our bodies, body parts and senses are 'loaded with cultural symbolism' and are 'socially constructed' and adds that self-change is more evident when 'the body-change is sudden and unexpected'. Cancer and medical treatment effects can negatively affect one's body/self image (Burt 1995) and self-esteem (Bottomley 1997), generating feelings of powerlessness and isolation (Colyer 1996) and loss of bodily ownership and control (Turner 1996).

Liminality can be associated with stigma and being perceived as potentially 'polluting' (Turner 1967: 97), 'untouchable and dangerous' (Van Gennep 1960: 114). Liminars 'dwell on and between the borders of our categories ... neither here nor there' (Myerhoff *et al.* 1987), and because they are difficult to classify they threaten order and can be designated as polluted or taboo (Douglas 1966).

Having cancer can be a stigmatizing experience (Muzzin *et al.* 1994; Colyer 1996; Flanagan and Holmes 2000), evoking 'separateness', 'alienation',

'distancing or loss of social familiars' (Little *et al.* 1998: 1488) and avoidance behaviour (Peters-Golden 1982). Physical disability can lead to perceptions of a 'grotesque body' (Waskul and Van der Riet 2002) and liminality
or a failure to be incorporated into society (Willett and Deegan 2001).
Cancer patients themselves 'may fear their potential to contaminate others'
(Schaverien 2002: 141). Cancer-related psychological problems (Holland
2002) and seeking help (Pandey and Thomas 2001) can be stigmatized.
Some patients feel they are being punished for something they have done –
bodies are inherently involved in discipline and punishment (Foucault
1991). Etymologically the word 'pain' derives from Latin and Greek words
meaning punishment and payment (Merriam-Webster 2004). Goffman
(1963) stressed the importance of the visibility element of stigma, and
therefore its bodily dimension.

Winnicott (1996: 36) suggests we can be patterned and 'cut into shapes
conceived by other people' and can develop a 'compliant false self', and in
contrast the 'true self' has the 'potential for the creative use of objects'
(p.102). Perhaps in fostering this potential, art therapy cultivates constructive relationship between the true self and appropriate presentations of self
needed in different contexts. This links to the concept of the 'false body'
(Orbach 1994) and body ego (Boadella 1989), which Freud (1923: 26, n.1)
suggests can be regarded as 'a mental projection of the surface of the body'.
Rowan (2000) suggests there are three approaches to the body in psychotherapy: body and mind separate; body and mind integrated; bodymind as
part of soul. Art therapy seems to feature the second and/or third approaches
and thus perhaps helps foster constructive relationship between the true
body and appropriate presentations of body needed in different contexts.

Paradoxically, Myerhoff *et al.* (1987) suggest that because liminars are
out of place they are also 'mysterious and powerful' and liminal beings or
states can be 'sources of renewal, innovation, and creativity'. Art therapy
can help patients move into a more active role and manage body image
changes relating to hair, weight and disfigurement (Wood 1998: 29–30) as
well as emotional trauma, interpersonal problems and spiritual dilemmas
(Malchiodi 1999). Therapeutic groups can modify self-perceptions and
internalized other-perceptions and lessen extreme feelings, thus balancing and integrating positive and negative self-aspects (Foulkes and
Anthony 1984: 150) and decreasing dependence on stereotyped behaviour
(Thompson and Kahn 1972: 116).

In many cases clients directly reported that artwork helped them express
issues relating to body/self image and/or stigma and sometimes helped a
movement toward greater acceptance of the new state.

During an artwork review of his pictures, one male client reported that
some seemed 'lopsided' and he related this directly to how he was 'lopsided'
due to a brain tumour affecting one side of his body. In one session he told
me that between sessions he had dreamed he was making a picture which

had 'lumps of chalk or wax pastel on both sides of the page . . . It was a dark page with vivid colours, beige, pink, yellow.' He reported feeling annoyed in the dream that 'something had got marked or spoiled and if you could get them off it would be back to normal'. He linked this to himself and proceeded to use the art to enable the 'marks' to be integrated and accepted into the picture. Fox and Lantz (1998) found that brain tumour patients reported themes including the 'stigma of a mind–body illness' and the tumour as an 'invasive disease of the self'. Another client reported other people's difficult reactions to seeing her disfigurement: 'It's kids especially just look and you can see their mouths just opening . . . I think it must look quite horrific to them . . . Whereas I can still see it but it's not as bad as it was. I've come quite a bit.'

Many clients reported that art therapy's non-judgmental approach toward client and art was beneficial in helping reduce stigma and promoting self-esteem and confidence. Typical written comments were:

> It's given me the chance to get certain issues into focus. It's also provided an uncritical environment of self-expression, relaxation and enjoyment.
> [To] . . . not feel like it was being judged at the end.
> I lost the self-conscious or fear aspect of making a fool of myself. Also helped me get out of myself.
> Time for me, time to express yourself . . . and a means to feeling good about yourself.
> Lift in mood over the weeks.
> I have a lot more self-confidence within myself.
> Improved my confidence in mixing with groups again.

Embodied boundaries

The outer boundaries of our bodies are thresholds between the world and us, particularly the skin (Prost 2004). Glover (1998) discusses how the body has been viewed as a 'container' and, by virtue of artwork's 'corporeality' and capacity to 'metaphorize the body', it too may be regarded as a container (Stokes 1978: 328; Wollheim 1987; Connell 1998: 44). Thus a key feature of bodily experience is 'containment and boundedness' (Johnson 1987: 21) and 'containment/constraint' (Sinha and Jensen de López 2000). Anzieu (1989: 17) asserts that even our skin is 'both permeable and impermeable'. Lawton (1998: 127) suggests that cancer patients particularly can be conceptualized as having an 'unbounded body' when their symptoms cause 'the surfaces of the patient's body to rupture and break down' allowing bodily substances normally 'contained' within the body to be uncontrollably 'leaked and emitted to the outside'. When this is not the case, patients could be deemed to have a 'bounded body'. Having 'complete' skin is perceived as important (Rudge 1998). Lawton (1998: 132) proposes that hospices can be places for the 'sequestration of the unbounded body' and she links this to Douglas's (1966) theories of 'dirt', 'pollution' and disorder of usual classifications.

Such threshold crossings are deemed inappropriate, especially when evoking disgust. Lawton (1998: 134, 141) argues that there is a 'current Western intolerance of bodily disintegration and bodily emissions' and a 'quest for firm bodily margins' (Bordo 1993: 191), yet some forms of bodily substance sharing are deemed appropriate as in consensual sexual activity. With cancer patients, unboundedness deemed inappropriate can escalate whilst unboundedness deemed appropriate can decrease due to the lack of sexual relations evident in liminality (Turner 1995: 104).

This is congruent with Turner's (1995: 109) view that liminars can be regarded as dangerous and he links this with Douglas's (1966) view that what falls outside usual classifications is regarded as 'polluting'. It links to Kristeva's (1982: 4) view of the 'abject' as that which relates to bodily emanations, is ambiguous and 'disturbs identity, system and order . . . does not respect borders, positions, rules'. Cancer can turn us inside out! Awareness of embodied liminality means acknowledging the permeable threshold of the body and addressing the otherwise sometimes unspeakable realities of bodily disintegration as part of human existence and no more shameful than other culturally acceptable bodily emanations. It is important to acknowledge how 'discourses of shame and dependence' affect the handling of 'unspeakable' bodily needs (Street and Kissane 2001: 169). Bodies have fluid boundaries and ignoring the 'volatile, messy, leaky' nature of bodies consigns them to the abject (Longhurst 2001: 23), thus it is important to extend social inclusion to the liminal threshold-crossing aspect of bodies.

Lawton's view of the hospice as a place of 'sequestration' might link to Foucault's (1986) concept of 'heterotopias of deviation', a less constructive variant of liminality meant for people regarded as different to the norm, discussed in Chapter 2. Indeed Lawton (1998: 131) draws on Van Gennep (1960: 18) and suggests hospices could be ' "fringe"/"liminal" spaces within which these "non-persons", wavering "between two worlds", remain buffered'. Yet paradoxically Lawton (1998: 131–2) suggests the very 'unboundedness' and disfigurement that leads to sequestration also contributes to cancer patients having a 'special social status' compared to others with chronic degenerative diseases.

Bodily containment seems related to our sense of identity and self-containment. Anzieu (1989: 98–108) proposes the concept of the 'skin ego' and suggests that its functions for the psyche parallel those of the skin's physical functions for the body.

Art therapy may provide a heterotopia of crisis rather than deviation (Foucault 1986). It is paradoxically a non-invasive treatment (Malchiodi 1999), yet allows symbolic unboundedness and boundedness through symbolic self-expression and projective and introjective processes. Esrock (2002) proposes that when viewing art we can lose our bodily boundaries and experience an 'imaginary fusion' of inner somatosensory sensations which through 'somatosensory *reinterpretation*' are perceived as qualities of the artwork. In this way the 'conventional boundary between self and object' is crossed. Esrock links this with psychoanalytic theory of projection and introjection. Milner (1977: 165) also suggests artists can experience a 'con-fusion of "me" and "not-me" '.

A number of clients reported using art materials to explore fears of lack of outer and inner body containment. One client described symbols in her art: 'They're like cells. That one has totally escaped because it doesn't have its boundary, it's seeping.' Another client, a woman in her forties diagnosed with cancer affecting her skin, made artwork about the impact on her skin. In one session she brought photocopied images of her hands and created a collage also depicting flesh coloured 'strips of skin' (Figure 4.2, on website). The background paper was reddish and she related this to heat sensations in her skin. She worked on feelings of 'I'm coming apart' and then linked the strips to 'bandages' keeping her together. Over the weeks she reported her self-image improved and she attended the last session without her wig, saying this was the first time she had gone out without it.

Perhaps another acceptable unboundedness is a sense of connection to the transpersonal or cosmos. One client reported that his art linked the microscopic, his cells and DNA, to the macroscopic, chaos and string theory. Perhaps relevant here is Turner's (1982: 27) view that liminars can experience a heightened importance of 'cosmological systems'. The client reported that his often interweaving abstract colours and shapes related to how 'everything is interlinked and interconnected, web-like or string-like'.

Inscribed body

Treatments for cancer have been described as the 'slash/burn/poison trilogy' (surgery/radiation/chemotherapy) and the marking of the body can be 'an additional source of stigma, often starkly visible and a challenge to body image' (Langellier 2001: 145–6). Facial disfigurement (Grealy 1995) and scarring can be particularly difficult because 'the face is a prime symbol of the self' (Synnott 2001: 2). Interestingly, terms like sharp, prick, stab, stitch, tattoo and stigma are etymologically linked (Pickett *et al.* 2000). Body scars can indicate 'an individual's membership of a social group', as can tattoos (Anzieu 1989: 105), and can be the mark of a survivor or warrior (Springer 1996). Some patients have transformed their scars by means of tattoos, such as of a tree (Metzger 1997: 91).

There are correspondences between skin, paper and bark and the tree can be an image of our condition (Cohen and Mills 1999). Trees were a re-emerging theme for some clients or could be significant even if only appearing once. One client rarely made figurative art but in one image he felt a tree appeared which he said was precarious as it could fall either way. I was reminded of Turner's (1982: 44) description of liminality as 'an instant of pure potentiality when everything, as it were, trembles in the balance'. This client also planned to get a tattoo that he felt would be a symbol of healing energy.

Cultural embodiment

Turner (1995: 103) suggests that those in liminality are a '*tabula rasa*, a blank slate' that can be 'inscribed' and 'whose form is impressed upon them by society'. We are not just an embodied self because inherently we are in intersubjective relationships (Cohn 1997: 25) with other embodied selves (Burch 1990). Art therapists must address interpersonal body experience (Diamond 2001), cultural influences on embodiment (Sinha and Jensen de López 2000; Chapple and Ziebland 2002) and the concept that we are 'culturally embodied' (Varela *et al.* 1993: 150). Hogan (1996) asserts that the artwork is not just a product of an individual, but rather it is embedded in, and influenced by, larger meaning systems.

Such intersubjective embodiment experience may be grounded in psychoneurobiology. Recent research indicates that body and emotional experiences are linked to consciousness (Damasio 2000). Schore (1999, 2003) proposes an 'inter-brain', 'brain–brain interactive perspective' which suggests that unconsciously we engage in 'adaptive self-regulating processes of the brain–mind–body' both within our self ('autoregulation') and with others ('interactive regulation'). Schore (1999) links this to unconscious 'affectively-charged transference–countertransference interactions between patient and therapist'.

Geertz (1973: 89) defined culture as a 'historically transmitted pattern of meanings embodied in symbolic form by means of which men communicate, perpetuate, and develop their knowledge about and attitudes toward life'. Culture may be viewed as having layers, like an onion, or like an iceberg with some being visible and others invisible, some conscious and some unconscious (Dahl 2003). This systemic perspective is developed by Hofstede (1991), Trompenaars and Hampden-Turner (1997) and Spencer-Oatey (2000). I have drawn on all these models in Figure 4.3 to speculate how intersubjective and cultural influences exist in reciprocal relationships between individual and society. Our motivational roots, values and basic assumptions are the foundations that drive our beliefs, then our behaving and expressing (art-making) and tangible products (art). Hawkins (1997: 426, Figs 2–3) uses the metaphor of water lilies for the cultural tangible products arising from the systemic layers.

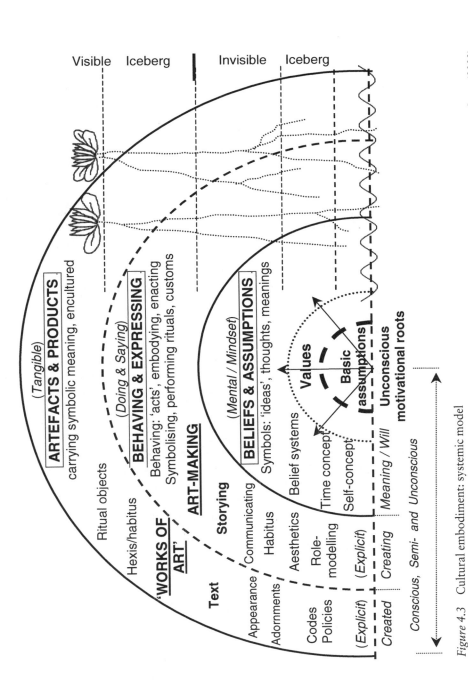

Figure 4.3   Cultural embodiment: systemic model

Source: Adapted from Dahl (2003), Hawkins (1997), Hofstede (1991), Trompenaars and Hampden-Turner (1997), Spencer-Oatey (2000).

The cultural influences on us can be portrayed by the body as suggested by Bourdieu's (1977) concept of 'habitus' or 'hexis'. This refers to the partly unconscious habitual beliefs and dispositions towards action of the 'socially informed body', manifested or '*em-bodied*' in a 'permanent disposition, a durable way of standing, speaking, walking, and thereby *feeling* and *thinking*' (Bourdieu 1977: 93, 124). Perhaps artwork, or lack of it, may mirror a client's habitus as it mirrors his/her body.

It is possible that some aspects of habitus/hexis are not necessarily permanent and perhaps art therapy is one approach that can enable a person to modify habitus, for instance from thinking and behaving in an 'I'm not creative' way to an 'I am creative' way. This might be a movement from a culturally imposed, constraining, false self-body to a more constructive relationsip with the true self-body. Importantly, this must respect the client's cultural diversity (Hiscox and Calisch 1998; Campbell *et al.* 2003), and must not be the therapist's own assumed-as-'right' cultural model imposed onto the client. Art therapists must have awareness of cultural influences and not let their own cultural views adversely affect professional practice (HPC 2003a, 2003b), thus ensuring multicultural competency (Lister 1999).

Sexual embodiment

The third dimension of liminal embodied experience that I will explore is *sexual embodiment*. This includes various aspects such as impact on sexuality and sexual relations (Turner 1982, 1995). Part of our cultural embodiment is that we are a gendered body (Chapple and Ziebland 2002).

Cancer can bring disturbances in sexuality, intimacy and sexual functioning (Bottomley 1997; Hughes 2000; Sundquist and Yee 2003) and altered embodiments of femininity and masculinity (Van der Riet 1998). Patients with advanced cancer can have altered sexuality and bodily functions yet also more significant need for physical intimacy and touching (Cort *et al.* 2004). Healthcare professionals need to address such sexual change issues and help attend to the patient's silence (Hughes 2000). Clients of both sexes reported that cancer and treatment could affect sources of their gender identity such as sexual organs and also hair.

Masculinity

Embodied experience of masculinity must be addressed in cancer care (Watson 2000: 3). Testicular cancer can impact on sexuality, gender identity and fertility and a study by Gurevich *et al.* (2004) found that a 'discourse of precarious masculinity' predominated, with 'disruption' interpolating with 'potentiality' and the 'link between anatomy and masculinity' being 'simultaneously asserted and disavowed'. Prostate cancer hormonal treatment can involve 'concurrent normalisation and deviantisation processes', thus subjecting patients to 'a liminal state . . . the inability to classify themselves into culturally available categories' (Navon and Morag 2004). Treatment can adversely affect libido and cause impotence, thus impacting on some patients' sense of masculinity, yet social constructions of masculinity such as 'men don't cry' can impair communication about such aspects (Chapple and Ziebland 2002).

One client, a male diagnosed with prostate cancer, created a series of paintings of male friends and their personality and bodily characteristics. On reviewing them he became emotional as he discovered that he had been reprocessing his *own* male identity.

Femininity

Body change can impact on the construction of feminine gender identity (Bordo 1989; Grosz 1994) and female cancer patients can experience compromised sexuality (Colyer 1996). Breast cancer is a 'life threat' (Arman and Rehnsfeldt 2003) that can affect women's relationship with 'our very selves' (Light and Brittingham 1994), as can ovarian cancer. Patient narratives indicate that breast cancer and its treatment 'suspend the narrator in a liminal state between life and death, a fear shared by all cancer patients . . . of recurrence' (Langellier 2001: 154).

Art therapists need to have awareness of gender and its cultural influences and the effects evident in art and verbal expression (Hogan 1996, 1997, 2002).

Sometimes in artwork issues of sexuality were deliberately worked on, but more often they appeared spontaneously in the art, such as a shape seeming 'breast-like' or a client suddenly realizing she was depicting the effect of cancer on her womb.

Hair

Leach (1967) explored hair as a prominent feature of rites of passage, suggesting it has cross-cultural libidinal (life-force) meaning. Hair can have 'magical' import as 'a public symbol' with 'explicitly sexual significance' (Leach 1967: 103, 89). The male beard can be a component in masculine gender identity, communicating manliness (Pellegrini 1973).

Hair loss can be an issue for both female and male cancer patients. Chemotherapy-induced alopecia, wigs and hair growing back different can negatively impact on sense of self and control (Williams *et al.* 1999). Hair loss is directly visible to others and can be a 'symbolic precursor to the loss of self' (Freedman 1994: 336). Art therapy can help patients come to terms with changes in body image such as hair loss and identity (Wood 1998:

29–30). Sometimes actual body parts such as hair can be used within art. One client brought her hair, cut before chemotherapy, to a session for me to witness.

The importance of hair and its loss appeared as a common theme for both female and male clients. One male client, diagnosed with neck cancer, drew an image of his face and spoke of how the loss of his beard before treatment was of huge significance to him. He said 'I'd had it ever since I became a man.' Another client, a woman in her forties diagnosed with bowel cancer, used art-making to deal with chemotherapy-related hair loss and the prospect of dying. In one session she used clay to express this by making a self-portrait featuring her hair as remembered and she spoke of how she was processing the impact on both her sexual and life identity (Figure 4.4, on website). In the next session she told me how, immediately after the clay-making session, she dreamed the clay-making session again. In the dream she re-experienced making the clay portrait and the same resulting feelings of absorption and well-being. She told me it was her 'first good night's sleep since the diagnosis'.

This might link to what Mohkamsing-den Boer and Zock (2004) call a '*rêve de passage*' (dream of passage) which, like ritual, may also have a 'transitional function' in crisis and change situations. In analysis a cancer patient's dreams can symbolically mark important times in the treatment progress and cancer state and also that the 'cancer condition and transference–countertransference reactions' are 'closely entwined' (Calogeras and Alston 2000). Taking account of terminally ill cancer patients' dreams is important and can counteract isolation (Welman and Faber 1992; Schaverien 2002) and acknowledge 'timelessness' *and* chronological time (Hartocollis 1980).

This client (Figure 4.4) was the same age as me and, after our sessions had ceased, I heard she was in a hospice and I visited her just before her death. When I was leaving, we embraced at the door as she turned to go back into the hospice. I found it emotional and, having had cancer myself, I also could not help wondering whether this would be my fate too some day. Such countertransference issues will be discussed in Chapter 16.

Liminal expression in embodied art

In the context of cancer experiences, art therapy and Turner's model, I have explored three dimensions of liminal embodied experience by means of discussing how a fourth – *expression* – relates to each. The dimension of expression in art therapy will now be explored further.

Rituals associated with rites of passage and liminality are 'performed' (Myerhoff *et al.* 1987; Turner 1982, 1988; Schechner 2003) and have 'a performed-for-an-audience aspect' (Turner 1988: 76). Therefore they are intrinsically associated with body expression. Turner (1982: 12–15) asserts that lived-through experience (*Erlebnis*) is 'pressed out' into expression that completes it and such expressions can be of three classes. These are: 'ideas'; 'acts', many of which can be viewed as 'expressing and fulfilling *unconscious purposes and goals*'; and 'works of art', in which the 'unconscious formative component' is even more important. Turner (1982: 15) regards such works of art as 'trustworthy messages from our species' depths, humanized life disclosing itself, so to speak'. Elsewhere, he asserts: 'Artists tend to be liminal and marginal people, "edgemen" . . .' and liminality frequently generates multivocal symbols, rituals and 'works of art' (Turner 1995: 128–9). Art therapy is a key approach that can facilitate and witness such expressions.

The embodied nature of art expression is important. Jung (1996: 173; para. 291) indicates that symbols are embodied: 'The symbols of the self arise in the depths of the body and they express its materiality every bit as much as the structure of the perceiving consciousness. The symbol is thus a living body, *corpus et anima* . . .'. Stokes (1978: 328) argues: 'There is a sense in which all art is of the body.' As suggested in Chapter 2, artwork might be a form of 'chronotope' (Bakhtin 2000: 84) or embodied 'time space' in which 'Time, as it were, thickens, takes on flesh, becomes artistically visible . . .'.

It has been suggested that transitional objects and their containing capacity function by a process of 'embodiment' where the 'continued existence of the therapist and the therapeutic relationship is given tangible form' (Arthern and Madill 1999, 2002: 384). Schaverien (1994: 79) asserts that an image can become 'embodied', i.e. when it holds powerful feelings that have been involved and expressed in its making (Skaife 1995: 4). An embodied image 'conveys a feeling state for which no other mode of expression can be substituted' (Schaverien 2000: 59). A client reported that his art seemed to express something beyond words and 'fundamental', almost more basic than even emotion.

Revelatory expression

Art therapy can be valuable in expressing that which has not been previously known or voiced. 'Silence' is a characteristic of liminality (Turner 1995: 103). Ritual can access 'knowledge of what would otherwise not be known at all' (Douglas 1966: 64) and it engages embodied knowledge not easily accessed by ordinary consciousness (Csordas 1994). The concept of 'threshold body' acknowledges felt knowledge of the body (Darroch-Lozowski 1999).

An inability to communicate is a feature of the cancer experience – sometimes 'language "collapses" in the face of the recollection of the incommunicable' (Little *et al.* 1998: 1486–8). Some aspects seem unspeakable, whilst some seem unhearable. Winaver and Slama (1993) suggest that there can be 'unspeakable' issues for women with breast cancer. This might include issues relating to sexuality, body unboundedness and fear of death.

Macquarrie (1973: 268) cites Jaspers (1931: 716) who suggests that 'the basic meaning of art is its revealing function', and Macquarrie adds: 'It reveals being by giving form to what we perceive.' Artwork can give form to the 'unspeakable' (Case and Dalley 1997: 97; Connell 1998: 75), enabling 'the unsayable to be said' and allowing acceptable ways to express 'anger, acceptance, or fear of death' (Miller 1996: 132–3). Lynch (1997: 128) suggests art is valuable when dealing with the 'silence of the limits', those areas of human experience where verbal language and thus verbal therapy are inadequate. Art can reveal personality aspects inaccessible through verbal therapy (Coleman and Farris-Dufrene 1996: 11). I believe art is also valuable in allowing expression relating to what Lynch calls 'the silence of oppression', and this might relate to aspects of stigma, shame and the unhearable. Sometimes it is less threatening to approach a difficult issue in the art where it can be initially spoken of in the third person perhaps before being owned (Wadeson 1980: 10).

Various written comments by clients participating in the research related to the capacity of art therapy to reveal and express:

> It has been a way of expressing things that are unspeakable, also emotions that you are sometimes not even aware of until they come out of your art.
> [To] . . . unearth hidden emotions and be able to express them in a safe environment.
> It stimulated thoughts and ideas which came to me outside the Monday sessions, helped me to tap into my creative, intuitive side.
> The art allowed me to express feelings that were hard to put into words. Sometimes there are no words and art is an unspoken expression.
> Using art as a powerful way of expressing and of approaching the cancer directly.
> They seem to be helping to get out some bits of communication about how you are feeling and the darker bits.
> Self-expression, giving 'picture' to the cancer experience.

Perhaps art therapy can help a person to reduce any perceived shame and thus find a voice. As well as being linked to the unspeakable and unhearable this also seems linked to the issue of gaze and dealing with any difficulties of being visible or unseeable. We can look at or away from portrayals of suffering (Radley 2002). This could link to shame and to feeling 'exposed' and 'self-conscious' (Erikson 1977: 227) and 'being looked at' (Lewis 1987: 18). Nathanson's (1992, 1995/2004) 'compass of shame' model suggests four defences against shame and perhaps some cancer patients can experience some from others or within self (Figure 4.5). The four points might also

WITHDRAWAL
Alienation, isolation, hiding, silence

ATTACK OTHER
Aggression, blaming

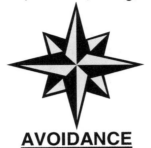

ATTACK SELF
Self-deprecation, passivity, deferential

AVOIDANCE
Distraction, addiction, disavowal

Figure 4.5 'Compass of shame': four defences/patterns of response (Nathanson 1995/2004).

relate to defences used by others and society in response to issues such as cancer. Such responses can potentially inflict 'symbolic violence' which is the imposition of values and meanings onto, or into, an individual or group so that they experience them as legitimate (Bourdieu 1977). In this way, a stigmatized view of cancer and its effects can be an oppressive social construction that can disadvantage, and can also potentially project such defence responses into those affected by cancer.

Art therapy is valuable in providing a metaphorical area where frightening aspects of the human condition can be faced and managed (Arnheim 1992: 170). Art therapy also has an important role to play because the principles underpinning its practice accommodate a holistic and social model of health and also integrate a postmodern embodied paradigm (Corker and Shakespeare 2002; Shakespeare and Watson 2002).

Therapeutic/creative process and rites of passage

Riskó *et al.* (1996) suggests that a cancer diagnosis can provoke a crisis, resulting in an increase of regression and defence mechanisms (splitting, projective identification, projection, denial, repression). Patients can regress to the object relational 'paranoid-schizoid' position that tends towards a polarized either/or, black-and-white perspective (Jarvis 2004: 111). Here, paranoid refers to how cancer patients can fear internal and external dangers (Riskó 2001) and death. Schizoid refers to how cancer and related feelings can be perceived as unbearable inner 'bad' objects (Bálint 1956; Dreifuss-Kattan 1994: 125) that patients attempt to get rid of through splitting and projective identification (Riskó *et al.* 1996, 1998). The projection is not owned, but is equated with its container, for instance a client stating that the 'it/he/she' in the art is terrified. Ehrenzweig (1968) compares the *paranoid-schizoid* position to the first phase of the creative process, '*projection*', in which fragmented unconscious material is projected onto/into the art. Perhaps we might also make a comparison with the rites of passage state of '*separation*' (Van Gennep 1960; Turner 1982, 1995) in which there can be a separation from society of that which is deemed ambiguous or problematic.

The transition to a new position involves *containment*. Projective identification (Klein 1946, 1975, 1988) serves to 'evacuate and 'communicate' (Bion 1959) intolerable 'undigested' aspects (Bion 1984: 6–7). The art therapist, the heterotopic (Foucault 1986) 'time space' (Bakhtin 2000: 84), and artwork function as 'containers' for these projections. Body-related claywork lends itself to such projective identification processes (Henley 2002: 75). Art therapy rituals (Skaife and Huet 1998: 12) such as contracting, opening, circular sharing, artwork reviews and closing also play a part in containment, thus art therapy involves *redefinitional rituals*. Healthcare professionals must be appropriately trained, for if containment is inadequate there can be a reintrojection of *unmodified* projections by which a patient can 'experience not the fear of dying made bearable, but a nameless dread' (Bion 1993: 116). When containment is adequate, projections can be 'modified' or 'digested', thus becoming 'tolerable', capable of reintrojection (Bovensiepen 2002: 245) and thinkable, thus 'food for thought' (Glover 1998). Ehrenzweig regards the creative phase of '*integration*' as vital in this transition as it allows multiple possibilities to be held and both chaos and a 'hidden order' to be experienced. This 'deeper order' features a sense of more fluid boundaries between self and the world (Milner 1977). Perhaps we might also make a comparison with the rites of passage state of '*liminality*' that features limbo, ambiguity, embodied experience, chaos, playing with multivocal symbols, expression and transition.

The person can move to the '*depressive position*' that tends to be a both/and perspective where ambivalent feelings can be tolerated. Creativity and symbolization are fundamental in the movement to this position (Glover 1998). The projection can now be *owned* and the container viewed as merely representing it (Klein 1975), for instance the client says the terrified figure in the art represents his/her *own* terror. Ehrenzweig (1968) compares the depressive position to the '*reintrojection*' phase in the art process in which the art's hidden substructure is reintegrated back into the artist's ego. Perhaps we might also make a comparison with the rites of passage state of '*(re)incorporation*' or reaggregation back into society and becoming relatively stable.

In this way art therapy, like psychotherapy, can be conceptualized as a process of 'assimilation of problematic experiences' in which one moves through the continuum of avoidance to insight and integration (Stiles 1999: 1021; Stiles 2002).

Constructive liminality in cancer care involves oscillations between these positions. Like liminality for cancer patients, movement through these positions is not simply linear. Creativity involves an inherent 'ego rhythm' (Ehrenzweig 1968: 79, 295) or an ongoing oscillation between the paranoid-schizoid and depressive positions (Bion 1984), thus developing a person's capacity for Keats' 'negative capability' (Rollins 1958: 193) and an ability to tolerate uncertainty (Glover 1998). Perhaps for cancer patients, experience of this in art therapy can strengthen the capacity to deal with the 'oscillating trajectory' between acute and sustained liminality (Little *et al.* 1998: 1493) and the 'shifting perspectives' dynamic of cancer experiences (Paterson 2001; Thorne *et al.* 2002: 449).

Cultural defence mechanisms

> We have, in our culture, an unspoken agreement not to speak about our own death . . . Without such a language we cannot integrate it. Integration requires metaphor and ritual. When as a group we are confronted with an image of dread, the group mind clangs shut . . . It is through the symbolic, the metaphors and rituals, that a group is able to integrate its fate collectively and individually.
>
> (Klement 1994)

Projective identification involves 'evoking in someone else aspects of the self which one cannot bear' (Segal 1995: 36) and perhaps this does not just apply to a client's potential splitting and projection of feelings into the art and the therapist. Perhaps society too can split off intolerable fears of cancer, the 'unbounded body' and, fundamentally, death. This could happen physically through sequestration into hospices (Lawton 1998). We could speculate that such defence mechanisms could also operate intersubjectively.

In this way, society could regard cancer, unboundedness and death as unbearable realities and therefore split and project them, for instance into cancer patients. Such dynamics could be a distortion of an adversarial type of play (*agôn*) (see Chapter 2), such as when vulnerability and unboundedness are regarded as a weakness, deviance and/or terrifying. They are thus disowned and projected into others who are then perceived as vulnerable and weak. Then, through the mechanism of projective identification, such feelings of terror and stigma could be evoked in cancer patients, thus inducing role play (*mimicry*) (Caillois 1962) whereby cancer patients identify with stigmatization. Such dynamics could also operate if healthcare professionals are not able to own the realities of their own unboundedness and death. This could be driven by the panic type of play (*ilinx*) (Caillois 1962) grounded in fears of weakness and mortality.

Pfeiffer (2002) suggests that the dominant Western ontology and epistemology tends towards dichotomies and stereotypes and these basic assumptions need to be critically evaluated in society and in research. An embodied liminality perspective that acknowledges illness and mortality as part of the human condition could be less likely to project denied vulnerability onto others (Shakespeare 1994; Shakespeare and Watson 2002). Turner (1988: 24–5) asserts that constructive liminality and the plastic arts promote the 'reflexive voice' and enable people to question basic assumptions and 'relations, actions, symbols, meanings, codes, roles, statuses, social structures, ethical and legal rules, and other sociocultural components which make up their public "selves" '. (See Figure 4.3.) This could promote restorying, social inclusion and reincorporation of the realities of our mortal embodied condition.

Conclusion

In this chapter, I have explored a fifth characteristic of liminality – *embodied experience* – and its relevance to cancer experiences and art therapy. I focused on three dimensions of liminal embodied experience – *physicality, structural inferiority/power*, and *sexual embodiment* – by means of discussing how a fourth, *expression*, relates to each of the first three. Consistent with Little *et al.*'s (1998) findings, it seems that the concept of liminality is a valuable lens through which to view cancer experiences and art therapy.

Turner (1982: 75–6) asserts that 'liminal reflexivity' is necessary if 'crisis is to be rendered meaningful' and he suggests that 'ritual procedures generate *narratives*' promoting the 'integration'. Narrative approaches, such as therapeutic 'emplotment' (Mattingly 1994), have been viewed as a form of expressive embodiment of experience (Brockmeier and Carbaugh 2001: 1). They can integrate illness into the life story and integrate patients in their social world (Cheshire and Ziebland 2004). Story-making can be beneficial during life-threatening illness (Bolen 1998: 95, 109; Murphy 1999: 24–42) and finding new voices can ease 'people's passages through times of transition' (Hedtke 2002: 286). Such narratives, 'told through a wounded body', give 'voice to the body, so that the changed body can become once again familiar in these stories' (Frank 1997: 2).

Viewing a person as a 'community of voices' (Honos-Webb and Stiles 1998), therapy can offer an opening to encourage previously unheard voice(s) to join the dominant voices, thus enabling a process of 'social inclusion' (McLeod 1999). An individual can become inclusive to previously projected material that can also be witnessed by an art therapist. Art therapy also accommodates various forms of expression and does not privilege verbal voice. Art therapy rituals and symbols have particular value in metaphorizing the body, thus enabling expression of emotions and bodily states including conscious and unconscious aspects otherwise deemed unspeakable, unhearable, unseeable and unthinkable. Perhaps this is helpful in redressing the structural inferiority of liminal situations.

Art therapy offers multi-sensory and verbal opportunities for symbolic reportraying. In this way the reconstruction of new narratives (Williams 1984; White and Epston 1990; McLeod and Balamoutsou 2000) can 'help patients to construct a meaningful narrative of disease' (Zollman and Vickers 1999). For cancer patients 'sustained liminality' can be a 'prolonged dialectic between body and self, in which a narrative is constructed to give meaning to the challenging and changing biographical, physical and existential phenomena in which illness and aging evolve in the locus of the body' (Little *et al.* 1998: 1493).

Art therapy offers an approach that addresses some of the criticisms of purely verbal narrative approaches in medical contexts (Lambert 2004). For instance, as noted in Chapter 2, art-making in art therapy can evoke and express a variety of time experiences, rather than just a linear approach to time; it values non-verbal expression and embodiment, rather than privileging the articulate and assuming language has primacy; it accommodates multiple shifting experiences, feeling there is no meaning and waiting for meaning, rather than implying that one meaning or truth has to be found.

Working with 'multivocal symbols' (Turner 1982: 27) in art therapy promotes and enables individuals to experience the oscillating nature of the creative process and ego positions in a containing environment. This perhaps strengthens the client's capacity to deal with the *multiple* narratives evident in a cancer experience – i.e. the 'oscillating trajectory' between acute and sustained liminality (Little *et al.* 1998: 1493) and the 'shifting perspectives' dynamic of cancer experiences (Paterson 2001; Thorne *et al.* 2002: 449).

Perhaps in art therapy in cancer care, through constructive liminality and containment, developmental oscillation between the paranoid-schizoid (separation) and depressive (reincorporation) positions can be achieved at the *individual* level. Thus splitting of self and body can be ameliorated and split projections of intolerable 'bad' objects can be contained, thus modified and made capable of reintrojection. A constraining habitus/hexis can be modified, fostering a more constructive relationship between the true body-self and appropriate presentations of self-body needed in different contexts.

However, constructive liminality and containment also needs to foster developmental oscillation at the *cultural* level to enable societal projections to be reincorporated. This could foster reflexive reconstruction of narratives of the 'unbounded body', stigma, shame, dichotomies of health and illness, and stereotyping. This could be less likely to view illness, unboundedness and death as intolerable, deviant or failures. Perhaps, at individual and collective levels, art therapy can play a valuable part in promoting a both/and perspective that is more able to deal with ambiguity, ambivalence, unboundedness, uncertainty and multivocal experience.

Note

1   My research motivation and methodology were outlined in Chapter 2. In brief, however, the auto/biographical art-based autoethnographic study was stimulated by my experiences of liminality in art-making and after cancer diagnosis. The research systematically investigated the relationship between key aspects of liminality and art therapy and my cancer experience and that of participating clients.

References

Anzieu, D. (1989) *The Skin Ego*. New Haven, CT: Yale University Press.

Arman, M. and Rehnsfeldt, A. (2003) The hidden suffering among breast cancer patients: a qualitative metasynthesis, *Qualitative Health Research*, 13(4): 510–27.

Arnheim, R. (1992) The artist as healer, *To the Rescue of Art – 26 Essays*. Berkeley and Los Angeles, CA: University of California Press.

Arthern, J. and Madill, A. (1999) How do transitional objects work? The therapist's view, *British Journal of Medical Psychology*, 72(Pt.1): 1–21.

Arthern, J. and Madill, A. (2002) How do transitional objects work? The client's view, *Psychotherapy Research*, 12(3): 369–88.

Bakhtin, M.M. (2000) *The Dialogic Imagination* (edited by Michael Holquist, translated by Michael Holquist and Caryl Emerson). Austin, TX: University of Texas Press.

Balint, M. (1956) *The Doctor, his Patient and the Illness*. London: Pitman Medical Publishing Co. Ltd.

Baron, P. (1989) Fighting cancer with images, in H. Wadeson, J. Durkin and D. Perach (eds) *Advances in Art Therapy*. NY: John Wiley & Sons.

Bion, W.R. (1959) Attacks on linking, *International Journal of Psychoanalysis*, XL: 308–15.

Bion, W.R. (1984) *Learning from Experience*. London: Karnac Books.

Bion, W.R. (1993) *Second Thoughts: Selected Papers on Psychoanalysis*. London: Maresfield Library.

Boadella, D. (1989) *Maps of Character*. London: Abbotsbury Publications.

Bolen, J.S. (1998) *Close to the Bone: Life-threatening Illness and the Search for Meaning*. New York: Touchstone/Simon & Schuster.

Bordo, S. (1989) The body and the reproduction of femininity: a feminist appropriation of Foucault, in A. Jagger and S. Bordo (eds) *Gender/Body/Knowledge: Feminist Reconstructions of Being and Knowing*. London: Rutgers University Press.

Bordo, S. (1993) *Unbearable Weight: Feminism, Western Culture and the Body*. Berkeley and Los Angeles, CA: University of California Press.

Borgmann, E. (2002) Art therapy with three women diagnosed with cancer, *The Arts in Psychotherapy*, 29(5): 245–51.

Bottomley, A. (1997) Psychosocial problems in cancer care: a brief review of common problems, *Journal of Psychiatric and Mental Health Nursing*, 4(5): 323–31.

Bourdieu, P. (1977) *Outline of a Theory of Practice*. Cambridge: Cambridge University Press.

Bovensiepen, G. (2002) Symbolic attitude and reverie: problems of symbolization in children and adolescents, *Journal of Analytical Psychology*, 47: 241–57, http://www.blackwellpublishers.co.uk/Joap/JOAP305.pdf (accessed 13 August 2004).

Brockmeier, J. and Carbaugh, D. (eds) (2001) *Narrative and Identity: Studies in Autobiography, Self and Culture*, pp. 145–84. Erdenheim PA: John Benjamins Publishing Co., http://www.benjamins.com/cgi-bin/booklist_ebrary.cgi (accessed 11 August 2004).

Burch, R. (1990) Phenomenology, lived experience: taking a measure of the topic, *Phenomenology & Pedagogy*, 8: 130–60. *Phenomenology Online*, http://www.phenomenologyonline.com/articles/burch2.html (accessed 14 August 2004).

Burt, K. (1995) The effects of cancer on body image and sexuality, *Nursing Times*, 91(7): 36–7.

Caillois, R. (1962) *Man, Play and Games*. London: Thames and Hudson.

Calogeras, R.C. and Alston, T.M. (2000) The dreams of a cancer patient: a 'royal road' to understanding the somatic illness, *Psychoanalytic Review*, 87(6): 911–37.

Campbell, J., Liebmann, M., Brook, F., Jones, J. and Ward, C.R. (eds) (2003) *Art Therapy, Race and Culture*. London: Jessica Kingsley.

Case, C. and Dalley, T. (1997) *The Handbook of Art Therapy*. London: Routledge.

Cash, T.F. and Pruzinsky, T. (eds) (2004) *Body Image: A Handbook of Theory, Research, and Clinical Practice*. London: Routledge.

Chapple, A. and Ziebland, S. (2002) Prostate cancer: embodied experience and perceptions of masculinity, *Sociology of Health & Illness*, 24(6): 820–41.

Cheshire, J. and Ziebland, S. (2004) Narrative as a resource in accounts of the experience of illness. Draft paper, Department of Linguistics, Queen Mary, University of London, http://www.modern-languages.qmw.ac.uk/research/linguisticstaff/jenny/Narrative%20form%20FINAL.pdf (accessed 14 August 2004).

Clark, D. (1999) 'Total pain', disciplinary power and the body in the work of Cicely Saunders, 1958–1967, *Social Science & Medicine*, 49(6): 727–36.

Cohen, B.M. and Mills, A. (1999) Skin/paper/bark. Body image, trauma and the diagnostic drawing series, in J. Goodwin and R. Attias (eds) *Splintered Reflections: Images of the Body in Trauma*. New York: Basic Books.

Cohn, H.W. (1997) *Existential Thought and Therapeutic Practice*. London: Sage Publications.

Coleman, V.D. and Farris-Dufrene, P.M. (1996) *Art Therapy and Psychotherapy: Blending Two Approaches*. London: Taylor & Francis.

Colyer, H. (1996) Women's experience of living with cancer, *Journal of Advanced Nursing*, 23(3): 496–501.

Comeau, T.B., Epstein, J.B. and Migas, C. (2001) Taste and smell dysfunction in patients receiving chemotherapy: a review of current knowledge, *Supportive Care in Cancer*, 9(8): 575–80.

Connell, C. (1998) *Something Understood. Art Therapy in Cancer Care*. London: Wrexham.

Corker, M. and Shakespeare, T. (eds) (2002) *Disability Postmodernity: Embodying Disability Theory*. London/New York: Continuum International Publishing Group.

Cort, E., Monroe, B. and Oliviere, D. (2004) Couples in palliative care, *Sexual and Relationship Therapy*, 19(3): 337–54.

Csordas, T. (ed.) (1994) *The Embodied Self: The Existential Ground of Culture and Self*. New York: Cambridge University Press.

Dahl, S. (2003) *An Overview of Intercultural Research*. Research paper, Middlesex University Business School, http://europacom.com/sdahl/intercultural/ (accessed 13 August 2004).

Damasio, A. (2000) *The Feeling of What Happens: Body and Emotion in the Making of Consciousness*. London: William Heinemann.

Darroch-Lozowski, V. (1999) *The Uncoded World: A Poetic Semiosis of the Wandered*. New York: Peter Lang.

Diamond, N. (2001) Towards an interpersonal understanding of bodily experience, *Psychodynamic Counselling*, 7(1): 41–62.

Dilthey, W. (1976) *Selected Writings*. London: Cambridge University Press.

Douglas, M. (1966) *Purity and Danger: An Analysis of Concepts of Pollution and Taboo*. New York: Frederick A. Praeger.

Dreifuss-Kattan, E. (1994) *Cancer Stories: Creativity and Self-Repair*. Hillsdale, NJ: The Analytic Press.

Ehrenzweig, A. (1968) *The Hidden Order of Art*. London: Weidenfeld & Nicolson.

Erikson, E.H. (1977) *Childhood and Society*. London: Paladin Grafton Books.

Esrock, E.J. (2002) Touching art: intimacy, embodiment, and the somatosensory system, *Consciousness & Emotion*, 2(2): 233–53(21), http://www. italianacademy. columbia.edu/pdfs/esrock.pdf (accessed 10 August 2004).

Flanagan J. and Holmes, S. (2000) Social perceptions of cancer and their impacts: implications for nursing practice arising from the literature, *Journal of Advanced Nursing*, 32(3): 740–9.

Foucault, M. (1986) Of other spaces, *Diacritics 16*, Spring, 22–7, http://www-unix. oit.umass.edu/~bweber/courses/foucaultspaces.html (accessed 7 August 2004).

Foucault, M. (1991) *Discipline and Punish: The Birth of the Prison*. London: Penguin.

Foulkes, S.H. and Anthony, E.J. (1984) *Group Psychotherapy: The Psycho-analytic Approach*. London: Karnac Books.

Fox, S. and Lantz, C. (1998) The brain tumor experience and quality of life: a qualitative study, *The Journal of Neuroscience Nursing*, 30(4): 245–52.

Frank, A.W. (1997) *The Wounded Storyteller: Body, Illness, and Ethics*. Chicago, IL: University of Chicago Press.

Freedman, T.G. (1994) Social and cultural dimensions of hair loss in women treated for breast cancer, *Cancer Nursing*, 17: 334–41.

Freud, S. (1923) The ego and the id, *Standard Edition of the Complete Psychological Works of Sigmund Freud*, Vol. XIX. London: Hogarth Press.

Geertz, C. (1973) *The Interpretation of Cultures*. New York: Basic Books.

Glaus, A. (1993) Assessment of fatigue in cancer and non-cancer patients and in healthy individuals, *Supportive Care in Cancer*, 1(6): 305–15.

Glaus, A., Crow, R. and Hammond, S. (1996) A qualitative study to explore the concept of fatigue/tiredness in cancer patients and in healthy individuals, *European Journal of Cancer Care*, 5(2 Suppl): 8–23.

Glover, N. (1998) *Psychoanalytic Aesthetics: The British School*. Online book,

Human-nature.com, Robert M. Young & Ian Pitchford, http://www.human-nature.com/free-associations/glover/index.html (accessed 8 August 2004).

Goffman, E. (1963) *Stigma: Notes on the Management of Spoiled Identity*. New York: Simon & Schuster.

Grealy, L. (1995) *Autobiography of a Face*. New York: Harper/Perennial Press.

Grogan, S. (1999) *Body Image*. London: Routledge.

Grosz, E. (1994) *Volatile Bodies: Toward a Corporeal Feminism (Theories of Representation and Difference)*. Bloomington, IN: Indiana University Press.

Gurevich, M., Bishop, S., Bower, J., Malka, M. and Nyhof-Young, J. (2004) (Dis)-embodying gender and sexuality in testicular cancer, *Social Science & Medicine*, 58(9): 1597–607.

Hartocollis, P. (1980) Time and the dream, *Journal of the American Psychoanalytic Association*, 28(4): 861–77.

Hawkins, P. (1997) Organizational culture: sailing between evangelism and complexity, *Human Relations*, 50(4): 417–40.

Hedtke, L. (2002) Reconstructing the language of death and grief, *Illness, Crisis and Loss*, 10(4): 285–93.

Henley, D. (2002) *Clayworks in Art Therapy*. London: Jessica Kingsley.

Hill, M.A. (2002) Healing grief through art: art therapy bereavement group workshops. *Drawn Together: Art Therapy for Groups*, http://www.drawntogether.com/healing.htm (accessed 13 August 2004).

Hiscox, A.R. and Calisch, A.C. (eds) (1998) *Tapestry of Cultural Issues in Art Therapy*. London: Jessica Kingsley.

Hofstede, G.H. (1991) *Cultures and Organizations: Software of the Mind*. London: McGraw-Hill.

Hogan, S. (ed.) (1996) *Feminist Art Therapy: Visions of Difference*. London: Routledge.

Hogan, S. (1997) *Feminist Approaches to Art Therapy*. London: Routledge.

Hogan, S. (ed.) (2002) *Gender Issues in Art Therapy*. London: Jessica Kingsley.

Holland, J.C. (2002) History of psycho-oncology: overcoming attitudinal and conceptual barriers, *Psychosomatic Medicine*, 64(2): 206–21.

Holley, S. (2000) Cancer-related fatigue. Suffering a different fatigue, *Cancer Practice*, 8(2): 87–95.

Honos-Webb, L. and Stiles, W.B. (1998) Reformulations of assimilation analysis in terms of voices, *Psychotherapy*, 35: 23–33.

HPC (2003a) *Standards of Conduct, Performance and Ethics*. London: Health Professions Council, http://www.hpc-uk.org/publications/brochures/HPC034HPCA5_Standards_of_conduct_performance_and_ethics.pdf (accessed 13 August 2004).

HPC (2003b) *Standards of Proficiency: Arts Therapists*. London: Health Professions Council, http://www.hpc-uk.org/publications/standards/Standards_of_Proficiency_Arts_Therapists.pdf (accessed 13 August 2004).

Hughes, M.K. (2000) Sexuality and the cancer survivor: a silent coexistence, *Cancer Nursing*, 23(6): 477–82.

Jarvis, M. (2004) *Psychodynamic Psychology: Classical Theory and Contemporary Research*. London: Thomson Learning.

Jaspers, K. (1931) *Philosophie*, cited in Macquarrie, J. (1973) *Existentialism: An Introduction, Guide and Assessment*. London: Penguin.

Johnson, M. (1987) *The Body in the Mind: The Bodily Basis of Meaning, Imagination and Reason.* Chicago, IL: University of Chicago Press.

Jung, C.G. (1996) *The Archetypes and the Collective Unconscious. Collected Works,* 9i. London: Routledge.

Klein, M. (1946) Notes on some schizoid mechanisms, *International Journal of Psycho-Analysis,* 27: 99–110.

Klein, M. (1975) Infantile anxiety-situations reflected in a work of art and in the creative impulse, *The Writings of Melanie Klein,* Vol. 1: *Love, Guilt and Reparation and Other Works.* London: Hogarth Press/Institute of Psychoanalysis.

Klein, M. (1988) *Envy and Gratitude and Other Works, 1946–1963.* London: Virago Press.

Kleinman, A. (1994) Pain as human experience: an introduction, in M.J. Delvecchio, P.E. Broswin, B.J. Byron and A. Kleinman (eds) *Pain as a Human Experience. An Anthropological Perspective.* Berkeley, CA: University of California Press.

Klement, V. (1994) An artist's notes on aging and death, *Art Journal,* Spring, http://www.findarticles.com/p/articles/mi_m0425/is_n1_v53/ai_15383251 (accessed 13 August 2004).

Kristeva, J. (1982) *The Powers of Horror: An Essay on Abjection.* New York: Columbia University Press.

Lambert, H. (2004) Proposer of the motion 'This house believes that narrative research is a passing fashion with no coherent theoretical rationale and no substantive or unique contribution to make in medical research or practice', Narrative Research in Health and Illness, conference 9–10 September, British Medical Association, London.

Langellier, K.M. (2001) 'You're marked': breast cancer, tattoo, and the narrative performance of identity, in J. Brockmeier and D. Carbaugh (eds) *Narrative and Identity: Studies in Autobiography, Self and Culture.* Erdenheim, PA: John Benjamins Publishing Co., http://www.benjamins.com/cgi-bin/booklist_ebrary.cgi (accessed 11 August 2004).

Lark, C. (2001) *Art Therapy Overview: An Informal Background Paper.* The Art Therapy Center, http://www.art-therapy.com/ArtTherapyOverview.htm (accessed 14 August 2004).

Lawton, J. (1998) Contemporary hospice care: the sequestration of the unbounded body and 'dirty dying', *Sociology of Health and Illness,* 20(2): 121–43.

Leach, E. (1967) Magical hair, in J. Middleton (ed.) *Myth and Cosmos.* Austin, TX: University of Texas Press.

Lewis, H.B. (1987) Introduction: Shame – the 'sleeper' in psychopathology, in H.B. Lewis (ed.) *The Role of Shame in Symptom Formation.* London: Lawrence Erlbaum Associates.

Light, R. and Brittingham, D. (1994) Breast cancer and body image, *Studies on Women and Gender Abstracts,* 24(10): 11.

Lister, P. (1999) A taxonomy for developing cultural competence, *Nurse Education Today,* 19(4): 313–18.

Little, M., Jordens, C.F., Paul, K., Montgomery, K. and Philipson, B. (1998) Liminality: a major category of the experience of cancer illness, *Social Science & Medicine,* 47(10): 1492–3.

Longhurst, R. (2001) *Bodies: Exploring Fluid Boundaries.* London: Routledge.

Lowenfeld, V. and Brittain, W. (1987) *Creative and Mental Growth*. New York: Macmillan Publishing.

Lynch, G. (1997) Words and silence: counselling and psychotherapy after Wittgenstein, *Counselling*, 8(2): 126–8.

McDaniel, R.W., Rhodes, V.A., Nelson, R.A. and Hanson, B.M. (1995) Sensory perceptions of women receiving tamoxifen for breast cancer, *Cancer Nursing*, 18(3): 215–21.

McGuire, D.B. (2004) Occurrence of cancer pain, *Journal of the National Cancer Institute, Monographs*, 32: 51–6.

McLeod, J. (1999) Counselling as a social process, *Counselling*, 10: 217–22.

McLeod, J. and Balamoutsou, S. (2000) Narrative processes in the assimilation of a problematic experience: qualitative analysis of a single case. School of Social and Health Sciences, University of Abertay Dundee, 28 November, http://shs.tay.ac.uk/shtjm/narrative%20coconstruction%20paper5.html (accessed 2 August 2004).

Macquarrie, J. (1973) *Existentialism: An Introduction, Guide and Assessment*. London: Penguin.

Magnusson, K., Moller, A., Ekman, T. and Wallgren, A. (1999) A qualitative study to explore the experience of fatigue in cancer patients, *European Journal of Cancer Care*, 8(4): 224–32.

Malchiodi, C.A. (ed.) (1999) *Medical Art Therapy with Adults*. London: Jessica Kingsley.

Mattingly, C. (1994) The concept of therapeutic 'emplotment', *Social Science & Medicine*, 38(6): 811–22.

Merleau-Ponty, M. (1962) *The Phenomenology of Perception*. London: Routledge and Kegan Paul.

Merriam-Webster (2004) *Merriam-Webster Online*, based on *Merriam-Webster's Collegiate Dictionary*, 10th edition. Springfield, MA: Merriam-Webster, Inc., http://www.m-w.com/ (accessed 13 August 2004).

Metzger, D. (1997) *Tree: Essays and Pieces*. Berkeley, CA: North Atlantic Books.

Miller, B. (1996) Art therapy with the elderly and the terminally ill, in T. Dalley (ed.) *Art as Therapy: An Introduction to the Use of Art as a Therapeutic Technique*. London: Routledge.

Milner, M. (1977) *On Not Being Able To Paint*. Oxford: Heinemann Educational Books.

Mohkamsing-den Boer, E. and Zock, H. (2004) Dreams of passage: an object-relational perspective on a case of a Hindu death ritual, *Religion*, 34(1): 1–14.

Morris, D. (1991) *The Culture of Pain*. Berkeley and Los Angeles, CA: University of California Press.

Morse, J., Bottorff, J. and Hutchinson, S. (1995) The paradox of comfort, *Nursing Research*, 44: 14–19.

Murphy, N.M. (1999) *The Wisdom of Dying: Practices for Living*. Shaftesbury: Element Books.

Muzzin, L.J. *et al.* (1994) The experience of cancer, *Social Science & Medicine*, 38(9): 1201–8.

Myerhoff, B.G., Camino, L.A. and Turner, E. (1987) Rites of passage: an overview, in M. Eliade (ed.) *Encyclopedia of Religion*, Vol.12. New York: Macmillan, http://www.clal.org/tb_rt001.html (accessed 12 August 2004).

Nathanson, D. (1992) *Shame and Pride: Affect, Sex, and the Birth of the Self*. New York: Norton.

Nathanson, D. (1995/2004) A conversation with Donald Nathanson. On Silvan Tomkins's affect theory. *Behavior OnLine, Inc.*, http://www.behavior.net/column/nathanson/index.html (accessed 13 August 2004).

Navon, L. and Morag, A. (2004) Liminality as biographical disruption: unclassifiability following hormonal therapy for advanced prostate cancer, *Social Science & Medicine*, 58(11): 2337–47.

Orbach, S. (1994) Working with the false body, in A. Erskine and D. Judd (eds) *The Imaginative Body: Psychodynamic Therapy in Health Care*. London: Whurr Publishers.

Pandey, M. and Thomas, B.C. (2001) Rehabilitation of cancer patients, *Postgraduate Medicine*, 47(1): 62–5.

Paterson, B.L. (2001) The shifting perspectives model of chronic illness, *Image: Journal of Nursing Scholarship*, 33(1): 21–6.

Pellegrini, R.J. (1973) Impressions of the male personality as a function of beardedness, *Psychology*, 10(1): 29–33.

Peters-Golden, H. (1982) Breast cancer: varied perceptions of social support in the illness experience, *Social Science & Medicine*, 16(4): 483–91.

Pfeiffer, D. (2002) The philosophical foundations of disability studies, *Disability Studies Quarterly*, 22(2): 3–23, http://www.dsq-sds.org/_articles_pdf/2002/Spring/dsq_2002_Spring_02.pdf (accessed 25 February 2005).

Picard, C. (1997) Embodied soul. The focus for nursing praxis, *Journal of Holistic Nursing*, 15(1): 41–53, Buddhist Digital Library and Museum, http://ccbs.ntu.edu.tw/FULLTEXT/JR-MDL/pichard.htm (accessed 14 August 2004).

Pickett, J.P. *et al.* (eds) (2000) Indo-European Roots Index, *The American Heritage Dictionary of the English Language*. Boston: Houghton Mifflin Company, http://www.bartleby.com/61/roots/IE498.html (accessed 2 August 2004).

Portenoy, R.K. and Itri, L.M. (1999) Cancer-related fatigue: guidelines for evaluation and management, *The Oncologist*, 4(1): 1–10.

Potter, J. (2004) Fatigue experience in advanced cancer: a phenomenological approach, *International Journal of Palliative Nursing*, 10(1): 15–23.

Prost, J.H. (2004) Skin: on the cultural border between self and the world, *Visual Anthropology*, 17(2): 191–2.

Prytherch, D. and McLundie, M. (2002) So what is haptics anyway? *Research Issues in Art as Design Media*, Issue 2, Spring, http://www.biad.uce.ac.uk/research/rti/riadm/issue2/riadmIssue2.PDF (accessed 10 August 2004).

Radley, A. (2002) Portrayals of suffering: on looking away, looking at, and the comprehension of illness experience, *Body & Society*, 8(3): 1–23.

Richardson, A. and Ream, E. (1996) The experience of fatigue and other symptoms in patients receiving chemotherapy, *European Journal of Cancer Care*, 5(2 Suppl.): 24–30.

Riskó, Á., Fleischmann, T., Molnár, Z., Schneider, T. and Várady, E. (1996) Influence of the pathological psychological state of cancer patients on their decisions, *Supportive Care In Cancer*, 4(1): 51–55, Onkopszichológia Online, http://www.oncol.hu/psicho/index.html (accessed 13 August 2004).

Riskó, Á., Deák, B., Molnár, Z., Schneider, T., Várady, E. and Rosta, A. (1998) Individual, psychoanalytically oriented psychotherapy during oncological treatment with adolescents suffering from malignant lymphoma. 4th International Congress of Psycho-oncology, Hamburg, Germany, 3–6 September, *Onkopszichológia Online*, http://www.oncol.hu/psicho/index.html (accessed 13 August 2004).

Riskó, Á. (2001) Close to the body. Lost Childhood International Conference, Ferenczi Sándor Society, Budapest, 23–5 February, *Onkopszichológia Online*, http://www.oncol.hu/psicho/index.html (accessed 13 August 2004).

Rix, B.A. (2000) Metaphors and power. A qualitative study of metaphorical thinking among Danish cancer patients, *Ugeskrift for Laeger*, 162(39): 5212–16.

Rogers, N. (1993) *The Creative Connection: Expressive Arts as Healing*. Palo Alto, CA: Science & Behavior Books.

Rollins, H.E. (ed.) (1958) Letter to George and Tom Keats, 21 December 1817, in *The Letters of J. Keats: 1814–1821*. Cambridge: Cambridge University Press.

Rowan, J. (2000) The three bodies in psychotherapy, *European Journal of Psychotherapy, Counselling & Health*, 3(2): 193–207.

Rudge, T. (1998) Skin as cover: the discursive effects of 'covering' metaphors on wound care practices, *Nursing Inquiry*, 5(4): 228–37.

Ruthrof, H. (1998) *Semantics and the Body: Meaning from Frege to the Postmodern*. Melbourne: Melbourne University Press.

Saunders, C. (1996) A personal therapeutic journey, *British Medical Journal*, 313: 1599–601, http://bmj.bmjjournals.com/cgi/content/full/313/7072/1599 (accessed 13 August 2004).

Schaverien, J. (1994) The scapegoat and the talisman: transference in art therapy, in T. Dalley, C. Case, J. Schaverien *et al.* (eds) *Images of Art Therapy*. London: Routledge.

Schaverien, J. (2000) The triangular relationship and the aesthetic countertransference in analytical art psychotherapy, in A. Gilroy and G. McNeilly (eds) *The Changing Shape of Art Therapy: New Developments in Theory and Practice*. London: Jessica Kingsley.

Schaverien, J. (2002) *The Dying Patient in Psychotherapy: Desire, Dreams and Individuation*. Basingstoke: Palgrave Macmillan.

Schechner, R. (2003) *Performance Studies: An Introduction*. London: Routledge.

Schore, A.N. (1999) The right brain, the right mind, and psychoanalysis, *Neuro-Psychoanalysis*, 1(1): 49–54, Commentary, University of California at Los Angeles School of Medicine. Included in Schore, A.N. (2003) *Affect Regulation and the Repair of the Self*. New York: W. W. Norton & Company, http://www.neuro-psa.com/schore.htm (accessed 13 August 2004).

Schore, A.N. (2003) *Affect Regulation and the Repair of the Self*. New York: W. W. Norton & Company.

Segal, J. (1995) *Melanie Klein*. London: Sage Publications.

Shakespeare, T.W. (1994) Cultural representations of disabled people: dustbins for disavowal?, *Disability and Society*, 9(3): 283–99.

Shakespeare, T.W. and Watson, N. (2002) The social model of disability: an outdated ideology?, *Research in Social Science and Disability*, 2: 9–28.

Sheets-Johnstone, M. (1990) *The Roots of Thinking*. Philadelphia, PA: Temple University Press.

Simon, R.M. (1992) *The Symbolism of Style: Art as Therapy*. London: Routledge.

Sinha, C. and Jensen de López, K. (2000) Language, culture and the embodiment of spatial cognition, *Cognitive Linguistics*, 11: 17–41, http://cerebro. psych. cornell.edu/chris/pdf/Language_Culture_Embod.pdf (accessed 13 August 2004).

Skaife, S. (1995) The dialectics of art therapy, *Inscape*, 1: 2–7.

Skaife, S. and Huet, V. (1998) Introduction, in S. Skaife and V. Huet (eds) *Art Psychotherapy in Groups: Between Picture and Words*. London: Routledge.

Slattery, P. (2001) The educational researcher as artist working within, *Qualitative Inquiry*, 20 June, 7(3): 370–98, http://www.coe.tamu.edu/~pslattery/documents/ QualitativeInquiry.pdf (accessed 2 August 2004).

Sontag, S. (1978) *Illness as Metaphor*. New York: Farrar, Straus & Giroux.

Spencer-Oatey, H. (2000) *Culturally Speaking: Managing Rapport through Talk across Cultures*. London: Continuum.

Springer, M. (1996) *A Tribe of Warrior Women: Breast Cancer Survivors*. Birmingham, AL: Crane Hill Publishers.

Stanley, L. (1992) *The Auto/Biographical I*. Manchester: Manchester University Press.

Stiles, W.B. (1999) Signs and voices in psychotherapy, *Psychotherapy Research*, 9(1): 1–21, http://www.users.muohio.edu/stileswb/readings/stiles1999.pdf (accessed 2 August 2004).

Stiles, W. B. (2002) Assimilation of problematic experiences, in J.C. Norcross (ed.) *Psychotherapy Relationships that Work: Therapist Contributions and Responsiveness to Patients*. Oxford: Oxford University Press, http://www.users.muohio. edu/stileswb/assimilation_model.htm (accessed 2 August 2004).

Stokes, A. (1978) *Critical Writings of Adrian Stokes*, Vol. III. London: Tavistock.

Street, A.F. and Kissane, D.W. (2001) Discourses of the body in euthanasia: symptomatic, dependent, shameful and temporal, *Nursing Inquiry*, 8(3): 162–72.

Sundquist, K. and Yee, L. (2003) Sexuality and body image after cancer, *Australian Family Physician*, 32(1–2): 19–23.

Synnott, A. (2001) *The Body Social: Symbolism, Self and Society*. London: Routledge.

Thomas, G. (1995) Art therapy and practice in palliative care, *European Journal of Palliative Care*, 2(3): 120–1.

Thomas-MacLean, R. (2004) Understanding breast cancer stories via Frank's narrative types, *Social Science & Medicine*, 58(9): 1647–57.

Thompson, S. and Kahn, J.H. (1972) *The Group Process as a Helping Technique*. Oxford: Pergamon Press Ltd.

Thorne, S. *et al.* (2002) Chronic illness experience: insights from a metastudy, *Qualitative Health Research*, 12(4): 437–52.

Trompenaars, F. and Hampden-Turner, C. (1997) *Riding The Waves of Culture*. London: McGraw-Hill.

Turner, B.S. (1996) *The Body and Society*. London: Sage Publications.

Turner, V.W. (1967) *The Forest of Symbols: Aspects of Ndembu Ritual*. Ithaca, NY: Cornell University Press.

Turner, V.W. (1975) *Dramas, Fields, and Metaphors: Symbolic Action in Human Society*. Ithaca, NY: Cornell University Press.

Turner, V.W. (1982) *From Ritual to Theatre: The Human Seriousness of Play*. New York: Performing Arts Journal Publications.

Turner, V.W. (1988) *The Anthropology of Performance*. New York: Performing Arts Journal Publications.

Turner, V.W. (1995) *The Ritual Process: Structure and Anti-Structure*. New York: Aldine de Gruyter.

UMCCC (2004) *Art therapy*. University of Michigan Comprehensive Cancer Center, Patient/Family Support & Services, http://www.cancer.med.umich.edu/clinic/art.htm (accessed 13 August 2004).

Van der Riet, P. (1998) The sexual embodiment of the cancer patient, *Nursing Inquiry*, 5(4): 248–57.

Van Gennep, A. (1960) *The Rites of Passage*. London: Routledge & Kegan Paul.

Varela, F., Thompson, E. and Rosch, E. (1993) *The Embodied Mind: Cognitive Science and Human Experience*. Cambridge, MA: MIT Press.

Wadeson, H. (1980) *Art Psychotherapy*. New York: Wiley-Interscience, John Wiley & Sons.

Waskul, D.D. and Van der Riet, P. (2002) The abject embodiment of cancer patients: dignity, selfhood, and the grotesque body, *Symbolic Interaction*, 25(4): 487–513.

Watson, J. (2000) *Male Bodies: Health, Culture and Identity*. Buckingham: Open University Press.

Welman, M. and Faber, P.A. (1992) The dream in terminal illness: a Jungian formulation, *Journal of Analytical Psychology*, 37(1): 61–81.

White, M. and Epston, D. (1990) *Narrative Means to Therapeutic Ends*. New York: W.W. Norton.

Willett, J. and Deegan, M.J. (2001) Liminality and disability: rites of passage and community in hypermodern society, *Disability Studies Quarterly*, 21(3): 137–52.

Williams, G. (1984) The genesis of chronic illness: narrative reconstruction, *Sociology of Health & Illness*, 6(2): 175–200.

Williams, J., Wood, C. and Cunningham-Warburton, P. (1999) A narrative study of chemotherapy-induced alopecia, *Oncology Nursing Forum*, 26(9): 1463–8.

Winaver, D. and Slama, L. (1993) Breast cancer: the unspeakable, *Contraception, Fertilite, Sexualite*, 21(4): 339–43.

Winnicott, D.W. (1996) *Playing and Reality*. London: Routledge.

Wollheim, R. (1987) *Painting as an Art*. London: Thames and Hudson.

Wood, M.J.M. (1998) Art therapy in palliative care, in M. Pratt and M.J.M. Wood (eds) *Art Therapy in Palliative Care: The Creative Response*. London: Routledge.

Zollman, C. and Vickers, A. (1999) ABC of complementary medicine. Complementary medicine and the patient, *British Medical Journal*, 319(7223): 1486–9, http://www.bmj.com/cgi/content/full/319/7223/1486 (accessed 13 August 2004).

Shoreline: the realities of working in cancer and palliative care

Michèle Wood

> I stand at the shoreline and build sandcastles.
> Picking up stones and shells I shape walls and a moat.
> Turrets with pebble armour stand firm against the ebbing
> and flowing waters.
> Tiny froth fingers stroke away at the sand.
>
> I stand at the shoreline and build sandcastles.
> Firming wet sand I make barricades embellished with filigree patterns.
> Ramparts and tunnels circle protectively the inner sand chambers.
> Seaweed gardens adorn my solid structures.
>
> I stand at the shoreline and build sandcastles.
> I have made something beautiful:
> An elevation and celebration of sand, shells, weed and stone.
> Satisfaction and pleasure orbit like seagulls.
>
> Now the froth fingers come
> Stretching out their hands and arms
> To rummage and rearrange
> And all is gone.

In thinking about my experience of working with people facing cancer, AIDS or other life-threatening and limiting conditions I am reminded of the ebb and flow of the sea on the seashore. The shoreline strikes me as a useful and rich metaphor for what is involved in working as an art therapist in this area. In a sense, when people receive a diagnosis of cancer and assume the role of patient they find themselves at the shoreline, where the firm ground of personal identity and certainty encounters the enormous unpredictable waves of illness with their power to disturb and destroy. It is at this shoreline that the art therapist meets patients and faces with them the challenge of reshaping their lives. This shoreline metaphor also describes the professional landscape in which the art therapist practises. On the one hand there is the expanse of beach full of big, round, hard pebbles of important scientific evidence, 'facts' and figures. On the other hand there is the open horizon of the creative arts, mysterious unfathomable practices with few clear boundaries and vast like the sea. Art therapy has emerged from the combination of these two different elements but finds itself challenged by both. In this chapter I wish to explore something of the realities of what it means to respond to the challenges of working at these metaphorical shorelines.

Arts activities and hard evidence

Arts activities have been present in UK healthcare settings since the 1940s when Adrian Hill, recovering in a tuberculosis sanatorium, discovered the healing properties of his own artwork and encouraged his fellow patients to paint (Waller 1991). Also at this time artists were beginning to be employed within psychiatric hospitals under the supervision of psychiatrists and psychoanalysts where the healing and diagnostic potential of art was beginning to be explored (Hogan 2001). Several decades later art therapy has emerged, melding the insights from these early roots into a state-registered profession that is practised in a wide range of health and social care settings. Alongside art therapists, artists continue to make an increasing contribution to healthcare. Their input can be found in projects that range from bereaved children's art workshops (Burroughs et al. 1992) and those that use video and computer technology with the terminally ill (for example see Rosetta Life website) to projects that transform the hospital environment from clinical to more person-friendly spaces (Kaye and Blee 1997). There is increasing recognition being given to the part played by the arts in promoting individual and community health in the widest possible sense. This interest is both academic and applied and can be seen in the development of departments and organizations in the UK such as the Centre for Arts and Health in Humanities and Medicine (CAHHM) at Durham University (www.dur.ac.uk/cahhm/), the Centre for Medical Humanities at University College London (www.pcps.ucl.ac.uk/cmh) and the National Network for the Arts in Health (www.nnah.org.uk/), as well as the investment by the present government in arts and culture ventures which promote social regeneration and counter the effects of social exclusion.

Despite having similar roots and overlapping interests, the relationship between artists and art therapists has not been an easy one (Learmonth 2002). Differences have centred on the purpose and function of the art object and the therapeutic significance of the relationship between professionals and their clients.

Many artists deplore therapeutic uses of arts, feeling that art is a pure form and should not be used in this way. Art therapists, on the other hand, have sometimes felt that artists without therapy skills should not work with patients.

(Gillie Bolton 2004: 79)

When working with an artist the patient is more likely to be described as a 'user', signifying a more collegial relationship. For the therapist, the label of 'client' or 'patient' indicates vulnerabilities and needs as well as the individual's desire for help and care from the therapist. In therapy the art form reflects something of the inner world of the patient, and the boundary of confidentiality that protects the safety of the work means the patient's artwork is usually kept private. By contrast, the work with the artist always has a public outcome even if the patient decides to keep viewing to a select audience. The quote from Bolton rather starkly describes the extreme positions that can be taken by artists and therapists, whereas the reality is that art therapists are more respectful of the patient's art form and process and do not simply view it as a means of extracting personal material, and artists will generally be employed for their sensitivity and interpersonal skills as well as their expertise. Both artist and art therapist may have empowerment, control and the development of the individual's personality amongst their goals, but it is the understanding of and ability to work with the interpersonal dynamics between the patient and art therapist that are critical to art therapy. Needless to say, any professional relationship with vulnerable people will have an impact, whatever one's role. While self-scrutiny and self-reflection are part of the tools of art therapy, artists may not have been educated to think in this way and even if they do they may not have access to the sort of supervisory support that art therapists have through the clinical supervision which is a requirement of their practice. A recent document (Pratt 2004), produced in consultation with arts therapies organizations and various artists in health enterprises, has set out guidelines to recommend the facilities, budget and support needed by the artist working in palliative care. It also attempts to clarify the differences between the work of art therapists and artists in this area and is aimed at managers who wish to include the arts in their services. In some settings, support for artists is provided by the art therapist and the knowledge and experience of each other's skills serves to enhance the contribution to patient care made by both. An example where artists and art therapists work alongside each other with the same patient/user population can be seen at Trinity Hospice in London (Thomas and Kennedy 1995).

Unless patients already enjoy their own art practice (at professional or amateur levels) prior to entering oncology or palliative care services, it can be a daunting prospect for them to be faced with the invitation to use art materials, and even more so when this is linked with the notion of 'therapy'.

Sometimes patients begin with art-making and are led towards therapy (Wood 2002) and on other occasions engaging in art therapy can ignite a desire for art outside the therapy space. This boundary has rightly been described as permeable and requires thoughtful and sensitive management.

Jacqueline Coote, an art therapist, describes one patient's discovery of painting as a result of art therapy that gave rise to the production of two distinct types of image (Wood 2004). The first was her private art therapy images that conveyed difficult and painful feelings and the second was her public pictures. The patient used her public pictures to portray her increasing skills and sense of empowerment, and these were given as gifts for staff and fellow patients. It is obvious that this art/art therapy boundary needs clear handling by the therapist and artists when they work with patients, but it is just as important for the staff team that the differences are clearly understood. Both can be seen to encourage the patient's creativity and enhance the milieu of the healthcare setting, but art therapy works with the emotional and psychological needs of the patient, including their difficulties with self-expression and their barriers to creativity. As indicated earlier, how this difference is articulated will depend in part on the context of practice and the nature of the options available for patients. One problem for the profile of art therapy is the confidential nature of the imagery and work with patients. This contrasts with the exhibitions that are the result of artists' involvement with patients. The art therapist must constantly educate and inform her colleagues about her work in a way that conveys its non-verbal and symbolic nature. However, permission to use the patient's work outside the therapy contract must be obtained, and the process for this involves sensitivity and adequate discussion with the patient. Deciding at which point in the therapeutic relationship to request permission is tricky; asking during the contract of sessions may seem like an intrusion of the therapist's needs and could alter how much patients are prepared to reveal about themselves. The most relevant point at which permission could be sought would be when the therapy has terminated. At this time discussions about consent to use the patient's artwork outside its original context may include taking decisions about the storage of the patient's work, and who the patient may want to have it should they die while it is left in the safe keeping of the therapist. Written consent is an essential way to document these discussions and is as relevant to the artist working with patients as it is for the art therapist. The task of representing art therapy to the world beyond the therapeutic relationship brings us to the importance of 'evidence'.

Evaluating art therapy in cancer care

There has been a gradual increase in the art therapy literature describing work with adults and children who have cancer and other life-threatening conditions in the last ten years. Table 5.1 provides an overview of the recent English language literature. This literature provides a reference point for those who wish to examine the evidence for art therapy. The table provides a snapshot that is not exhaustive but aims to provide a sense of the range of practices or research projects undertaken by art therapists who have worked at the shoreline, where therapeutic encounters are opened up in response to the call for evaluation.

The following outcomes of art therapy have been identified in this literature as:

- better communication;
- development of a creative attitude by patients towards their circumstances;
- an increased sense of control;
- wider range of expressive capabilities;
- increased insight into patients' own behaviour;
- body image issues addressed;
- increased self-esteem;
- increased quality of life;
- a cathartic release of emotive issues;
- increased ability to confront existential questions and relieve spiritual distress;
- development of positive coping strategies;
- reduction in experiences and reports of physical pain.

Although it is encouraging to see such a breadth of practice and out-comes, most of the literature is anecdotal and difficult to compare and verify because of its diversity. It is also interesting to note that several papers have been written by art therapists about their clinical work as trainees (interns). One such paper is by Heywood (2003), who portrays a successful pilot project introducing art therapy to a cancer hospital in Manchester. Despite its success and the support from staff at the hospital, what is not reported is the fact that an art therapy post was not established when the project came to its end. Perhaps the measure of any institution's commitment to art therapy is found in its purse? This raises questions about the type of evidence needed to convince an organization to employ an art therapist.

The modernization of the National Health Service (NHS) in England is the most radical development in healthcare since its formation. As part of this process the government has set out its NHS Cancer Plan (DoH 2001), from which a Supportive Care Strategy has been developed. This strategy will set the standards for quality in supportive and palliative care against which services will be monitored, and it will significantly influence their funding. One key element of the strategy is the development of a guidance document for these services produced by the National Institute for Clinical Excellence (NICE).

Table 5.1 Overview of recent literature on art therapy with cancer and other life-threatening illnesses

Diagnosis/reason for referral to art therapy	Location of therapy	Relevant details of study	Evaluation/presentation of material	Reference
Acute lymphoblastic leukaemia	USA children's hospital	Work included a strategy for dealing with family dynamics	Description of practice with nine-year-old girl	Teufel (1995)
AIDS	UK hospice	Single session where patient presents himself as the artwork	Case study	Wood (1998)
AIDS dementia	UK hospice	Seven years analysed	Qualitative analysis	Wood (2002)
AIDS/HIV	UK day care	Drop-in art history group	Description of practice	Bartholomew (1998)
AIDS/HIV	UK prison	Closed art therapy group	Description of practice	Beaver (1998)
Bone marrow transplant	USA	Individual sessions with patients in isolation	Description of practice and some qualitative analysis	Gabriel et al. (2001)
Cancer	UK patients' homes	Individual and family art therapy	Description of practice	Bell (1998)
Cancer	UK specialist cancer hospital	Art therapy – individual and group sessions; group notebook	Descriptions of a range of practices using patients' pictures	Connell (1992), Connell (1998)
Cancer	Sweden day centre	Expressive art and music therapy	Description of short-term practices	Olofsson (1995)
Cystic fibrosis	USA private practice	Art therapy with young people	Description of practice	Farrell Fenton (2000)

Table 5.1 – continued

Diagnosis/reason for referral to art therapy	Location of therapy	Relevant details of study	Evaluation/presentation of material	Reference
Melanoma	UK	Patient reports on art therapy and other resources used	Personal account	Morley (1998)
Mixed diagnoses	i) UK hospice	Art therapy group	Description of practice	Mayo (1998)
	ii) UK hospice	Pain control mentioned as one outcome of art therapy	Description of practice. Art therapy presented alongside artist in residence	Thomas and Kennedy (1995)
	iii) UK hospice	Individual work	Description of practice	Coote (1998)
Multiple myeloma	USA	Individual work	Qualitative case study	Zammit (2001)
Niemann Pick's disease	UK day centre	Individual work and referral to music therapy	Description of practice	Stevens and Lomas (1995)
Pain control	USA hospice with adults	Art and music therapy	Theoretical discussion illustrated by case material	Trauger-Querny and Haghighi (1999)
Post-treatment cancer	USA outpatients	Short-term group work	Qualitative analyses using questionnaires and follow-up interviews	Luzzatto and Gabriel (2000)
Rheumatoid illness	Germany day care	Art therapy group work	Description of practice	Dannecker (1991)
Working practices of art therapists in cancer care	USA, New York Metropolitan area	Survey to determine demographics and practice of art therapy	Survey 10% of NY work	Bromberg (2003)
Cancer	UK hospice	Six-month project art therapy in day therapy unit	Pre-post intervention questionnaire	Wilson and Morris (2003)

Condition/Setting	Country	Description of work	Type	Reference
Palliative care	UK hospital-based	Group work	Brief description of service accompanied by clients' work	Jones (2000)
Leukaemia and oncology ward	UK hospital	Short-term pilot project undertaken during postgraduate art therapy training	Illustrated description of project	Heywood (2003)
Multiple sclerosis and uterine cancer	USA	Individual work undertaken as art therapy internship	Case study	Sutherland (1999)
Leukaemia	Italy	Art therapy used as part of a technique to prepare children undergoing painful medical procedures	Report of technique	Favara-Scacco et al. (2001)
Myelofibrosis	USA	Work with a male patient in isolation undergoing stem cell transplantation during internship	Case study	Greece (2003)
Laryngeal cancer	USA	Art therapy provision pre and post surgery as part of team approach	Case examples presented	Anand and Anand (1997)
Cancer	USA	Art therapy used to promote coping strategies	Case study	Borgmann (2002)

The NICE guidance document is an important document that provides:

> evidence-based recommendations on how best to ensure patients receive high quality information, communication, symptom control, psychological support, social and spiritual support. The guidance will cover care given in the community, in hospitals and in hospices. It will also cover the needs of carers both during a patient's illness and after bereavement. The evidence relating to the benefits of complementary therapies will also be reviewed. (Department of Health 2001, section 7.5)

The Cancer Plan establishes a commitment to a holistic view of the person with cancer and, by implication, to a multidisciplinary team of professionals who are competent to meet the needs of patients and their carers. The NICE guidance was published in March 2004 and although a range of psycho-social interventions has been included there is no reference to art therapy. Unfortunately this was due to the late registration of the British Association of Art Therapists as a stakeholder in the consultation process (this has now been rectified), and may have been due in part to the low profile of art therapy in supportive and palliative care organizations. The next NICE consultative round is due to occur in 2007 by which time art therapists will be invited to submit their evidence for consideration. The challenge for British art therapists is to formulate the evidence needed, taking into account that the quality of evidence will be assessed systematically and graded at four levels as follows: Grade I is for 'strong evidence' obtained from randomized controlled trials, Grade II is for 'fairly strong evidence' provided by prospective studies with a comparison group or good observational studies, and Grades III and IV constitute 'weak evidence', such as that gathered from professional consensus or cross-sectional studies. One attempt to gather professional consensus is being planned as I write (Wood and Low, in preparation).

The systematic study of the artwork made by people with cancer and other life-threatening illnesses is beginning to be undertaken as art therapists develop research methodologies that are most appropriate to their work, for example Gabriel *et al.* (2001) who used a thematic analysis of patients' images. However, this challenge is not unique to present-day art therapists, as four decades earlier Susan Bach (Bach 1968) was pioneering a diagnostic approach to the pictures made by terminally ill children. Her approach has been emulated and developed by some since then (Bertoia 1993; Weldt 2003). The tradition of using art therapy as an assessment and diagnostic tool is perhaps more developed in the USA (Kaplan 2000). While this approach has not been embraced in the UK, the idea of art therapy primarily as a form of interpretation made by the therapist about the patient's work still remains a common misconception here among the general population. The NHS Cancer Plan is bringing enormous challenges to all healthcare providers and art therapists are not the only professional groups facing pressures (economic and otherwise) for evidence to explain themselves. Thus art therapists working in cancer care find themselves walking along a demanding shoreline where the examination of professional identity and efficacious practice is intensifying.

In the poem that introduced this chapter the art therapist's task is described as engaging with both land and sea in the creative act of building sandcastles. On one level the sandcastles represent the work with patients; on another they represent structures created by the art therapist within which the therapeutic work can occur. It is true to say that the procedures and interventions that each art therapist develops evolve from the clinical environment in which he or she is employed and also from their personalities and interests.

My sandcastles

In order to give a feel of how I have responded to my professional and clinical shorelines I would now like to present the 'sandcastle' structures of my own practice. I work as a part-time art therapist in a Marie Curie Hospice Specialist Palliative Care Unit in London. I am part of a team comprising a family therapist/counsellor, social workers, a chaplain and a children and young people's counsellor who is a trained play therapist. Together we form the psychosocial provision of a larger multi-professional team of medical staff, physiotherapists, occupational therapists, complementary therapists and volunteers. The hospice has two in-patient wards and a day therapy unit that offers a unique model of rehabilitative care (Tookman *et al.* 2004). Although I work part-time, my remit extends across the entire unit. I provide an art therapy service to an ever-changing population of patients. This is due to brief admissions (on average two or three weeks), fluctuations in health and patients being discharged when they are so well they no longer need our support or, sadly but inevitably, when they die. The ebb and flow at the shoreline is to be recognized here. In the face of the continual change and loss that characterizes the day-to-day reality of hospice work I have found it essential to create a framework within which I can articulate to others (my colleagues and patients) and to myself exactly what I do (especially at times when I feel beached on the sharp cold stones of scientific and medical jargon or when I feel the undertow of waters that demand pictures for decoration and distraction). This framework is set out in Table 5.2.

What is notable about our day therapy unit is the individualized programme of care it offers patients. Patients come in specifically for their appointments (with the nurse, doctor, counsellor or therapist), and although relationships do develop with other patients there is no official expectation or encouragement for social groups. This means that I have not been able to develop the sort of groupwork described by other art therapists working in cancer care (Connell 1998).

Table 5.2   Different levels of art therapy intervention at MC Hospice Hampstead

Intervention	Access	Location	Aims	Outcome
Loan of materials for individual art activity	All patients and relatives	Off-site, own room or bay	Self-reflection Recreation	An end in itself or as an initial link with art therapist
Mobile graffiti board	All patients and relatives in attendance on the day	In-patient areas, room and bay	Integration of patient and relatives into community life of hospice Increase communication with team and within families Introduction to art therapy	Identify concerns/ issues for patients and relatives and take appropriate action Referral on as appropriate Contribution to hospice in-house publication
Open art therapy studio	All ambulant or wheelchair patients from Day Therapy Unit (DTU) and wards May be accompanied by volunteers or relatives	Art therapy room every Thursday 11.30a.m.–12.30p.m.	Introduction to AT Time away from medical or ward areas Creative activity Opportunity to socialize	Artwork is stored and not used for display Referral on to AT or team as appropriate
Individual art therapy sessions by appointment	Non-ambulant in-patients Ambulant in-patients DTU patients	Own room or bay In art therapy room In art therapy room	Exploration of personal and emotional issues concerning changes in health Psychological support for process of readjustment following changes in health	Contributes to patient's care plan Contract of sessions is agreed Artwork made is confidential and stored

Intervention	Access	Location	Aims	Outcome
Evaluation and research	Information and consent form Participation in hospice documentation	Hospice	Educational use of patients' artwork Closing summaries	Consent discussed fully before being obtained Audit of practice Opportunities to develop collaborative research projects

Consequently I have adapted two art therapy interventions in order to create a notional group space where some of the benefits found in groups (promoting connections and support between people who might otherwise feel rather isolated) can be realized, albeit on a very limited scale. These are the mobile graffiti board and the open art therapy studio.

Mobile graffiti board

This idea is a version of Connell's group notebook (Connell 1998) and the group images made by patients at New York's Sloan Kettering Memorial Hospital (Luzzatto and Gabriel 2000). The mobile graffiti board provides an invitation to patients or their visitors to record a thought, comment, doodle or picture on a shared sheet of paper. All in-patients are given the opportunity to make a contribution to this joint piece of work that reflects any aspect of their experiences or that relates to their stay in the hospice. Contributions can be in the form of written comments or images, drawings or simply smudges of colour. Most people are curious to see what others have written or drawn and are pleased to be invited to make their own marks. I carry a small toolbox containing a range of art materials and a large pad of paper and my interactions with patients can be brief (five minutes) or much longer. It is made clear to all who add something that the final piece has a communal endpoint – it will be seen by patients and staff – and it may be incorporated into the hospice newsletter as and when appropriate. This has proved to be an excellent way of introducing myself and the art therapy service, and also introduces me to the full range of people admitted each week.

The development of this intervention comes out of the implementation of clinical governance within my hospice. Clinical governance is another manifestation of the modernization process of the NHS in which increasing emphasis is being placed on patients as partners in the process of improving services (Scally and Donaldson 1998). In addition to the formal committees and working parties at the hospice we have set up graffiti boards to encourage more informal feedback as part of this clinical governance process. These boards are in the dining room and day therapy corridor. They are digitally photographed at periodic intervals and their contents are noted and discussed by the user perspective and senior management groups. Where appropriate, action is taken in response to comments arising from the boards. The mobile graffiti board was conceived as an extension of these boards for in-patients, especially those who were bed-bound. The mobile graffiti board aims to provide a relatively straightforward and comfortable way for patients to connect with the community of other patients and staff of which they are a part. However, it is more than another form of patient survey for it invites participants to reflect on their own experiences in a playful and creative way. The boards provide a snapshot of some people's experiences of the hospice and both patients and their visitors are invited to contribute. Staff views are not included in the boards for obvious reasons. I have found that even the most frail patients have been keen to make a mark and that sometimes visitors will either make a contribution with the patient or will write a message to the hospice or the person they have come to see. On one occasion the mobile graffiti board provided the focus for a terminally ill patient's six adult children to share their differing responses to their grief. Each made their own marks and as the eldest daughter's image was altered by her younger sibling they joked about how they had unwittingly reproduced their family dynamics on paper. It is clear to see how participating in the mobile graffiti board project can be an introduction to art therapy.

Open art therapy studio

The open studio is a well-established approach in art therapy and one that has been used in medical settings as well as psychiatric ones for some time now (Adamson 1984; McGraw 1999).

In my own context I have found it helpful to have a weekly drop-in open studio for one hour where patients can come to use the art therapy room. This hour provides regularity for the staff team to direct anyone who may not as yet warrant a 'proper' referral but who is interested to find out more about art therapy. There is the potential for a one-off group to occur or for individuals to work in parallel. It is also open to carers and the drop-in nature means that patients can determine how much time they want or are able to stay. On one occasion two rather sceptical elderly in-patients decided to venture in. After a brief welcome chat with me the older woman decided to use chalks to make a sphere of gold that opened into a distant path. She talked of these as symbols representing her deeply spiritual approach to life.

The other woman listened, a softening expression appearing on her face, and she viewed the range of materials on offer. Eventually she too joined in the making and long after her fellow patient had returned to the ward she was still working in clay, laughing with surprise at her own playfulness. Paradoxically the sculpture that emerged was full of her pain and her representations of the roots of all suffering. As we talked, her daughter – in search of her mother – joined us and was amazed at her mother's abilities and her work. In subsequent studio sessions this patient's entire family were invited by their mother to view her work and to make their own. This introduction led on to several individual art therapy sessions with me on each of her subsequent admissions. Our final session was held in her room on the ward and included her adult son three days before she died. This illustrates the way in which attendance at the open studio can lead into the next type of intervention: individual art therapy sessions.

Individual work

My individual work with patients is where art therapy takes on its depth. It is at this level that the more usual formal systems of referrals and contracts are established with patients and other members of the multi-professional team. For in-patients the contract will usually be brief with an average of only two or three sessions in the course of the patient's admission. For those attending our day therapy unit the length of contract will be determined according to the patient's need, although there will always be an end point of review and termination. This fits into the goal-setting aspect of the rehabilitation model and is appropriate for this population where ongoing contact with the unit indicates fluctuations in health.

Individual work with patients can take place at the bedside, in a shared bay or single side room or in the art therapy room. Location depends of course on the health of the patient and once again requires flexibility from the therapist to ensure the conditions are adequate for optimal therapeutic engagement. This may involve consulting the physiotherapy, occupational therapy and nursing staff to ensure a suitable working environment.

Art therapy opens up people's emotions and reveals their psychological realities through physical symbolic expression. The very act of physically making a mark or squeezing and smoothing clay engages affective and cognitive processes and links these together through behaviour within the interpersonal context of a therapeutic relationship. Through this active engagement with the art materials patients are made aware of their own vitality, accentuating an awareness of their embodied selves. This is art therapy's unique contribution to the psychological care of people with physical and chronic illness for it places the complexity of personal biography and selfhood literally within the person's hands. In my experience there are two recurrent themes found in-patients' explorations in art therapy. The first is existential in nature and is characterized by a search for meaning; the second has to do with making adjustments to one's self-image in order to survive the threat posed by illness. The artwork that emerges can often apprehend experiences that are out of view and beyond the reaches of language. The importance of the connectedness of mind and body that is intrinsic to art therapy is also being explored by other disciplines, for example psychoneuroimmunology, medical sociology and recent psychoanalytical literature, and I find it helpful to consider my practice from these viewpoints.

Evaluation and research

Evaluation should be a routine part of the art therapist's reflections on her work. Being able to identify whether one has enabled patients sufficiently to address their reasons for embarking on art therapy is a critical skill for safe and effective practice. There are several means by which this should take place, for example documentation, discussion with colleagues and clinical supervision. These also allow other members of the multi-professional team to learn about the art therapist's contribution to patients' care. I have found the writing of closing summaries for the patients' files a valuable discipline for clarifying the focus of my work with patients and for bringing it to closure, even if I anticipate working again with a patient some time in the future. The significance of documentation of one's practice in an area characterized by transience was brought home to me when I conducted a small-scale qualitative research project on art therapy with people who had AIDS-related brain impairment (Wood 2002). One outcome of the study was the way in which my case notes were very much part of my own emotional engagement and disengagement with patients.

The personal motivation for writing as a way of processing what can be intense and powerful encounters with patients has been noted by other arts therapists such as Schaverien (2002) and Lee (1996), who have turned their clinical experiences into books. Similarly many sufferers of cancer have used writing to examine, explore and explain their own stories (Picardie 1998; Diamond 1999). One author, Stacey (1997), reflects on her motives for writing a cultural study of cancer that is both academic and personal. She suggests that writing may be a symptom of returning to health and of recovery, rather than an indication of disease and dying, and she wonders at her inner desire to complete the manuscript, suggesting 'I must still be alive, I am producing – "I write therefore I am"?' (Stacey 1997: 242). This is an interesting thought, especially on a professional/institutional level where I would suggest that documentation may be one way in which the art therapist's contribution cannot get 'lost' as patients move on and take their experiences with them.

Returning to the notion of clinical governance and the increasing value being placed on incorporating patients' views into service development, the practice of some art therapists of formally including patients in the evaluation process is an interesting one (Caryl Sibbett, personal communication).

I have included research within my framework for it fits with the culture of my hospice setting and also with my own curiosities. It is universally agreed that art therapists in all areas of health and social care need to participate in the research agenda (Reynolds *et al.* 2000). This does not necessarily mean conducting research projects (for which a whole other set of skills is required), but it does mean being cognizant of the rationale for any interventions undertaken with patients and whether, why, or how these improve patients' lives, in order to gauge one's own practices and to participate in critical debates with colleagues.

The importance of ending

One of my first patients in my present post was a young woman with metastatic cancer. She came to see me weekly and used our sessions to express both an increasing physical exhaustion and her frustration with her partner who, although caring, was unable to recognize or accept her increasing deterioration. Her images were gently executed and conveyed her desire for rest. She attended the agreed contract of six sessions and when our review session came I went into it confident that, since she had engaged so well, and given the struggles with her health, it would be appropriate to offer her a further contract. As part of the review we looked through her artwork and discussed and reflected on our time together. I asked whether she wished to continue and was surprised when she said no. She spoke of finding the art therapy valuable but of wanting a break. It seemed important to understand what she meant by 'break', and as we talked it was clear that she wanted an ending, though found it hard to say so. When I said that while I would be more than happy to work with her again it seemed more fitting to identify our ending as such, she looked relieved. This young woman was quietly letting go of life – something that had been evident in her pictures but of which I had not been fully aware. There was a part of me that, like her partner, found it unbearable to think of an end and the sadness of her imminent untimely death. By acknowledging her desire for an end, and in naming it, we were able to render the process of ending tolerable.

This patient taught me an important lesson that day. For although our building and shaping of services and procedures are valuable and our empathy, attentiveness and support are crucial, in the end they are only temporary. Paradoxically this is their essential benefit – that they can hold something precious ... for a time. The process of building up and letting go of relationships is intrinsic to working in cancer care, and in the end we must be satisfied with this, creating sandcastles on the beach.

References

Adamson, E. (1984) *Art as Healing*. London: Coventure.

Anand, S.A. and Anand, V.K. (1997) Art therapy with laryngectomy patients, *Art Therapy*, 14(2): 109–17.

Bach, S. (1968) *Life Paints its Own Span: On the Significance of Spontaneous Pictures by Severely Ill Children*. Einsiedeln, Switzerland: Daimon Verlag.

Bartholomew, A. (1998) A narrow ledge: art therapy at London Lighthouse, in M. Pratt and M.J.M. Wood (eds) *Art Therapy in Palliative Care: The Creative Response*. London and New York: Routledge.

Beaver, V. (1998) The butterfly garden: art therapy with HIV/AIDS, in M. Pratt and M.J.M. Wood (eds) *Art Therapy in Palliative Care: The Creative Response*. London and New York: Routledge.

Bell, S. (1998) Will the kitchen table do? Art therapy in the community, in M. Pratt and M.J.M. Wood (eds) *Art Therapy in Palliative Care: The Creative Response*. London and New York: Routledge.

Bertoia, J. (1993) *Drawings from a Dying Child*. London and New York: Routledge.

Bolton, G. (2004) The healer's art, *Progress in Palliative Care*.

Borgmann, E. (2002) Art therapy with three women diagnosed with cancer, *The Arts in Psychotherapy*, 29(5): 245–51.

Bromberg, E.L. (2003) The demographics and practices of art therapists working with cancer patients in the New York Metropolitan area, *Art Therapy*, 20(4): 219–25.

Burroughs, A.G., Tyler, J., Moat, I.B. and Pye, S. (1992) Griefwork with children – workshop days at Pilgrims Hospice Canterbury, *Palliative Medicine*, 6: 26–33.

Centre for Arts and Humanities in Health and Medicine (CAHHM) website: www.dur.ac.uk/cahhm/

Centre for Medical Humanities website: www.pcps.ucl.ac.uk/cmh

Connell, C. (1992) Art therapy as part of a palliative care programme, *Palliative Medicine*, 6: 18–25.

Connell, C. (1998) *Something Understood. Art Therapy in Cancer Care*. London: Wrexham.

Coote, J. (1998) Getting started: introducing the art therapy service, in M. Pratt and M.J.M. Wood (eds) *Art Therapy in Palliative Care: The Creative Response*. London and New York: Routledge.

Dannecker, K. (1991) Body and expression: art therapy with rheumatoid patients, *American Journal of Art Therapy*, 29 May: 110–17.

Diamond, J. (1999) *C: Because Cowards Get Cancer Too . . .* London: Vermillion.

DoH (Department of Health) (2001) *The NHS Cancer Plan: A Plan for Investment, A Plan for Reform*. DoH and www.doh.gov.uk/cancer/cancerplan.htm

Farrell Fenton, J. (2000) Cystic fibrosis and art therapy, *The Arts in Psychotherapy*, 27(1): 15–25.

Favara-Scacco, C., Smirne, G., Schiliro, G. and Di Cataldo, A. (2001) Art therapy as support for children with leukaemia during painful procedures, *Medical and Pediatric Oncology*, 36(4): 474–80.

Gabriel, B., Bromberg, E., Vandenbovenkamp, J., Walka, P., Kornblith, A.B. and Luzzatto, P. (2001) Art therapy with adult bone marrow transplant patients in isolation: a pilot study, *Psycho-oncology*, 10(2): 114–23.

Greece, M. (2003) Art therapy on a bone marrow transplant unit: the case study of a Vietnam veteran fighting myelofibrosis, *The Arts in Psychotherapy*, 30: 229–38.

Heywood, K. (2003) Introducing art therapy into the Christie Hospital, Manchester, UK, 2001–2002, *Complementary Therapies in Nursing and Midwifery*, 9: 125–32.

Hogan, S. (2001) *Healing Arts: The History of Art Therapy*. London: Jessica Kingsley.

Jackson, C. and DeJong, I. (2000) *Achieving Effective Health Care Integration: The Essential Guide*. Brisbane: Mater University of Queensland Centre for General Practice.

Jones, G. (2000) An art therapy group in palliative cancer care, *Nursing Times*, 96(10): 42–3.

Kaplan, F. (2000) *Art, Science and Art Therapy: Repainting the Picture*. London: Jessica Kingsley.

Kaye, C. and Blee, T. (1997) *The Arts in Health Care*. London: Jessica Kingsley.

Kennett, C. (2000) Participation in a creative arts project can foster hope in a hospice day centre, *Palliative Medicine*, 14: 419–25.

Learmonth, M. (2002) Painting ourselves out of a corner, *Newsbriefing, Newsletter of British Association of Art Therapists*, June: 2–5.

Lee, C. (1996) *Music at the Edge: The Music Therapy Experiences of a Musician with AIDS*. London: Routledge.

Luzzatto, P. and Gabriel, B. (2000) The creative journey: a model for short term group art therapy with post-treatment cancer patients, *Art Therapy: Journal of the American Art Therapy Association*, 17: 265–9.

McGraw, M.K. (1999) Studio-based art therapy for medically ill and physically disabled persons, in C. Malchiodi (ed.) *Medical Art Therapy with Adults*. London and New York: Jessica Kingsley.

Mayo, S. (1996) Symbol, metaphor and story: the function of group art therapy in palliative care, *Palliative Medicine*, 10: 209–16.

Mayo, S. (1998) The story board: reflections on group art therapy, in M. Pratt and M.J.M. Wood (eds) *Art Therapy in Palliative Care: The Creative Response*. London and New York: Routledge.

Morley, B. (1998) Sunbeams and icebergs, meteorites and daisies: a cancer patient's experience of art therapy, in M. Pratt and M.J.M. Wood (eds) *Art Therapy in Palliative Care: The Creative Response*. London and New York: Routledge.

National Network for Arts in Health website: www.nnah.org.uk/

NICE (2004) *Improving Supportive and Palliative Care for Adults with Cancer*, www.nice.org.uk

Olofsson, A. (1995) The value of integrating music therapy and expressive arts therapy in working with cancer patients, in C. Lee (ed.) *Lonely Waters: Proceedings of the International Conference, Music Therapy in Palliative Care UK 1994*. Oxford: Sobell Publications.

Picardie, R. with Seaton, M. and Picardie, J. (1998) *Before I Say Goodbye*. London: Penguin.

Pratt, M. (1998) The invisible injury: adolescent griefwork group, in M. Pratt and M.J.M. Wood (eds) *Art Therapy in Palliative Care: Creative Response*. London and New York: Routledge.

Pratt, M. (2004) *Guidelines for the Arts Therapies and the Arts in Palliative Care Settings*. London: Hospice Information.

Reynolds, M.W., Nabors, L. and Quinlan, A. (2000) The effectiveness of art therapy: does it work?, *Art Therapy: Journal of the American Art Therapy Association*, 17(3): 207–13. Rosetta Life website: rosettalife.org

Scally, G. and Donaldson, L.J. (1998) Clinical governance and the drive for quality improvement in the new NHS in England, *British Medical Journal*, 4 July: 61–5.

Schaverien, J. (2002) *The Dying Patient in Psychotherapy: Desire, Dreams and Individuation*. Basingstoke: Palgrave Macmillan.

Sheppard, L., MacInally, F., Rusted, J., Waller, D. and Shamash, K. (1998) *Evaluating the Use of Art Therapy for People with Dementia: A Control Group Study*. A report commissioned by the Brighton Branch of the Alzheimer's Disease Society.

Stacey, J. (1997) *Teratologies: A Cultural Study of Cancer*. London and New York: Routledge.

Stevens, G. and Lomas, H. (1995) Working with the unknown: music and art therapy with a young man with Niemann Picks Disease, in C. Lee (ed.) *Lonely Waters: Proceedings of the International Conference, Music Therapy in Palliative Care UK 1994*. Oxford: Sobell Publications.

Sutherland, J.I. (1999) Art therapy with a woman who has multiple medical conditions, *American Journal of Art Therapy*, 37: 84–98.

Teufel, E.S. (1995) Terminal stage leukaemia: integrating art therapy and family process, *Art Therapy: Journal of the American Art Therapy Association*, 12(1): 51–5.

Thomas, G. and Kennedy, J. (1995) Art therapy and practice in palliative care, *European Journal of Palliative Care*, 2(3): 120–3.

Tookman, A.J., Hopkins, K. and Scharpen-von-Heussen, K. (2004) Rehabilitation in palliative medicine, in D. Doyle, G. Hanks, N. Cherny and K. Calman (eds) *Oxford Textbook of Palliative Medicine*, 3rd edition. Oxford: Oxford University Press.

Trauger-Querry, B. and Haghighi, K.R. (1999) Balancing the focus: art and music therapy for pain control and symptom management in hospice care, *The Hospice Journal*, 14(1): 25–37.

Waller, D. (1991) *Becoming a Profession: A History of Art Therapists 1940–82*. London: Routledge.

Weldt, C. (2003) Patients'responses to a drawing experience in a hemodialysis unit: a step towards healing, *Art Therapy: Journal of the American Art Therapy Association*, 20(2): 92–9.

Wilson, A. and Morris, F. (2003) Evaluation of art therapy intervention as an aid in the elevation of patients' psychological and emotional distress following a diagnosis of advanced cancer, *Lung Cancer ISLAC*, 41, supplement 2: 48–9.

Wood, M.J.M. (1998) The body as art: individual session with a man with AIDS, in M. Pratt and M.J.M. Wood (eds) *Art Therapy in Palliative Care: The Creative Response*. London and New York: Routledge.

Wood, M.J.M. (2002) Researching art therapy practice with people suffering from AIDS-related dementia, *The Arts in Psychotherapy*, 29: 207–19.

Wood, M.J.M. (2004) The contribution of art therapy to palliative medicine, in D. Doyle, G. Hanks, N. Cherny and K. Calman (eds) *Oxford Textbook of Palliative Medicine*, 3rd edition. Oxford: Oxford University Press.

Wood, M.J.M. and Low, J. (in preparation) Survey of art therapists working in supportive and palliative care.

Zammit, C. (2001) The art of healing: a journey through cancer. Implications for art therapy, *Art Therapy: Journal of the American Art Therapy Association*, 18(1): 27–36.

Further reading

Bint, J. (2000) A report on the exploration of arts therapies in palliative care, cancer, AIDS and bereavement. Unpublished report, The Omega Foundation.

Haldane, D. and Loppert, S. (eds) (1999) *The Arts in Health Care: Learning From Experience*. London: King's Fund.

Malchiodi, C. (1999) *Medical Art Therapy with Adults*. London and New York: Jessica Kingsley.

Pratt, M. and Wood, M.J.M. (1998) *Art Therapy in Palliative Care: The Creative Response*. London and New York: Routledge.

6 A woman with breast cancer in art therapy

Elizabeth Stone Matho

> As long as my unconscious continues to produce images, I know that I am alive.
>
> Mrs Verdier (a pseudonym), a woman with breast cancer.

In this chapter I shall discuss how art therapy helped one woman through the final stages of her illness as she sought to understand herself, fortify her identity, come to terms with family relationships and prepare for death. Her deep pleasure in tasting life enabled her to confront the conflict of her inner world so that she could live the last months of her life more freely. The experience of working with her has touched me at least as profoundly as she was touched by art therapy.

In spite of increasing fatigue, Mrs Verdier continued using creative expression to soothe herself, to resolve more of her past, to engage the resources of her body that could still function and, importantly, experience the pleasure of the art materials which were of great comfort to her, particularly the gouache and the pastels. A woman courageously determined to come to terms with her femininity, carve out her identity after having been devastated by illness and loss, she also worked to claim what was for her a lost voice. Lost along the way to becoming a woman, much of her work was also about the evolution of her femininity. Mrs Verdier's way of engaging in art therapy clearly demonstrates M.J.M. Wood's description of Erskine and Judd's notion of 'the interdependence of mind and body working together as a dynamic unity rather a duality (mind versus body) . . .'. Wood rightly points out that such a melding of mind and body tends to be the unusual occurrence in our work (Wood 1998).

I shall offer some session extracts of the eight months of our work together in the Centre Hospitalier Universitaire de Grenoble and then the

Centre Medical de Pneumonologie Henri Bazire, St Julier de Ratz, France. Due to space limitations and confidentiality requirements, certain aspects of this case were condensed or disguised. I have sought to keep the content linking one session to another as intact as possible, so as to convey how the therapeutic development of central themes evolved.

Mrs Verdier was pleased to offer her personal experience in art therapy as a way to benefit professionals and other patients.

Session 1: Beginning art therapy

Mrs Verdier, age 50, petite and attractive, recovered from ovarian cancer twenty years ago, but has battled breast cancer for the past five years. A large tumour on her right breast, visible wearing normal clothing, has rapidly metastasized. Separated from her second husband, she has adult children from her first marriage. Before becoming ill, she had been a mental health professional and had been in previous psychoanalysis.

In our first session, she described feeling as if her breast were on fire and thought she might want to represent fire. Coughing often, she said she used words too much. Almost dazzled by the colourful art materials, she finally chose clay. By squeezing and massaging the clay, she pushed so hard that pushing hurt her. She felt the pain in her breast. Since she wanted to continue, I suggested that she take a smaller piece of clay. She still felt the sore spot, but insisted it was no longer painful. She enjoyed the sensation of working the clay and found herself able to relax. By adding water as the clay became drier, she discovered she could touch and caress the clay with softer movements. Finally, she became tearful and didn't know if she wanted to make anything at all or just play with the clay in the same pleasurable way she had started to do. Then, almost immediately, she made a breast (Figure 6.1, on website). She commented that she felt secretly pleased to have a larger breast, even knowing that it was due to a tumour. Her comment reflected the traumatic assault she experienced on her femininity as reaction formation helped her to negotiate a way to make it bearable.

Working with the clay evoked visits to her grandmother at 12 years of age, when she dug clay from a stream and sculpted when there was nothing else to do. Her pleasure in handling the clay in our session recalled that carefree moment. In retrospect, I believe that this pleasant memory indicated that, for her, creativity exists within that part of the psyche Hartmann described as the conflict-free ego sphere, which resides outside intrapsychic conflict (Hartmann 1958).

Now menopausal for twenty years since her surgery, the cusp of her pubescence was brought to mind by using clay, along with a lifelong dissatisfaction with her small breasts that she considered pre-adolescent. She fondly recalled pregnancy, which had made her feel very round, very pleased with her form, she had maintained a few extra pounds for several years until her first cancer. At the end of the session she decided that next time she would make the other breast. She felt that working with the clay relieved the pains in her stomach that she had when she came to the session. As Luzzatto commented regarding work with cancer patients, 'The body suddenly becomes very important in the therapeutic relationship' (Luzzatto 1998: 170).

Session 2: Clay figure of a woman

Mrs Verdier remembered having created the left breast in clay during the previous session rather than the inflamed right one. Ego defence in the service of adaptation to the exigencies of illness protected her fragility (Blanck and Blanck 1975). The use of defence was in the service of restoring lost narcissistic supplies and bolstering body image (Stone 2003). That her creativity resided outside conflict did not prevent the unconscious *content* of her imagery from embodying considerable conflict. Nevertheless, she told me that after our session she felt physically much better and she could 'let go'.

She wanted to make a woman nude to the waist opening her arms and allowing her two normal breasts to be seen. She worked on this figure in almost complete silence throughout the session. She found the clay difficult to manipulate and expressed confusion about how to proceed. I suggested making the parts and assembling them afterwards. Imperatively, she needed to pull the entire figure out of one piece of clay. Foremost was her need for a sense of inner cohesiveness, a unity of her body image to offset her anxiety of fragmentation (Kohut 1971). Making a figure out of one piece of clay would help her feel more whole. At first she was displeased that her figure looked masculine, but as she kept working on it, smoothing it, it became more feminine. She called it her little woman (Figure 6.2, on website). Using a gesture to smooth the clay upwards, she got a better feeling, a sense of more movement. Afterwards, she claimed that her own head and neck felt better, that again she had let go of something that was holding her back.

In this session the seeds that would become the major themes of our work together became apparent: body image, femininity/masculinity and identity. We have also seen how remarkably her ego defences revised a memory about the previous session, similar to the secondary revision in dream work (Freud 1900). She remembered sculpting a left instead of a right breast, when it was, indeed, the other way around.

Therefore, in spite of her conscious willingness to delve into feelings about her illness, unconscious revision, in the form of defence, altered her story, as it does with almost everyone. The need for protection in the form of ego defences is always operative and must be respected, often fostered, even when a patient insists on working directly on the deepest issues. Awareness of defences was always present in my mind and probably played an important role in helping Mrs Verdier therapeutically.

Session 3: Expressing grief

She came in with oxygen to help her breathe as her lungs were involved in the cancer. Feeling depressed, she sat down and began to cry – then wanted to use the clay to calm down. She didn't want to return to her figure from last time, but only wanted to feel the clay and not make anything special with it. At first the clay became a breast, as in the first session, though this one was hollow, a bit lumpy and hard to make solid. She crushed it and began to make a ball that gave her pleasure. She enjoyed rolling the ball and making it perfectly round. She told me that she wanted to have two equally sized breasts but didn't know how. She had a lot of pain under her right arm, which was partly what made her cry, and couldn't wear a bra. Her left breast was smaller and she wanted to do something about it, but didn't know what – no implants or anything like that. When her prognosis worsened three years ago her second husband quickly found a girlfriend and asked for a separation. He continued to be dutiful, but would not give of himself in a sharing way. He promised to assist Mrs Verdier to the 'end', which hurt her even more as she wanted to be valued in life. She felt her husband could no longer value her femininity; he could only see her in terms of death. Although their sexual relationship continued, it was not the same as before due to her lack of trust.

Session 4: A few drops of blood

Now she experienced the clay as too heavy, but was extremely pleased to see that her unfinished sculpture of a woman was still intact and had retained its moisture over the week. She was in a crisis and told me that the mass had pressed so heavily upon her breast that a few drops of blood came through her skin. She cried as she said it revived puberty and the onset of her menses. She remembered her mother telling her very matter-of-factly about how her body would change, but recalled no gentleness. She wasn't told why she would bleed, nor what reproduction was all about, only the mechanics of bleeding and to be careful of boys. She described her mother as a hard worker who didn't know how to offer tenderness; she was too busy eking out a living. Mrs Verdier felt like going into a cocoon, where she could feel surrounded and protected. Thinking about everything she had to do on her own, she felt sad. She felt she managed in much the way her mother did by putting up a good front about being independent, but missed her husband who was away on vacation. He had offered her his house in the mountains (her former house), which she gladly took.

Seeing the blood made her realize her vulnerability as a woman and she felt that her entrance into puberty had been brutal. Becoming a woman was experienced as dangerous and linked somehow to her father. When asked how he had greeted her entrance into womanhood, she said that there was something repudiating in his reaction. And now her femininity was linked with disease. Complicating everything was the rejection of her femininity by her husband that echoed what she experienced earlier from her father. As a woman, she could not be good enough.

Seeking soothing through the art materials, she made light gestures on paper with lots of water and pastel-coloured paint. Dipping her brush into blue paint, she enjoyed the back and forth rhythmic motion while tracing a few horizontal lines. Curves began to appear, though the circles remained open. We recalled her need to be contained and encircled, perhaps symbolized in these concentric curves. Urgently she added a purple curve that she thought resembled a uterus and which pleased her. She wanted to find a way to represent her father too and expressed relief in the loosening of tension between her shoulder blades.

Session 5: Feelings concerning her father

More tired than before, she told me that the long parabolic curve of her painting from last time reminded her of her father's money pouch. Though not rich, her father was described as counting every penny. Last week, this image had reminded her of a uterus. Concentrating hard, she wanted to bring out the feeling of the pouch being tied. She dipped her brush into dark greenish paint and closed the neck with a string-like shape. I reminded her about the cocoon-like, protective shape from the last session. She agreed that this must be part of her image, but her anger with her father took precedence. She rebuked him for always grilling each family member, her mother especially, on how each penny should be spent. Then she added little round floating money-like shapes. An ambiguous image, a breast with a series of tumours is also suggested (Figure 6.3, on website).

Taking another paper, in one grand swoop, she sketched an upside-down parabola in pale red paint (Figure 6.4, on website). Afterwards, she released a long outpouring of breath and said she had the desire to expel the 'bad' from within her by breathing it out. She felt tired afterwards but much better. By enlisting the action of her body in creating the image, she was trying to achieve an internal transformation. At the end, she did look much brighter and at peace with herself. I commented that her inner world appeared so active and alive. She said that if she didn't have her inner life she couldn't see how she could stay alive, after all she had gone through.

In attempting to come to terms with her anger at her father, she could not see how angry she felt toward her husband. In the eight months we worked together, she never touched her relationship with her husband in her artwork, while she worked assiduously on many other aspects of her suffering. In spite of her conscious awareness, sadness and occasional anger at the loss of her marriage, she somehow needed to deny its impact unconsciously. Because her body image and bodily integrity were compromised, because her sense of femininity was betrayed, because she was deserted emotionally by her husband, all this was experienced as a deep traumatic narcissistic blow to her sense of self-esteem and to the intactness of her sense of self. I suspected that it was less dangerous to confront deep feelings toward her father than those toward her husband. As her work in art therapy developed, more unforgiving feelings toward her father were expressed. Ambivalent conflicted feelings toward him had early roots and she looked for ways to keep him at a distance, which may have also shielded other complicated feelings about closeness.

Session 7: Feelings concerning her mother

She came to the session telling me that she wanted to confront her feelings about death and felt sad that people 'wrote her off' because of her illness. She reported that friends rallied when she was in the hospital, but distanced themselves once she was back on her own, treating her as if she were already gone. This reminded her of feelings that neither parent was sufficiently nurturing emotionally throughout her life. She gave the following example, an incident that occurred a few days before. Mrs Verdier had invited her mother and brother for dinner and felt hurt when her mother brought her own food, explaining that her brother only liked *her* food. Certainly this devaluation of Mrs Verdier's cooking capabilities resonated symbolically with other profound denigrations of her femininity.

She began by 'painting' with only water, using her hands. The motion of touching the paper with her fingers on the downswing felt good, but on the upswing, she could feel the grain of the paper and it wasn't pleasant. The grain of the paper was, in reality, of minimal tooth, but for this woman of extraordinary suffering, discomfort was easily imparted in a touch – her sensitivity was that sharp. As we talked about touching the wet paper, she told me that she felt I was attuned to her in a way she hadn't experienced before – that I was attentive to her brush strokes and ways of using the paint, which helped her feel contained and safe (Figure 6.5, on website). In subsequent sessions, she referred to this session as being about her mother, about tenderness and the exploration of maternal feelings. The session ended on a very different note from the way it began.

Session 8: Learning that her cancer was inoperable

She felt she had lost her taste for life in the past few weeks or months. She had little energy, which distressed her, and she wanted to get back her zest for life. She had always been a very active person, though also thought of herself as someone who holds things inside. Now she wanted to expel whatever was blocking her. This week she learned that her cancer was inoperable. She said that when she originally had ovarian cancer, twenty years before, it was deep inside. Her current cancer was on the exterior of her body, on her breast, which she thought would be better, closer to being out and away. She expelled breath to show me what she meant, as if by breathing out she could get rid of it. Somehow this brought to mind the sac-like shape she drew a few sessions ago that could contain something, even air. Then she began talking about aggressively getting rid of the negative and her anger at not being able to do it.

She thought of the aggression of men who slaughter animals so easily and described a vivid memory of her uncle who slaughtered a pig on a special holiday once a year. She always remembered the cry of the pig being slaughtered and the sight of blood all around. She was about eight at the time and felt that what was so hard to reconcile was that she loved her uncle. Her father also participated, but it was the memory of her uncle that stood out most in her mind, surely a cover memory concealing the aggression that she could not bear to be aware of in her father. I suggested that what was hard to accept was, perhaps, that he was the same beloved uncle (analogously, father) as he who could kill. Now more than ever she identified with the pig, with its vulnerability, its innocence and the fact that no matter how much it protested, it would lose its life.

She wanted to use paint to express the 'getting rid of' feeling and started with red gouache, placing a dot rather aggressively on the paper. She used black too and hit the paper with the paintbrush. She began using her whole body to strike the paper (Figure 6.6, on website). Her body was energized by this rhythmic activity which was almost frightening to watch in its urgency. I worried about her getting overwhelmed with emotion and using too much of her energy. I considered slowing her down but realized as I watched her that she was in complete control, that the rhythmic bending and striking, even if it looked as if she was chopping the paper with an axe, was in the service of gaining control of unspeakable dread. Here she identified with all the men who had power – her husband who had left her and now her surgeon who had just told her that her cancer was inoperable. And at the same time she was enraged with them. Afterwards she told me how well she felt, and asked me whether I noticed that she was now able to breathe freely on her own, inhale deeply. Normally she had a lot of difficulty breathing, due to the fact that the cancer had metastasized to her lungs, and had to use an oxygen tank. What she created was splotches, lots of thrown random paint. She said that this was so different from what she usually did, which pleased her. She sat looking at it for a while, smiling.

Finally she did a second painting (Figure 6.7, on website) using similar colours but with more modulated movement, still with a lot of aggressive energy but less direct anger. The painting was more structured and she felt better afterwards, saying it was a good way to end the session.

Session 10: Enactment

Hardly able to breathe, she needed a minute to catch her breath after over-exerting herself climbing a flight of stairs instead of using the elevator. She had awakened in the night with an idea of what she wanted to do in our session. Her idea, again, was to chop. She took her hand and sliced through the air. She said she didn't know what material she wanted to use but she knew she needed to do that. She said she was glad to have had this thought since it came from her unconscious. She imagined a yellow arrow darting through a ball – and thought about the ball of clay she had formed in an early session. She wanted to slice it symbolically and thought of it as a breast or tumour. She began to make the gesture of slicing, as though she was getting ready. I questioned whether using that kind of energy might tire her out too much and she said she'd be fine. I was uneasy anyway. She was then sure that she wanted to use paint, though couldn't decide between the gesture of slicing and the gesture of 'whooshing' upwards and out. She decided it was the whooshing that she preferred.

Mrs Verdier commented that the way she was working now was different from what she had done in psychoanalysis before and that she had changed since she'd been coming to art therapy. I asked her in what way she had changed and she said that she was raised to be good, to be small, never to be noticed, never to stand out. Now she felt that image didn't fit her anymore.

She wanted the paint to be thick so I added white glue, making an unctu-ous homemade acrylic. She dabbed green in the centre. Not sure how to make violet, she made a muddy violet, then a brighter one which outlined the green central area; then bright red became wavy lines. With the side of her hand, she sliced up from the centre in a whooshing vertical movement, smushing the colours into a thin line out of the circle area, as though released in a vertical spurt upwards (Figure 6.8, on website).

Afterwards she told me about how much better this painting made her feel, but it tired her out incredibly. She explained the sensation of feeling something alive, growing inside her breast, as the tumour had enlarged to an extraordinary size. She felt as though serpents were inside and she mimicked a groaning sound to convey her terrible awareness of their being there and growing. Afterwards, she wanted to bring some light to the paint-ing and surrounded the circle with yellow paint going outward. She said it looked like a sunflower and added some orange flame-like shapes to the yellow.

Session 11: 'Puissance' (Power)

Appearing more fragile and tired, she arrived with the oxygen tank. A new bandage on her breast prevented blood from leaking out of her very stretched skin. She wanted to create an image of flying, thinking of wings she had once drawn, but was concerned about not making a butterfly since she regarded it as a traditional symbol of impending death.

She said an image came to her this week from her unconscious that she wanted to work on, a horse and tightrope walker. She reminded me of feeling her right leg like the haunch of a horse when she was standing in an energized position over a recent painting, but didn't know how the idea of a tightrope walker occurred to her. She demonstrated, bending on her right leg as if to use it as a springboard for taking off, feeling her own sense of power in her muscles as though she could really enact the power of a horse. She wanted to draw the horse abstractly, to represent its energy more than visual verisimilitude. She returned to the whooshing movement, the upward and outward motion of getting rid of something, as last time, but now experienced it as a desire to feel power. From the bottom of the paper, she drew upward in brown crayon as if drawing a tree, then some lines expanded outward as though branches. Each line was drawn with meticulous concentration, as she attempted to get the feeling just right. She explained the brown at the bottom represented earth that grounded her image (Figure 6.9, on website).

Afterwards, she wrote 'Puissance' and told me it represented feelings about her father who was a very cautious driver. He followed all the rules exactly, held himself back. She added underneath: 'Stay within the white line', as though she were reminding or admonishing him. She thought of his feelings toward her as overly charged with sexuality, even if they were never acted upon nor even hinted at overtly by him. Her own feelings toward him continued to remain unrecognized, but this Oedipal territory had to be entered very slowly, given that the trauma of illness was still in the forefront of our work. I mentioned that she had often said that she felt herself to be someone who was restrained. She said: 'Yes, like my father and everyone I have ever known from the countryside, those who equate restraint with being "good" '. But now she would start to feel her own power. She had a good feeling at the end of this work and said that the words she wrote came to her out of nowhere; she had no predetermined intention of writing them.

We spoke about how important it was for her to please her father and be seen favourably in his eyes. As an adolescent, she was concerned that she might have been more valued as a boy than as a girl and felt the devaluation as a kind of castration. I suggested that perhaps in some ways it was safer to identify with a boy than a girl because as a girl one could be desirable, so there could be worry about being desired. She confirmed that this was so and said that even now she was uncomfortable that her father brought her flowers when she was sick, since he never brought flowers to her mother. She wished he hadn't brought them to her as, for her, this act confirmed his unconscious wishes toward her.

We talked about her own feelings of guilt and she said that she believed having had cancer was her way of dealing with issues of her femininity, almost as a punishment for finally becoming a woman, a woman who could be desirable and who could desire. She said she always believed her cancer was a psychosomatic response to these issues. Although with my knowledge of science I found the notion unacceptable that cancer could be fabricated as an unconscious way of dealing with conflict or guilt, I realized only after-wards that her cancer as a psychosomatic response was woven deeply into the fabric of her adult identity due to having been a cancer patient for the last twenty years.

Session 13: Goblet filled with pleasure

She came to this session more tired than ever with a more powerful oxygen tank. She was wearing glasses for the first time, was coughing a lot and barely able to speak. She had been in the hospital and was just being dis-charged. She wanted to do an image that would just bring her pleasure, nothing more. She began to outline a cup, a goblet, in yellow. Her idea was to fill it with differently coloured 'pebbles of life', an abstract symbol which was to represent all that had meaning for her. For most of the time, she worked in silence. She worried about returning to her apartment later in the day because she didn't know how capable she would be of caring for herself.

An upside-down heart was painted next to circular shapes and a string of pearls (without the string) was also formed. Next to the heart, she placed a tiny black pebble that she realized right away resembled a tumour. She hadn't wanted to place anything in her painting that was unpleasant, and yet she did. She quickly painted exploding lines saying that they, too, were part of the picture. They were painted next to the heart just as her own tumours had metastasized toward her own heart, making surgery impossible. She was upset at having placed them so close together (Figure 6.10, on website).

She began crying that her husband had told her that as long as she was alive, he couldn't live; he could not go on with his own life. She said that recently she had been unable to stand her father, unable to look at him, found him hostile and repugnant. Surely a splitting mechanism had to be operating. It must have been her husband's rejection of her in her illness that revived her pubescent rejection of her own body as a burgeoning woman, which she felt her father both rejected (because she wasn't a boy) and desired. Hating her father protected her from hating her husband too much.

She painted rain falling into the trophy, the cup. She said that she wanted to breathe freely and wrote 'whoosh' on both sides of it, as if to show that she wanted to expel the negative. We talked some more about where she got her energy to face all that she had to face.

Session 16: 'Papa, I see life in colours'

This time she came to our session by ambulance from the pulmonary rehabilitation centre where she was now residing. She could no longer care for herself independently and was feeling very fragile. Though our sessions tired her, she felt dealing with the material that was emerging was necessary.

This time she wanted to use paint and chose a large paper. She stood in front of her paper with her oxygen tubes, steadying her position, planting her feet carefully, feeling her balance, feeling the weight of both legs, feeling the energy of her body, which, by the way, appeared formidable, in spite of her tiny size. I experienced her as artist standing before me, as one in charge of her body, one who is poised to use her energy completely. And this was so. She began by feeling the sensation come to her fingers and used the paintbrush to express it. She wanted to make violet and asked how to do it. When she got the shade she sought, she dipped her brush into the paint and in a quick, almost calligraphic stroke, made the 'whooshing' of the kind of strokes she made before, but this time without the sound. It was an upward swirling motion, repeated several times. The paintbrush unfortunately didn't hold enough paint to get to the end of her stroke as the paint was thick. Unconcerned, she said that whatever traces she put down she would leave just that way. She would not redo that moment in time (Figure 6.11, on website). She continued to make a number of upward but wavy strokes and the effect was rather random because the paint did not fully follow her gestures. Toward the lower right corner, she placed a number of red lines near each other and later said that they looked like a hand. She was then reminded of the red nail polish she tried to paint her fingernails with as a teenager, that her father forbade her from wearing. She said that since then she had never really worn nail polish, except on her toes. She took the pointed end of the paintbrush and scratched fingernails into the red paint, clearly delineating a hand. She had the desire to write something on her painting but she didn't know what. Thinking for a moment, she took the brush and scratched in the word 'Papa'. Not sure why she wrote it, she was thinking about how her father was always afraid of everything, afraid to dare, always sticking to the rules. She thought of him as very 'grey', very colourless. She said he even smoked, maybe that was also why she associated him with the colour grey. Then she decided to paint in some light grey to be a background but actually only painted a smoky grey around the hand. Then, in incrementally larger letters, she finished her phrase, 'Papa, moi, je vois la vie en couleurs' ('Papa, I see life in colours'). Smiling, she was very pleased.

She told me that her mother often said: 'My poor daughter, how much you suffer.' She responded that her illness has taught her so much about life, even if it meant that she hadn't been able to live normally for the past ten years. She said she had seen a side of the richness of life that she never would have known otherwise, a side of the inner world, her own inner world that she probably wouldn't have encountered.

Session 18: Motions reaching upward

She came by ambulance today with the oxygen tank and said just preparing herself to come, showering, dressing, tired her out. She wanted to use paint again on large paper, but was too fatigued to start from the standing position she enjoyed so much. She sat and dipped the fingers of both hands into paint, blue on the left and green on the right. She made swirling motions and the movement of her arms was like a dance both on paper and in the air. There was a kind of upward reaching with her arms and a taking in of air as she worked. Her arms moved symmetrically and rhythmically, looping around on paper and shooting outwards diagonally as the gesture came to finality. Once again, I felt her intense desire to shoot all the bad out of her body and her painting gesture was linked to that, but also to her sexuality, of which she was equally very aware (Figure 6.12, on website).

She was very pleased with the new colours she was learning to mix. The smallish loops on the bottom resembled breasts and the outreaching diagonal strokes, quickly executed, arms. A loop in between resembled a head. I thought she might comment about this, but she did not. Taking red, with a forceful gesture she made what looked like fire coming or shooting out of the right breast-like loop, by abruptly flicking the paint with her fingernails. Adding orange, she gave it a very fiery look. She saw this as her sexuality, and could feel the sensation in her genital area. She wanted to mix brown as an 'anchoring' colour next to this fire and we worked on how the deep chocolate brown that she wanted could be mixed. Whether this part of the image referred symbolically to her inflamed, enlarged breast, or had overtones of anality, she did not draw a connection. Although she was someone who welcomed insight, one must be aware that only so much insight can be useful therapeutically in any one session. The best insight tends to be that which the patient arrives at herself. After completing this painting the knot of tension that she felt upon arriving was gone; she felt this was due to the act of painting, coupled with the understanding she gained related to her body.

Session 19: Confronting death

Arriving in a wheelchair this time, she looked very tired, but happy to be here. She began by telling me that so far she had not confronted death though she knew she should do it. Before, she felt she neither knew how nor wanted to, but a change came over her during the past few weeks when a patient in the next bed died at the rehab centre. She said that she had just been discovering many things about herself and had so many ideas, particularly for images, paintings and collages that she'd like to make. But she could not because she lacked the energy. I commented that I understood how hard it must be for her to confront death since so much about her is so vital, creative and alive.

She wanted me to know that after last week when she painted with her arms, she had the impression that our work had actually opened her left lung. But a new X-ray revealed that her left lung was still not functioning. Although she often felt a physical easing of tension at the end of our sessions, it is beyond my competence to offer further understanding about how this occurred, except to transmit my observations and unanswered questions.

Probably induced by her disappointment in the lack of improvement in her lung, she wanted to do a drawing about death. Her image was to be the earth with all the people who have died and who die. She used coloured pencils because they required less energy. She drew a large circle and put in a map of Japan – to denote a ritual where parents had their teeth pulled out and were left to die, their bodies were burned and floated down a river. She showed Africa where people died out in the open and their skeletons could be found. She spoke of these horrifying ways to die in rather euphemistic terms. Then she drew crosses for cemeteries in France and remembered all the deaths of people close to her: an older sister, grandparents, and so on (Figure 6.13, on website). Then she thought of her father with whom she was so angry and said he was only interested in money. I think the anger she has successfully mobilized toward him has kept her grief at bay.

Session 24: Working from the rehabilitation centre

Now we worked together from her bed at the rehab centre, as she could no longer make the trip to the hospital. She requested large paper. Leaning on a large board, she was able to use her upper body and arms freely. Very frail, she began drawing with difficulty that was uncharacteristic of her, almost as though she didn't know how to use a pastel.

Pressing hard with her pale orange pastel, she began to scrawl the beginning of a spiral in a wobbly line going from the centre outwards. Around and around she went until she picked up her stride and loosened up, ending up with her usual free, joyful and sure line going out of the spiral. This time she had more energy than the last time. At the end, her face had more colour than when I arrived. She felt the energy and told me that the work we do is really about the energy of her body, about her body being engaged in a special way. She felt an opening up that she said was profound. She didn't know what it was but she could feel it in her body all the way down to her genital area. She thought it had to do with reproductive organs, and where her illness began, but also where life began (Figure 6.14, on website).

Conclusion

Although Mrs Verdier has since weakened, she has been determined to continue art therapy. I would like to add a few further comments about the limits and extent of our work together. At the core of our work, the creative art process and therapeutic process were so intertwined that one could not have yielded the same results without the other.

Notwithstanding how much has been addressed through art therapy, more was yet to be done. It was not yet possible for Mrs Verdier really to come to terms with conflicts regarding her father, not only because these issues required more time but also because, due to her illness, she unconsciously experienced him as not having protected her existence. She often remarked how illness made her feel like a little girl. Certainly, early conflicts were evoked and conflated with newer circumstances, engendering a plenitude of meaning. I felt we were working against time to understand her feelings toward him, yet awareness of the lack of time was fuelling her anger.

Some aspects of her relationship with her parents are still unresolved, in particular her angry feelings. We have seen that distancing herself from her father through anger served several unconscious purposes. I see her anger as her way of detaching from her parents in order to be able to say goodbye. She had told me that if she were to allow her parents, who lived at a great distance in the mountains, to visit her every day, they would be there. Keeping them at bay was probably her way of remaining in control of her grief at leaving them, a way to separate. As in many parent/child relationships, no matter what the age, the struggle for optimal psychical distance in the sense of Mahler's *optimal distance* (Mahler *et al.* 1975) weaves its way throughout all the stages of life.

Another example of an issue that needed more work was her feeling that the dinner she prepared was rejected by her mother, who brought her own meal to Mrs Verdier's house. It is plausible that her mother, who was probably also traumatized by her daughter's suffering, wanted to save her daughter the trouble of exerting extra energy in cooking and attempted to surreptitiously conserve or control her daughter's energy by bringing the meal. This was a mother who hadn't the language of emotional communication and perhaps awkwardly only made matters worse by suggesting that the meal be for her son. Of course, speculation is really useless because we can never know, but it is important to remember that other family members are also traumatized by serious illness (Riley 1999). Her father's bringing flowers was another case in point. We don't know whether this father, traumatized and in desperation to be of help to his declining daughter, may have thought of flowers, a gesture dramatically out of the norm for him.

Months earlier in our work, Mrs Verdier told me that once a nurse had described her as 'a little mouse', in a similar way to the way she saw her mother, as though, like her mother, she did not have the right to ask for anything in life. I mention this incident because six months after her fiftieth birthday Mrs Verdier was finally able to ask her parents for the birthday gift she really desired – a very large box of beautiful pastels. She had enjoyed using pastels in our sessions and an artist friend had loaned her such a box when she began living in the rehabilitation centre.

When her parents arrived with the box, Mrs Verdier wanted their presence at the opening of the gift. But instead of surrounding her bedside, each of them was busy doing something else in her room, with their backs toward her. She felt a repetition of old disappointment. To make matters worse, the box of pastels proved to be of an inferior quality than she expected, only intensifying her disappointment. When she showed the pastels to me, she commented that the colours looked almost garish, not fine and subtle. She wondered whether to simply keep them and not upset her parents or to ask for an exchange. In this case, I encouraged her more openly than I normally would to opt for the exchange, pointing out that she was an adult and that exchanging the pastels for those she really wanted was only a practical matter.

Finally she did so and, when she explained the problem to her mother, her mother disclosed that she too had been disappointed upon seeing them. Her mother's admission was the surprise rapprochement Mrs Verdier had always sought. She had thought of her mother, of both parents, as unconcerned with aesthetic or cultural matters. Now her mother revealed that she could appreciate what Mrs Verdier also appreciated. What is more, the admission bespoke of gentleness, a tender aspect of her mother that Mrs Verdier thought her mother either lacked or couldn't share. This propitious moment permitted her to make a special peace with her mother. She received the emotional response she sought because she didn't hold back, but asked for what she needed. Mrs Verdier had taken the step to speak to her mother as one adult to another and her mother responded with more than Mrs Verdier expected.

Patients entering an end-of-life phase require extra strengthening of their inner resources in order to affirm their sense of humanity and own a self-identity that is larger than the name of their illness. Mobilizing creativity during a time of physical illness fortifies the life-giving inner resources that may still be intact and offers a patient an antidote to the forces that work against life. It is the continuous affirmation of being on the side of life that fosters a sense of health. Art therapy offers a specially adapted alternative means of personal expression when words alone do not suffice.

Note

I wish to thank l'AGARO (l'Association Grenobloise d'Aide à la Recherche en Oncologie) for its continued generous support in creating and sustaining a part-time art therapy position at the Centre Hospitalier Grenoble. Particular thanks go to le Professeur Mireille Mousseau, Dr Jacqueline Léger and Dr Mireille Bost for their unwavering interest and collaboration in the project.

References

Blanck, G. and Blanck, R. (1975) *Ego Psychology: Theory and Practice*. New York: Columbia University Press.

Freud, S. (1900) *The Interpretation of Dreams*, Standard Edition 5. London: Hogarth Press and the Institute of Psycho-Analysis.

Hartmann, H. (1958) *The Ego and the Problem of Adaptation*. New York: International Universities Press.

Kohut, H. (1971) *The Analysis of the Self*. New York: International Universities Press.

Mahler, M.S., Pine, F. and Bergman, A. (1975) *The Psychological Birth of the Human Infant*. New York: Basic Books.

Riley, S. (1999) External stress: the impact of illness on the family structure, in C.A. Malchiodi (ed.) *Medical Art Therapy with Adults*. London: Jessica Kingsley.

Stone, E. (2003) Body image in art with a focus on trauma and loss, in R. Hampe, P. Martius, A. Reiter, G. Schottenloher and F. von Spreti (eds) *Trauma und Kreativität: Therapie mit künstlerischen Medien*. Dokumentation zur 13. Jahrestagung der IGKGT an der Universität Salzburg. Bremen: Universität Bremen.

Wood, M.J.M. (1998) Art therapy in palliative care, in M. Pratt and M.J.M. Woods (eds) *Art Therapy in Palliative Care: The Creative Response*. London: Routledge.

Further reading

Cane, F. (1983) *The Artist in Each of Us*, revised edition. Craftsbury Common, VT: Art Therapy Publications.

Casement, P. (1985) *On Learning from the Patient*. London: Tavistock Publications.

Colarusso, C.A. (2000) Separation-individuation phenomena in adulthood: general concepts and the fifth individuation, *Journal of the American Psychoanalytic Association*, 48(4): 1467–89.

Freud, A. (1952) The role of bodily illness in the mental life of children, in *Psychoanalytic Study of the Child*, Vol. 7. New York: International Universities Press.

Gabriel, B., Bromberg, E., Vandenbovenkamp, J., Walka, A., Kornbluth, B. and Luzzato, P. (2001) Art therapy with adult bone marrow transplant patients in isolation: a pilot study, *Psycho-oncologie*, 10: 114–23.

Greenacre, P. (1958a) Early physical determinants in the development of the sense of identity, in *Emotional Growth: Psychoanalytic Studies of the Gifted and a Great Variety of Other Individuals*, Vol. I. New York: International Universities Press.

Greenacre, P. (1958b) Toward an understanding of the physical nucleus of some defense reactions, in *Emotional Growth: Psychoanalytic Studies of the Gifted and a Great Variety of Other Individuals*, Vol. I. New York: International Universities Press.

Hoffer, W. (1950) Development of the body Ego, *Psychoanalytic Study of the Child*, Vol. 5. New York: International Universities Press.

Jacobson, E. (1964) *The Self and the Object World*. New York: International Universities Press.

Kaplan, L.J. (1995) *No Voice is Ever Wholly Lost: An Exploration of the Everlasting Attachment Between Parent and Child*. New York: Simon & Schuster/ Touchstone Books.

Leiberman, J.S. (2000) *Body Talk: Looking and Being Looked at in Psychotherapy*. Northvale, NJ: Jason Aronson.

Lussier, A. (1980) The physical handicap and the body ego, *The International Journal of Psycho-Analysis*, 61(2): 179–85.

Luzzato, P. (1998) From psychiatry to psycho-oncology: personal reflections on the use of art therapy with cancer patients, in M. Pratt and M.J.M. Wood (eds) *Art Therapy in Palliative Care: The Creative Response*. London: Routledge.

Luzzato, P. and Gabriel, B. (1998) Art psychotherapy, in J. Holland (ed.) *Psycho-oncology*. New York, Oxford: Oxford University Press.

Mahler, M.S. (1966) Notes on the development of basic moods: the depressive affect, in *The Selected Papers of Margaret S. Mahler, Vol. II: Separation–Individuation*. New York, London: Jason Aronson.

Schilder, P. (1950) *The Image and Appearance of the Human Body*. New York: International Universities Press.

Winnicott, D.W. (1971) *Playing and Reality*. New York: Basic Books.

Art therapy as Perseus' shield for
children with cancer

Cinzia Favara-Scacco

Introduction

Children diagnosed with cancer are suddenly exposed to a life-threatening
experience. They are unexpectedly taken away from their 'normal' lifestyle
and expected to face significant changes in their settled daily routines: at
home, within the family, at school, and in their comforting play rituals. The
child is exposed to diagnostic procedures involving numerous medical tests
and visits to unknown hospital settings and machines, to frequent alarming
interventions and, progressively, he becomes the unwilling witness of his
body metamorphosis. The experience of cancer is extremely intense. The
child perceives a parallel growth of good and bad within his own body, even
if he is very young (two years), and a sense of impotence starts to dominate.
Chemotherapy reinforces such emotional experience because it is injected to
destroy illness, but at the same time it shows how cancer is intertwined with
the child. In this status of autogenous war, the parallel, encumbering emotional distress stays still, unexpressed. It crouches in the soft, fragile young
patient's internal world. The child finds great difficulty in expressing the
emotional experience generated by cancer. Enormous defensive barriers are
built, blocking any possibility for the emotion to move, to be 'touched'. It is
too dangerous; the patient is paralysed.

Childhood is a very important and delicate period of life during which
each child develops physically as well as psycho-emotionally towards a
stronger sense of self (Jung 1959: 390) and capacity to adapt (Piaget 1967:
135). Continuity and rituals define a safe space for the child, protecting him
from the anxious, fearful unknown. Sudden changes, especially traumatic
experiences, cause risks to a child's balanced growth (Boggs *et al.* 1991;
Prager 1995; Scudder 1995) and children with cancer have to face such
risks, which have the capacity to influence their developmental process.

The importance of *curing* children with cancer through an holistic approach, emotionally as well as physically, is a right for them and a duty for us. When a child is unable to organize the experience of illness and release it into the external world, illness can become the cause of unbearable internal feelings (Masera *et al.* 1996). These days a very high percentage of children (over 70 per cent) (Blatt *et al.* 1993) are cured after a reasonable period of time and they will need all their energies to construct a positive orientation for future development (Jenney *et al.* 1995), to express their identity and build towards personal as well as social success.

Through the creative process the child is helped to take an active role in the fight for life, rather than becoming a passive 'victim' of events. In our Paediatric Oncology Unit in Catania in Italy, the intention is to assure continuity in the child's psycho-emotional development by facilitating adjustment; reinforcing the ego structure; stimulating the release of anguishing experiences (Figure 7.1, on website); helping children recognize and declare proper needs; living the present, as well as offering a parallel support to parents.

Art therapy to help children control cancer-related pain

Children with cancer have to face a long-term therapeutic programme and specific steps are experienced by the child and the family as very traumatic, often resulting in a crisis (Jannoun and Chessels 1987; Kazak 1998). These cause prolonged psycho-emotional discomforts. The value of 'holding' (Winnicott 1958: 381) the child during these steps is essential, specifically at children's first arrival in the oncology unit during which intrusive diagnostic procedures are commonly performed. These might be bone marrow aspiration (BMA) and lumbar puncture (LP); central venous catheter application through surgery; during prolonged hospitalizations due to therapy side effects; and during the terminal phase.

Since September 1996, the Paediatric Haematology-Oncology Unit of the Polyclinic of Catania has offered a continued and structured psycho-emotional support to children and parents, using art therapy (AT) modalities. AT implies the use of creativity and symbolism to allow individuals to express their severe anxiety about their experiences, in a non-traumatic way (Figure 7.2, on website). Through non-verbal communication, it facilitates empathy, comprehension, therapeutic relationship, reassurance and emotional equilibrium (Malchiodi 1999: 194). It intensifies the brain's right side activities (Arieti 1976: 352; Deri 1984: 347; Robbins 1986: 203), stimulating imagination, giving continuity to thoughts and actions which do not stop simply because of illness. The child can play alternative roles without being trapped in the specific one of 'the patient'. In fact, AT is particularly efficient for a hospital setting because its different modalities make it adaptable to children's different personalities. It is also capable of offering support for their fears. Through stimulating the imagination, AT facilitates children's natural capacity to engage in playful activities while improving their quality of life. This enables the child to relax and reduce corporeal hypersensitivity (Collins *et al.* 1995). Furthermore, the child is given the opportunity to choose, to express his will about which creative activity to undertake and which materials to use. But he is also given a chance to say 'no' to something within the hospital setting. Decision making facilitates children's capacity to maintain their identity, helping them feel more in control. In the creative process, the child is free to be; he defines his own space. An opportunity is provided which gives continuity to psycho-emotional development (Montesarchio and Sardi 1989: 114).

It is imperative that we define a model of intervention which can reduce children's psycho-physical experience of pain. We will present our method of supporting the child during two of the former listed invasive treatments, specifically how to protect the child from pain during LP–BMA and during the terminal phase using art therapy modalities.

Children with cancer have to face periodic painful diagnostic and therapeutic procedures. Entering an oncology unit, children feel an instinctual fear, anxiety and hostility due to this new mysterious environment. Their whole physical perception is known to be highly influenced by their psycho-emotional condition (Solomon and Saylor 1998: 2.1–2.20). They become hypersensitive and their level of tolerance is low. In this state, children experience any diagnostic or therapeutic procedure as excessive, overwhelming and above all, *painful*. Cancer, long-term therapy and pain cause a crisis for parents as well. They feel threatened, knowing that their child is in danger, and desperate, feeling helpless, useless and, often, irrationally guilty for failing in a parent's basic role of protecting their own child from suffering, not having been able to prevent illness. In this state of internal turmoil, parents usually see their child's pain, or absence of pain, as an indicator of good or bad quality of treatment and, consequently, develop resistance towards therapy, or faith in it, and directly influence their child (Mechanic 1994; Perrin *et al.* 1993). To support the child we have to help parents to use their energy productively. Through creativity, parents can engage in a lively dynamic interaction, and sense again during this life-threatening time the essential, active role they have in stimulating their child's well-being (Figure 7.3, on website).

The delicate issue of supporting children during the stressful LP and BMA has been faced in different ways in various hematology–oncology departments. Some offer total anesthesia, with its associated risks and expenses in terms of time and money (American Academy of Pediatrics 1992; Cote *et al.* 1995; Murphy 1997); others offer generic support; and still others offer no preparation at all. The modes of AT before, during and after these punctures were as follows: clinical dialogue to calm children and help them cope with painful procedures; visual imagination to activate alternative thought processes and decrease the attention towards overwhelming reality and raise the peripheral sensitivity-gate; medical play to clarify illness, eliminate doubts, and offer control over threatening reality [Figure 7.4, on website]; drawing to contain anxiety by offering a structured, predictable reality (the drawing) that was controllable by children; free drawing to allow children to externalize confusion and fears, and dramatization to help children accept and reconcile themselves to body changes.

(Favara-Scacco *et al.* 2001)

To clarify the experience, we will present two cases. The names of the children have been changed to maintain confidentiality.

Case 1

Felicia was a two-year-old girl of enchanting beauty, with soft, red curls, big green eyes and freckles that moved each time she smiled. Because she was so young, during the first clinical dialogue (CD), the art therapist (ATst) used a puppet named Gnomy. Felicia seemed to be delightfully surprised by Gnomy's sudden ability to speak. A few minutes later a doctor entered the room to apply the local anesthesia for Felicia's next BMA. Her smiling face immediately became still, she resisted being touched by the doctor and started to cry. So Gnomy started the fantasy-based storytelling (through the ATst voice) and asked Felicia to be a mountain to climb. Meanwhile the doctor applied the local anesthesia. Gnomy's storytelling soon involved butterflies and bees that landed on the mountain and that sometimes, unwittingly, might pinch the mountain. Felicia continued to be totally involved in the story and followed Gnomy to the treatment room as part of the game. She kept her attention focused on the story during the entire BMA procedure with a few exceptions, at which times her mother's intervention was very helpful. Constantly looking at the art therapist, Felicia's mother would put her mouth very close to Felicia's ear and whisper lovely details about the story. Eye contact with the ATst showed that her mother needed to be reassured that she was doing the right thing. It is important for a parent to feel helpful at such a traumatic time and to overcome any possible sense of guilt. Once Felicia had returned to her room, she went back to her play activity and soon her good mood returned. As her therapy cycle was continuing, dramatization became the most appropriate modality for allowing continued therapeutic release of her inner feelings. When Felicia's hair was cut, to save her from having to see it constantly falling out, her mother reported that Felicia expressed no emotional reaction and this continued until playing with a doll gave her a chance to express how intensely this had affected her. Dramatization uses characters which provide the necessary emotional distance such that a person's feelings belong to the characters. After a long time spent caressing the doll's hair, she laid the doll down with her face towards the bed saying that the doll was sick. Felicia was recreating, in front of our eyes, the drama of her experience. She was starting to free herself from its weight by releasing her inner trauma into the external world. The intensity of the experience soon became overwhelming and Felicia suddenly stopped speaking and started seeking eye contact with her mother. She kept this contact for a few seconds as if she wanted to ask for something that she couldn't express because of her limited vocabulary. She then stretched her little, fragile arms towards her mother and started touching her hair. She was 'telling' us that she needed time to process the whole experience. What she needed at that moment was to escape from threatening feelings and to be held in the comforting embrace provided by the warmth of her mother's touch.

Case 2

Rita's melancholy little face was quite shocking, being far too sad for an eight-year-old girl. She had the reputation of being a difficult patient, having adopted many 'negative behaviours'. Entering her room, one felt an illusionary calmness that concealed an unconscious choice of being passive and submitting to events. During the first clinical dialogue, Rita was uncomfortable and resisted verbal communication, while her mother kept repeating that Rita was lazy and useless. Rita appeared to be indifferent to any of the proposed creative activities. The proposal to draw seemed to be attractive but scary at the same time. Staring at the white sheet, she dared not put a mark on the paper. Rita needed to engage in a reassuring, controllable activity that might awaken her faith in herself and gradually generalize this faith to include the therapeutic process. The mother also needed to commit to this because she seemed to have initiated a process of resignation and of emotional distancing from a daughter whom she saw as already condemned. Structured drawing was the most appropriate modality to engage Rita's active self. She had just started colouring when suddenly the timer on the intravenous drip started beeping. Rita froze, she stopped breathing and her eyes opened wide: the beeping was the threatening sound of danger. Rita followed the nurse's every movement. Her eyes became shiny, her breathing was now rapid; it was clear that she wanted to give up and weep. When the nurse left the room, the tension was finally dissipated and Rita started to cry. Fantasmagorical, life-threatening images had sneaked into her young mind. Rita needed detailed explanations about her treatment, which were given in the following sessions through medical play. The negative behaviours expressed her anger at having no control over her existence. The clinical director felt that she needed a visual task to focus her imagination, and that the freeing of her imagination would open a door to all her suppressed fears. Control and empowerment were necessary. With the doctor's cooperation, some control was possible since Rita was allowed to count up to 100 seconds during the LP to decide the duration of her procedure. The child's mother seemed able to understand that her daughter had the right to speak out about her needs and to have her needs satisfied. When the procedure began, Rita started counting clearly and loudly. With the exception of a few facial expressions of pain, the procedure went very smoothly. Furthermore, a sense of satisfaction, engendered by the empowerment, stimulated a sense of complicity with the medical staff and allowed her to cope better with the LP.

Art therapy to support children in the terminal phase

Long-term therapy for cancer is energy-consuming; to keep hope and faith constantly alive is hard and yet essential. At times it can be extremely difficult, at others almost impossible, such as in cases when we have to recognize the specific tremendous power of the cancer and the impossibility of saving the child. All we can experience is uselessness and failure. For such reasons the psycho-emotional dynamics that the terminal phase evokes need to be deeply comprehended so that we can treat every single case in the most appropriate way. When medicine has to give up, facing a too aggressive neoplasia (tumour), the child understands this, although adults try to deny it; parents start to experience boundless loss, an emotional gulf filled with rage and desperation; the whole team is filled with sadness and has to face its limits since it is no longer possible to restore health and life. When this state of total pain is established, chaos and tension dominate. In the attempt to offer support in this extremely difficult moment, it is essential to respect specific rules.

In our unit we utilize AT modalities to reach our goals. Through AT we no longer have a bipolar therapeutic relationship (Bellani *et al.* 2002) that implies the patient and the therapist. Art therapy gives a third element, 'the creative process', that in the case of terminally ill patients acquires a profound value. Comparable to Winnicott's 'transitional object', through using symbolic elements, art therapy helps the child and the family cope better with the terminal phase. We observed how the tripolar field, patient–creativity–therapist (Luzzatto 1989), annuls the fight between the two extremes of life and death, utilizing the creative process as a lightning conductor. When medicine declares its impotence in the face of specific cases, death seems to be invited into a dimension to which it does not yet belong, because life is still present. The team, parents, and consequently the child are trapped within this unrelenting fight of the shrill tension of opposites crystallizing the space around. To enter this dimension is to freeze and it is the cause of pain. This is why it is so difficult to stay by the child in this phase, and this is particularly so for the parents who feel totally impotent. It is necessary to recognize the existence of specific tools that can help us to face and overcome this immobilizing state of mind: respect the child by not encumbering their remaining life with death; live the present; open a symbolic, spiritual dimension. AT allows us to use creativity as Perseus' shield, to face and defeat Medusa without becoming the immobilized victim, petrified by fear.

To clarify the experience, we will present another case, related to a previous experience in the United States of America.

Case 3

A sense of impotence was what one immediately perceived when entering Davis' room. His young parents were sitting in a corner of the room, far away from the child. The mother was staring into space, while the father was holding his head in his hands. Davis was six weeks old, recovering at the intensive care unit after a bone marrow transplant (BMT). The continuous, rhythmical beeping of the medical instruments that surrounded him would immediately dispel the illusion that the baby was simply sleeping. 'What can I possibly do?' For just an instant Medusa's look caught me unprepared and trapped me in the desire of immobility. The physical distance that the parents were keeping was a way of protecting themselves from the harsh reality of the situation. The death power that was overwhelming the room had to be weakened, and we had to recognize that Davis continued to have basic needs which had to be satisfied, and to offer to parents the 'tools' to enable them to stay by their baby, actively involved. To give Davis' needs a voice, 'Smile faces' were drawn and attached on the room walls, suggesting the most delightful sensorial perceptions that Davis had to continue receiving (Figures 7.5, 7.6, 7.7, on website). To help Davis' family overcome the sense of helplessness and keep a sense of intimacy, a tree made of hard paper was attached to one of the walls of his room and a notebook was placed beside it in which 'the tree' had expressed its wish to know more about the baby in front of him (Figure 7.8, on website). To write things on the paper leaves to satisfy the curiosity of the tree would make it bigger. In the following days the energy within the room totally changed: all around you could see toys; a Mickey Mouse tape recorder played soothing lullabies. His mother was by his side, caressing him and expressing delight as she noticed how Davis' heart rhythm would change each time she whispered in his ear. The paper tree was filled with new paper leaves and on each of them were written blessings. On the notebook parents and family members started writing things about Davis (Figure 7.9, on website). The father kept giving thanks. The creative activity allowed everyone to recognize that Davis was still alive and needed to be respected on a physical as well as on an emotional level. Unfortunately, a few days later Davis got worse and died, but his parents were able to assist him because they re-engaged their essential parental role of support and being a source of well-being. Through the symbolism within the creative activity, they became capable of overcoming that sense of impotence and uselessness that initially had immobilized them.

Conclusion

There is no possibility of denying the overwhelming sadness that we face, as practitioners, in working with children who have cancer. In particular, as I have tried to show, it is devastating when all medical treatments have failed and they are going to die. Art therapy can offer some release to children during the frightening clinical procedures which accompany diagnosis and treatment, and it can help to ease the suffering of the child and his parents during the terminal phase of the illness. We can engage the creative process to ease the pain of the losses that are experienced throughout, and for those children who are able to recover, we can help them to overcome the trauma of their struggle with the illness.

References

American Academy of Pediatrics (1992) Committee on drugs, section on anesthesiology. Guidelines for monitoring and management of pediatric patients during and after sedation for diagnostic and therapeutic procedures, *Pediatrics*, 89: 1110–15.

Arieti, S. (1976) *Creativity*. New York: Basic Books.

Bellani, M. *et al.* (2002) *Psiconcologia*. Milan: Masson.

Blatt, J., Copeland, D.R. and Bleyer, W.A. (1993) Late effects of childhood cancer and its treatment, in P.A. Pizzo and D.G. Poplack (eds) *Principles and Practice of Pediatric Oncology*. Philadephia, PA: Lippincott Raven.

Boggs, S.R., Graham-Pole, J. and Miller, E.M. (1991) Life-threatening illness and invasive treatment. The future of quality of life assessment and research in pediatric oncology, in J.H. Johnson and S.B. Johnson (eds) *Advances in Child Health Psychology*. Gainesville, FL: University of Florida Press.

Collins, J.J., Grier, H.E., Kinney, H.C. *et al.* (1995) Control of severe pain in children with terminal malignancy, *The Journal of Pediatrics*, 126: 653–7.

Cote, C.J., Alderfer, R.J., Notterman, D.A. and Fanta, K.B. (1995) Sedation disaster: adverse drug reports in pediatrics – FDA, USP, and others, *Anaesthesiology*, 83: 1183.

Deri, S. (1984) *Symbolization and Creativity*. Madison, WI: International Universities Press.

Favara-Scacco, C. *et al.* (2001) Art therapy as support for children with leukemia during painful procedures, *Medical & Pediatric Oncology*, 36 (4): 429–506.

Jannoun, L. and Chessels, J.M. (1987) Long-term psychological effects of childhood leukemia and its treatment, *Pediatric Hematology and Oncology*, 4: 292–308.

Jenney, M.E.M., Kane, R.L. and Lurie, M. (1995) Developing a measure of health outcomes in survivors of childhood cancer: a review of the issue, *Medical and Pediatric Oncology*, 24: 145–53.

Jung, C.G. (1959) *The Archetypes and the Collective Unconscious*. New York: Princeton University Press.

Kazak, A.E. (1998) Post-traumatic distress in childhood cancer survivors and their parents, *Medical and Pediatric Oncology*, Suppl. 1: 60–8.

Luzzatto, P. (1989) On the relationship between art and therapy, *Inscape*, Journal of BAAT, 5: 31.

Malchiodi, C. (1999) *Medical Art Therapy with Children*. London: Jessica Kingsley.

Masera, G., Chesler, M., Jankovic, M. *et al.* (1996) SIOP Working Committee on Psychosocial Issues in Paediatric Oncology: guidelines for care of long-term survivors, *Medical and Pediatric Oncology*, 27: 1–2.

Mechanic, D. (1994) The influence of mothers on their children's health attitudes and behavior, *Pediatrics*, 33: 444–53.

Montesarchio, G. and Sardi, P. (1989) *Dal teatro della spontaneità allo psico-dramma classico*. Milan: Franco Angeli.

Murphy, M.S. (1997) Sedation for invasive procedures in paediatrics, *Archives of Disease in Childhood*, 77: 281–6.

Perrin, E.C., Ayoub, C.C. and Willett, J.B. (1993) In the eyes of the beholder: family and maternal influences on perceptions of adjustment of children with a chronic illness, *Journal of Developmental and Behavioral Pediatrics*, 14: 94–105.

Piaget, J. (1967) La construction du réel chez l'enfant, in Neuchatel, Delachaux and Niestlè (eds) *L'Enfant*. Paris: Folio.

Prager, A. (1995) Pediatric art therapy: strategies and applications, *Artherapy*, 12: 32–8.

Robbins, A. (1986) *Expressive Therapy*. New York: Human Sciences Press.

Scudder, T. E. (1995) Terminal stages leukemia: integrating art therapy and family processes, *Artherapy*, 12: 51–61.

Solomon, R. and Saylor, C.D. (1998) *Pediatric Pain Management: A Professional Course*. Michigan, MI: Michigan State University.

Winnicott, D.W. (ed.) (1958) *Through Pediatrics to Psycho-analysis*. London: Tavistock Publications.

8 | The efficacy of a single session

Jacqui Balloqui

Introduction

I work within the Oncology Department of a large British district hospital as part of the Palliative Care Team in a National Health Service Trust. Due to a shortage of beds it is hospital policy to turn people around and discharge them into alternative care as quickly as possible; consequently I frequently only see patients for one or two sessions before they die or are transferred to home, nursing home or hospice. This has led me to question and evaluate what can be achieved in the time available. I draw on case studies to demonstrate how the therapist's approach can enable working within the transference relationship even in a single session and how this can help patients to address emotional and spiritual concerns. To help me to place this work in the context of other work going on in Britain, and to see what has been written about brief therapy, I have looked at the literature written by art therapists working in cancer care, and to open my chapter I will summarize this for the reader.

Literature review

British literature on art psychotherapy in cancer care does not refer specifically to brief psychodynamic psychotherapy. Skaife (1993), Schaverien (2000), Luzzatto and Gabriel (1998), Wood (1998), Thomas (1998) and others acknowledge that art therapists tend to develop different styles and models of working in response to the needs of medically ill patients. Joan Woddis (1998), in exploring the professional context of art therapy in *Something Understood* (Connell 1998), explains that art therapy cannot remain 'a homogenised service with the same experience offered to all patients' but has to adapt to the needs of different client groups. Whilst this is so, it is important not to lose sight of the analytic framework that guides art therapy practice. Luzzatto and Gabriel (1998) maintain that the three communicative dimensions of expressive–creative, cognitive–symbolic and interactive–analytic are always present in art therapy and may be activated at different times. This would indicate that it is possible to keep a psychoanalytic orientation, whilst adopting a flexible approach which can facilitate art therapy in a myriad of different settings. (This is a point shared and developed by David Hardy in Chapter 13 of this book.)

Brief psychodynamic psychotherapy can be particularly appropriate to working with cancer patients and is readily adapted within art therapy. It maintains the focus on the psychodynamics of the relationship whilst exploring existential concerns in a more directive way. Time limits, enforced by the patient's illness, can increase the sense of urgency to work through and resolve individual issues, thus making an intense piece of work possible.

David Hardy (2001) states, and I agree, that: 'any contact between a client and a therapist, with or without a picture, necessarily involves a degree of reciprocity, which in turn infers a transference reaction'. Caroline Case (1998) speaks of 'the intense transference that can be present in an assessment, both person to person and through the images made'. In my experience this also happens within a single session. Case asks several questions regarding transference and countertransference, which have helped me to formulate my own thinking. Jackie Coote (1998), in her discussion on the 'one-off' session, suggests that people facing their own mortality often feel compelled to plunge in and address unresolved issues so that one session may be all that is needed. Her case vignettes demonstrate how a close monitoring of the countertransference allows her to stay with patients whilst encouraging them to step over the threshold into previously unexpressed feelings. Michèle Wood (1998) confirms that there are times when a single session can be useful. She describes a situation where physical, emotional and social changes gather momentum and she is guided by the unconscious exchanges that occur between herself and her patient. Schaverien (1998, 1999, 2000, 2002) emphasizes how an understanding of transference and countertransference should inform the process of art therapy, whatever approach is adopted and whether or not this knowledge is interpreted to the patient. Byers (1998) considers an understanding of transference and countertransference part of personal as well as professional development and links it to issues of difference. Campbell et al. (1999) insist that art therapists own and acknowledge individual and cultural experiences in order to creatively inform both personal and professional relationships and avoid the risk of detachment and/or imposition upon others. In assessing my own practice I recognize that experiences of transference and countertransference are at times, in the words of Camilla Connell (1998), 'profound and difficult to put into words'. The above authors have contributed significantly to my understanding. To illustrate these points, I will now discuss some work I have carried out with patients suffering from cancer.

Case studies

Amanda

Amanda had been known to the service for a long time. She had a slow growing brain tumour, deteriorating physical health, and was no longer able to look after herself. I was told she had social problems and might benefit from spending time with me whilst she was in hospital having her medication adjusted.

In our initial meeting Amanda sat in a chair being washed by an auxiliary nurse. I noted the familiar bloated look which suggested that Amanda was on steroids, and she had lost much of her hair. Although quite a large woman, I was aware of a childlike quality about her. I introduced myself and gave her an information sheet on art therapy. I explained that if she wanted to have a go, we could either set up in the day room or she could sit in the chair by her bed. She looked at the sheet I had given her. I thought at first she was reading it but realized she was staring at it vacantly, so I sat with her and went through the sheet explaining each point. She appeared to listen intently. I experienced Amanda as being of a congenial disposition, eager to please. I noted that I had made an assumption that she could read and understand what I had written and reminded myself that assumptions underlay most mistakes. After I had explained the process, Amanda said she would like to draw something. I arranged to see her in the afternoon.

When I returned Amanda had visitors. There was a look of wonder and excitement on her face as she tried to guess the contents of a large parcel on her bed. I did not disturb them.

On my next visit Amanda was eager to draw. She experimented with different art materials whilst she talked about her ex-husband who had been physically and emotionally abusive towards her, eventually leaving her for a much younger woman. Amanda said she had found losing her home and being separated from her children very hard. Amanda had explained to her children why she could no longer look after them but did not know how much they really understood. She was worried about what would become of them, especially the youngest, and felt that social services ignored her concerns for their welfare.

Amanda drew a big pink heart in oil pastel and wrote underneath in rainbow coloured felt tips 'Kids, love you all'. She asked if she could keep the picture as she would like to put it in a box of things she wants her children to have when she dies.

She was very appreciative of having this opportunity to talk about her problems and make something for her children. She held my hands and thanked me with tears in her eyes. I felt deeply moved that she had appeared to gain so much from such a short encounter.

Reflections

In the transference I had recognized a childlike quality in Amanda and responded to her vulnerability, automatically slotting into the role of nurturing parent which she unconsciously required of me. This, I believe, had led Amanda to trust me, a stranger, with her story. In the countertransference I was aware of how some of Amanda's experiences echoed my own. I think my empathy allowed her to look at her relationships with her ex-husband and children, mourn her losses and find a lasting way of letting her children know she loved them within this single session.

Eve

Eve was in her late seventies. Her diagnosis was cancer of the uterus; she also had a tear in the wall of her vagina with bowel seepage. I was informed she had poor insight into her prognosis. Eve had been put in a side room because of the smell, which she was acutely aware of, and felt lonely and frustrated.

Having had previous experience of working with adults who were incontinent, I was able to acknowledge Eve's distress and not allow the smell to interfere unduly with our relationship. Although bedridden and unable to move unassisted, Eve was chatty and playful and said she got very bored. She asked me about what I did and the sort of things people drew. I responded to her playfulness and explained that I encourage people to experiment with the art materials to see what happens. She said she used to like art at school and would like to have a go. She was unable to sit up unsupported so I propped her up with pillows and held the board for her whilst she drew. This took Eve a considerable amount of effort. She drew a tree and a dog in green oil pastel (Figure 8.1, on website). Eve told me about her dog, which was pining for her. She explained that her grandsons would be visiting her the following day and she would tell them she had been drawing. Eve asked me to take the picture and do what I want with it; she did not want her grandchildren to see it. She also asked me to call in to see her again. When I did so, she was too ill to move, so I sat with her whilst she talked about her grandchildren and the possibility that she may be transferred to a small hospital near her family soon.

Reflections

I responded to Eve's chatty, playful disposition by tuning in to it. My unconscious response to her invitation to play was 'OK let's play', child to child. The images that she drew could be seen as images of self and, to hold the transference of her illness, the tree with the gap, trunk and branches as a reflection of diagnosis, the dog as an image of self falling out of the frame (dying?). I would suggest that through the process of playful drawing she was able, if only for a few moments, to face at a conscious level her unconscious awareness of her illness and mortality.

Sharon

I was informed that Sharon was used to coping on her own and resistant to help. She had cancer of the cervix and was receiving palliative care. Nursing staff had found her quite prickly and it was assumed that she may have unfinished business or spiritual concerns that needed attention but she had rejected an approach from the chaplain.

I introduced myself to Sharon who greeted me enthusiastically with the statement 'I like art'. She was about to have physiotherapy so I said I would return later. On my return Sharon said 'I need to draw how I feel – a black flower, I don't know why.' She used charcoal and drew boldly in the centre of the sheet of paper (Figure 8.2, on website). Sharon appeared confident with the materials and visibly relieved by the process. She said she enjoyed this and found it relaxing. She asked me to pin the drawing up above her bed and said she may add some colour to it or develop it in some way during the week.

On my next visit Sharon told me she had never felt worse in her life and just wanted to sleep. The flower remained unchanged. When I returned later in the week, Sharon had been moved, but had left the picture behind.

Reflections

I thought the timing of our contact was particularly important. Sharon had an image in her mind that she needed to express and I was able to facilitate use of the art materials. The striking image of a black flower held for me in the countertransference a conflict between the delicate ephemeral quality of the flower and the darkness of its representation. Flowers are a symbol of transition and, as such, are included in the rituals of birth, marriage and death. I was reminded of the alchemical process of *nigredo* – 'germination in darkness', and of St John's *dark night of the soul*. Was this the 'unfinished business' that had been identified by nursing staff or the cancerous growth within her? I hoped that in the days after Sharon had drawn this image she might complete the transition she was making and find peace.

Fiona

'Fiona appears to have suffered a lot' were the words on the referral form. Fiona had lung cancer; however, the 'suffering', according to the consultant, referred to social problems rather than physical.

I visited Fiona on the ward. She said she would like to do some art therapy. She chose a green felt tip pen and drew in silence: a stream with ragged banks, fir trees and animals (Figure 8.3, on website). She said: 'It isn't very good.' I explained that it was not about artistic merit but what it did for her. She explained the picture as a place of peace which she had found whilst drawing and asked why I hadn't come before. She asked if I could visit her at home. I explained that wasn't possible. She said she had some pencils and would perhaps do some more drawing on her own. She asked: 'Why couldn't I have had this earlier?' I got the sense that there was much she would have liked to have happened earlier. She did not wish to keep the picture.

Reflections

Fiona saw her drawing as a place of peace. Looking at it, my countertransference reaction was that it appeared to reflect transference of her unconscious acceptance of her illness onto a conscious plane. Like Eve, who had chosen the same colour to work with, it had given her a fleeting glimpse of the reality of her diagnosis. I wondered if her feeling that this was a place of peace was also linked to her spiritual convictions. Her verbal comments indicated that the session I facilitated, which had been conducted in almost complete silence, had been of value. As Malcolm Learmonth (1994) explains, the silent, attentive therapist who resonates with the patient is a valuable witness to his or her experience. There are, however, times when we find ourselves inadvertently reacting to what the patient brings.

Richard

Richard was referred to me as an outpatient who was shut off from his feelings. His diagnosis was cancer of the bowel, terminal and inoperable. He had been given six months to live two years ago. I saw him for an individual assessment session so that we could decide whether we wanted to work together.

Richard described himself as an organized person; his career training ensured that he did not take risks.

His images were two-dimensional line drawings (Figures 8.4 and 8.5, on website). The first was of a setting sun over sea, with a strong sea defence wall, a figure pushing a wheelbarrow full of rocks, five palm trees in the foreground. The second was of a bowl of fruit on a table with a chair either side. The bowl of fruit is disproportionately large. To the upper right is a vase with four flowers in. In the foreground is a boy with a dog on a lead.

I remarked on the similarities between the two pictures: the linear style, the single figure holding on, the strong defences, the sense of containment, and how this appeared to reflect his experience. Richard appeared to find my remarks intrusive. He was seeking distraction activities and found art therapy too exposing. He said: 'We all have an allotted time span; I will go when my time is up. I'm not going to waste time thinking about it now.' I accepted that his way of coping appeared to be working for him at the moment and suggested the option of joining the open group some time in the future if he changed his mind.

Reflections

I found Richard pleasant but inflexible, determined and challenging. He kept me at arm's length and I struggled to connect with him. Richard provided an unspoken challenge – prove to me art therapy is safe. In the countertransference I missed the challenge and felt I needed to prove my ability as a woman and an art therapist. Richard's defensiveness was projected into the images he drew and, whilst I respected his need to maintain these boundaries as a coping strategy, I felt an unconscious pressure to interpret his drawings which I inadvertently responded to. This let him know I was aware of his defences and could therefore be a potential threat to his stability – art therapy wasn't safe! Unfortunately in a single session it is not always possible to reflect upon and repair one's mistakes. On reflection, a softly-softly approach which resisted the pressure to interpret may have been more helpful in engaging Richard in the process.

Conclusion

The timing of a session can be seen as crucial to its effectiveness. The images created by the patient contribute to understanding by both the patient and therapist through the transference and countertransference, which may or may not be verbalized.

The value of the session depends on its ability to meet the requirements of the patient, whether this is to express the previously unexpressed or to reinforce boundaries. I have attempted to demonstrate the therapist's obligation to be constantly aware of personal thoughts, feelings and bodily sensations, as well as visual, verbal and bodily clues from the patient, so that both the conscious and unconscious needs of the patient can be recognized and responded to appropriately within the time available. There will be times when, however we present what we have to offer, it is not what the patient wants, and times when we simply get it wrong.

I would emphasize the importance of regular psychodynamic supervision, personal art-making and therapy as essential components in developing understanding and articulating experience of transference and countertransference issues to inform art therapy practice.

Transference and countertransference are by nature highly subjective experiences, influenced by issues of difference such as race, culture, class, gender, sexuality, age and ability and therefore open to criticism. Whilst discussion may broaden our understanding, each person's experience will be different and therefore difficult to interpret or evaluate. Malcolm Learmonth (1994) advocates the practice of suspending judgement and waiting in attentive silence for the story to be revealed. It is then that we can understand the experience of the patient whilst staying in touch with our own experience, and differentiate between the two. Maybe as authors and as critics we need to remember that transference and countertransference are not limited to the therapeutic relationship but are evident in all interactions including those with the written word.

References

Byers, A. (1998) Candles slowly burning, in S. Skaife and V. Huet (eds) *Art Psychotherapy Groups*. London: Routledge.

Campbell, J., Liebmann, M., Brooks, F., Jones, J. and Ward, C. (eds) (1999) *Art Therapy, Race and Culture*. London: Jessica Kingsley.

Case, C. (1998) Brief encounters, *Inscape*, 3(1): 26–33.

Connell, C. (1998) *Something Understood: Art Therapy in Cancer Care*. London: Wrexham.

Coote, J. (1998) Getting started: introducing the art therapy service and the individual's first experiences, in M. Pratt and M.J.M. Wood (eds) *Art Therapy in Palliative Care: The Creative Response*. London: Routledge.

Hardy, D. (2001) Creating through loss: an examination of how art therapists sustain their practice in palliative care, *Inscape*, 6(1): 23–31.

Learmonth, M. (1994) Witness and witnessing in art therapy, *Inscape*, 1: 19–22.

Luzzatto, P. and Gabriel, B. (1998) Art psychotherapy, in J. Holland (ed.) *Psycho-oncology*. New York, Oxford: Oxford University Press.

Pratt, M. and Wood, M.J.M. (eds) (1998) *Art Therapy in Palliative Care: The Creative Response*. London: Routledge.

Schaverien, J. (1998) Individuation, countertransference and the death of a client, *Inscape*, 3(2): 55–62.

Schaverien, J. (1999) *The Revealing Image*. London: Jessica Kingsley.

Schaverien, J. (2000) The triangular relationship and the aesthetic countertransference in analytical art psychotherapy, in A. Gilroy and G. McNeilly (eds) *The Changing Shape of Art Therapy*. London: Jessica Kingsley.

Schaverien, J. (2002) *The Dying Patient in Psychotherapy*. Basingstoke: Palgrave Macmillan.

Skaife, S. (1993) Sickness, health and the therapeutic relationship, *Inscape*, Summer: 24–9.

Thomas, G. (1998) What lies within us, in M. Pratt and M.J.M. Wood (eds) *Art Therapy in Palliative Care: The Creative Response*. London: Routledge.

Wood, M.J.M. (1998) The body as art: individual session with a man with AIDS, in M. Pratt and M.J.M. Wood (eds) *Art Therapy in Palliative Care: The Creative Response*. London: Routledge.

Art therapy with a late adolescent cancer patient: reflections on adolescent development, separation and individuation, and identity form

Kathryn Horn Coneway

This chapter will describe the developmental tasks of late adolescence and discuss ways in which a cancer diagnosis may impact on this developmental stage. The case material focuses on a client diagnosed with lymphoma at age 19. Her work in art therapy reflected her developmental stage and the difficulties of achieving the goals of this stage due to her illness and treatment. The artwork reflects a progression from a passive, dependent and depressed emotional state to a more active, autonomous and related state.

The case material and discussion explores active and passive stages of creative activity, the way creativity can aid in the process of individuation and the role of the art therapist as a witness and guide in creative therapy. The therapy took place in a large hospital in Washington, DC. We met weekly for individual sessions over a period of seven months, during the time of the client's active chemotherapy treatment and in the months immediately following her treatment. The work described combines the use of traditional art materials with photographs created within the sessions. Treatment goals focused on issues concerned with adolescent individuation and identity formation in relation to the challenges of the lifestyle changes required by her diagnosis.

Theories of adolescent identity development, separation and individuation

Meeks and Bernet (2001) described late adolescence as extending from ages 17 to 20. He wrote: 'The developmental emphasis during this time is on autonomy from parents; emotional investment in a significant relationship with another person; and commitment to a general career area' (p. 7). Muuss (1988) wrote about Blos' theory of a second individuation process in adolescence:

> Blos stresses the separation experience from parental dependencies and familial love objects as a crucial task for normal adolescent development, an idea he refers to as the second individuation process (Blos 1979). This developmental process of adolescence requires a partial regression to earlier stages of development, which is necessary not as a defense mechanism but in the service of adolescent development (Blos 1979).
>
> (Muuss 1988: 87)

The role of the peer group becomes increasingly important for adolescents and often replaces the family as a primary support group.

> The peer group can become an emotional alternative to the family, a substitute family. One danger is that the family dependencies will be replaced by permanent peer group dependencies, with emotional independence remaining unresolved.
>
> (Muuss 1988: 91)

According to Blos, late adolescence is the period in which the ego is stabilized and organized and part of this process involves gaining a sense of autonomy and separation from the parents (Muuss 1988).

Erikson's description of the adolescent stage of development relates to Blos' ideas about the organization and stabilization of the ego. Erikson refers to the conflict of the adolescent phase of development as identity versus identity confusion; this is a time when an individual establishes a sense of personal identity (Muuss 1988). Identity is not given to an individual but must be achieved through effort. Muuss describes Erikson's theory that 'unwillingness to work actively on one's identity formation carries with it the danger of role diffusion, which may result in alienation and a sense of isolation and confusion' (p. 60).

These psychoanalytically based theories of adolescent development are reflected in the work of the client I will describe. Additionally, theories from the object relations approach relate to the process of separation and individuation and are applicable to my relationship and work with the client. According to Malchiodi (2003),

> Therapists who subscribe to an object relations approach to treatment believe that humans have an innate drive to form and maintain relationships and it is through our relationships with people around us that shapes our personality . . . Helping clients with issues of separa-

tion and individuation, dependence and independence, and intimacy
are intrinsic to this approach.

(Malchiodi 2003: 53)

Malchiodi further describes the role of art-making in this approach. 'Art
adds a dimension to therapist–client interactions because it creates a setting
in which individuation and separation can be witnessed, practiced, and mas-
tered through creative experimentation and exploration' (p. 54). These ideas
relate to Winnicott's (1953) concept of transitional space and the function of
the therapist as creating a safe holding environment for material the client
wishes to explore during the session.

Case material

Mary [a pseudonym to protect client confidentiality] was a 19-year-old
Caucasian female who was diagnosed with lymphoma in August. She began
chemotherapy in September and came to the hospital for chemotherapy treatments every three weeks. She met weekly with me for individual art therapy
at the hospital, beginning in October. I also visited her during her last two
chemotherapy treatments and worked with her before, during and after her
infusion. A chaplain, who was meeting with Mary's mother for spiritual
counselling, referred Mary to the paediatric team. She was concerned about
meeting Mary's psychosocial needs; Mary's mother had expressed concern
about Mary's depressed affect and angry physical outbursts at home.

Mary seemed to enjoy art therapy and was comfortable expressing herself
with the materials. Many of her issues focused around questions, fears and
anxiety about her illness and treatment. Additionally, lifestyle changes
required by her treatment had been difficult. She had to adjust to living at
home and being dependent on her parents again after a year away at college.
Her former college boyfriend had begun dating one of her friends and she
felt upset that her friends' lives seemed to go on so easily without her. Mary
reported that her mother had a history of depression and was taking anti-
depressants. She and her mother seemed to have a close, emotional and often
conflicted relationship. She expressed that both she and her mother felt
regret and responsibility for not having gone to the right doctor earlier so the
cancer could have been diagnosed and treated sooner.

Mary's work progressed through several phases in the time I worked with
her. Initially she created mandalas that seemed to contain and depict her
sense of despair, hopelessness and helplessness. Using the circular form of
the mandala, she created watercolour faces, expressing sadness and frustration about having to live at home and longing for the previous year when she
had been healthy and had an active life away at college. It was clear from our
discussion that her relationship with her mother was also a source of stress

and her mother was frustrated with her for wanting to be back at college; she continually reminded Mary of the times the previous year that had not been as positive and of how her friends had let her down.

A second phase of imagery related to Mary's feelings about her friends from college whom she still visited on weekends when she was feeling well. She created bold abstract designs depicting intense feelings particularly about her former boyfriend and her friends who still associated with him. These images seemed to mark a shift from more passive to more active emotions, from hurt and despair to anger, which spurred her to action. She began to look for things she could do to fill her time at home so as not to spend time dwelling on past hurts. Her increased activity seemed to be affirming and helped her to feel more connected to others in spite of being isolated by her illness.

Throughout this time, my role was mainly that of a witness and guide, offering space and time to create and reflect on her images. Additionally, I served a role of mirroring and reflecting her emotions and concerns, helping her to express and process them through the artwork and through our inter-actions. Incorporating photography into our work together seemed to be a way to encourage further self-reflection and a way to reflect on aspects of her identity. I presented Mary with the idea of taking pictures as a way of exploring her sense of identity and showed her images created by women who had worked with photographer Wendy Ewald (1998). I explained that she could pose in the images herself or could bring in objects to stand in for her or to pose with to create images.

The following week, Mary brought in a collection of objects from home and as she described each one I was able to learn more about her support system and her relationships with family and friends; I was able to see more of her strengths through this process. Many of the objects were things people had given her as tokens to represent their thoughts, prayers and care after her diagnosis. She also brought in objects depicting things she was proud of, such as getting into college and performing in a school play. Mementos of her grandmother prompted her to tell the story of her grand-mother's death a few months earlier and objects representing her mother gave me insight into the family's religious and spiritual practices. The objects Mary brought in enabled her to symbolically bring her family and friends into the session and allowed me to see the strengths she had in her relationships to others.

Mary first arranged her objects and photographed them in different configurations. I offered to take pictures for her if she wanted to pose with the objects. We spent the majority of the session acting as photographer and subject; I took pictures and she posed to depict different emotions or held objects to represent her relationships with different people. This photo ses-sion seemed to represent another shift in our work, one in which Mary was putting more of herself into the images literally and symbolically. I took a more active role as a co-creator and the relationship required a deeper level of trust between us. I was conscious of using my creative and artistic skills in framing her poses and creating sensitive portraits. Through the photographs, I hoped to be able to help her further reflect on her identity and her emotions. I was also sensitive to the dynamic created with me as the photographer and she as the subject. I wanted her to feel ownership of her portraits and encouraged her to direct me as I operated the camera.

In the following session, Mary worked with Xerox copies of the photographic images and created a collage (Figure 9.1, on website) depicting different emotions. She worked more slowly on this project and seemed less confident and decisive than in her earlier work. She said it was more difficult working with images of herself. In the end Mary decided on a circular form, depicting eight different emotions, with an image of her hand holding a cross in the centre, symbolizing her faith. She described the emotions as different levels and manifestations of sadness, confusion and anxiety and said she felt she cycled through these emotions frequently. The form seemed reminiscent of her early mandalas, although the configuration of this circle seemed to indicate more movement and more of a sense of wholeness. At the time Mary created her image, she was halfway through her chemotherapy. She felt it was unfinished and at the end of the session she suggested she might want to add more to it later. She took additional copies of the pictures with her to work with at home and also reported that she had purchased soft chalk pastels and had begun creating pictures outside the session. It was several weeks before she returned to the collage but she reported back to me about the artwork she was doing with the photographs in her journal. She seemed to like the photos but shared that she felt more pressure to 'get it right' when working with them. It seemed it was more comfortable for her to do some of this work privately in her journal. The opportunity to self-reflect encouraged another shift in Mary's artwork; she began to bring more of herself and her immediate feelings about her situation into her drawings and paintings.

Three images created shortly after Mary began her collage relate specifically to her struggle with separation and individuation as an adolescent. This work was done on the infusion floor before and during her chemotherapy treatment. Mary had reported that her past chemotherapy treatments had been upsetting and anxiety-provoking for her and I hoped that I might be able to assist her by being present. When I arrived she was alone and crying behind a curtain, still waiting for her medications to be ready. She was frustrated about the timing of her treatment just before a holiday and was anxious about receiving the infusion. Her mother stopped by to say she was leaving to run an errand and, as soon as she left, Mary decided she would like to draw her mother and chose to work with oil pastels. Her image (Figure 9.2, on website) depicted her mother as a large head covering the second floor of her home. The trees on either side of the house appear to grow together over it and she described them as adding to the overall trapped feeling of being in her house and with her mother. A second image (Figure 9.3, on website) depicted a round face with a question mark in place of features. Around it were four sets of features showing different expressions; the features of these faces seemed old and wrinkled. Mary described this image as relating to her feeling about being so young when most of the others around her receiving treatments were much older. She said she felt that others looked at her with sadness and pity or that seeing her made them want to ask how this could happen to someone so young. It seemed these questions also related to Mary's own feelings and concerns about her illness and why it happened to her at such a young age. She created a third image (Figure 9.4, on website), a mandala, depicting her feelings of anger and sadness. She explained that the dark blue shapes depicted sharp tears and the red represented anger. The sharp tears were more serious and painful than tears she used to cry over 'silly things' like worrying about a test. She said the black shape depicted a shutter she had broken when she threw something out of anger at home. The mandala seemed to help her contain and recognize intense emotions. This was the first time she had told me about her outbursts of anger at home in which she threw things. Our session ended abruptly when the nurse came with her chemotherapy and Mary, her nurse, a friend and I shared conversation as she worked on taking deep breaths and relaxing her body during the infusion. Using the art to express and contain emotions before her treatment seemed to help Mary relax and this seemed to help things to go more smoothly with the infusion.

It was interesting to me that Mary's work shifted in this way and that she made such personal images in a somewhat public setting on the infusion floor of the hospital. The chairs for patients were arranged into alcoves but there were interruptions throughout her process from medical staff and from patients and visitors walking past. Her ability to focus and express herself in this space seemed to relate to the fact that we had established a therapeutic alliance so she could use our relationship and the art materials to create a transitional space even within this different environment.

These three images seemed particularly related to Mary's process of individuation and identity formation. The image of her mother and home was the first she had made about her mother and seemed prompted by her mother's presence in the setting. Her mother was clearly a source of stress during her infusions. Drawing her mother connected in this way to her home seemed to relate her mother to a source of nurturance but one that was overpowering; she felt trapped in her house and with her mother. The trees appeared sickly and added to the overall feeling of being trapped and smothered. Even the door outlined in red seemed to reflect anger and hurt that began upon entering the house. Creating this symbol for her relationship with her mother seemed to help Mary to calm herself and she seemed to find a sense of satisfaction and even some amusement in the drama of the image.

In the second image, Mary placed herself in the centre but she has a question mark instead of a face. The hair around the face is different from her natural hair or her wig and seemed to suggest a child much younger than she with babyish curls. This seemed to reflect identity confusion and uncertainty. She described the faces around her as all older than her and said she felt they stared at her and questioned her. Being treated in the adult clinic of the cancer hospital, the patients around Mary were mostly much older than she. Having been separated from her peer group by her illness, she recognized she clearly did not fit in with this new peer group of other cancer patients.

The third image contained both anger and sadness; the shutter referred to how she sometimes impulsively acted on these intense feelings. This image seemed important because it was the first time Mary had told me about the incidents that had initially caused her mother to request help for her. She seemed to feel comfortable enough to share this part of herself and her image also suggested she was starting to feel more able to contain and express this sort of feeling. In subsequent sessions we brainstormed ways Mary might use art materials to express and discharge anger when she felt like throwing something.

Wilson (1985) described how art therapy could help patients to see and understand their emotions and to represent them symbolically, decreasing impulsive behaviour. She wrote:

> As art therapists, when we ask our patients to make pictures or sculptures when they are under pressure to act or behave impulsively, we are seeking to help them delay peremptory drive discharge and instead put their feelings, thought, or fantasies into visible form. We do so by attempting to impose a conscious intervening factor that allows the patient to momentarily 'see' what is in his mind.
>
> (Wilson 1985: 129–30)

Mary was able to create images depicting how she felt trapped and uncertain of herself in her first two images. Her third image seemed to be an expression of her ability to contain the impulse to act on her anger and frustration. The artwork served to help her see her feelings, making them less intense and decreasing her drive to act on them. By containing the emotions in the artwork, she was able to calm herself and to have a more positive experience during her chemotherapy treatment. When I visited Mary during her last treatment three weeks later, she had chosen to bring a friend along instead of her mother and remained composed and calm throughout the procedure. This decision seemed to reflect an ability to integrate and learn from the earlier experience and to begin to assert some autonomy by asking that her friend attend instead of her mother.

Minar (1999) described how cancer patients often create symbolic images in their work.

Cancer patients in individual or group art therapy often create images of 'the hurter' living in their house and 'the healer,' an image which helps the person begin to heal or help the hurt. 'Hurter' images may be of the disease itself, of their feelings as they work through their personal grief, or of the ways in which their lives have been changed.

(Minar 1999: 229)

In her three images, Mary explored different facets of that which was hurting her: her suffocating relationship with her mother, her own insecurity and uncertainty, her disease, and the difficult emotions she felt in response to her illness. As her treatment neared its end, she also began to be able to create more healing images and to begin to explore her feelings and options for the immediate future when treatment was complete.

In our next session, Mary spontaneously created an image depicting how fragmented she felt and she contrasted this to the time before her illness when she had felt more whole. I suggested Mary create two images – one of her internal critic, the voice in her head when she feels hurt and depressed and the other of a safe and nurturing voice or place. I suggested exploring some of the parts of her self in order to possibly envision a new whole.

She began with the inner critic (Figure 9.5, on website), creating the image with white pastel on black paper. She identified the dot as herself and described the fingers as pulling her in to the mess and chaos inside where she would get lost. She felt the fingers related to others' opinions of her and her doubts about her own ideas. Mary described this image as representing times when she was with others but felt invisible and withdrawn. She felt this way in particular in response to a particular group of friends at her college, those associated with her ex-boyfriend. Mary added the red hammers, saying they represented the way her sense of self got crushed once it was pulled inside. She identified messages from the inner critic, including 'you're not good enough', 'you don't matter' and 'you should just get over it'. I expressed my concern for the small dot and asked if she could create another image depicting a safe place for the dot, somewhere it felt supported and affirmed.

In describing her second image (Figure 9.6, on website), Mary explained that the dot was in the centre with a circle of yellow figures around it representing her family and close friends, people who affirmed and supported her. The blue wavy lines represented her relationships and connections with these people and the outer white circle depicted how she felt she was able to expand. The finger-like shapes on the right and left were reminiscent of the fingers in the inner critic and they again represented others' opinions. In this image, these are outlying and available to her but do not overtake her or even surround her. She called the image 'Growth, positive, expanding' and said the messages coming from it included: 'You are strong', 'You will get through this', and 'You are worth it'. In discussing these images, Mary was able to recognize how different situations and relationships activated her in different ways. Creating the images and externalizing different parts of herself seemed to help Mary to explore these parts and gain greater awareness of their influence on her.

It was interesting that in these images, the client's mother and other family members were identified in the circle of support, representing a change from an earlier view when they were seen as a source of stress. This seemed to reflect a more balanced view of her family members and her relationship to them. There was also a more balanced view of her peer group. She seemed able to recognize that some friends were closer and more supportive than others and this reflected a move toward a more individual sense of judgement and identity. The first image again depicted an aspect of what hurt her while the second image represented a move toward a more healing symbol.

An image of a tree (Figure 9.7, on website) that Mary created in our next session during her final chemotherapy treatment also reflected growth and represented a contrast to the earlier trees in the image with her mother. She described the image as a tree with two branches and as a divided path. It represented her future after her treatment and two potential paths, one in which she would return to her college in another part of the country and another in which she would attend college near the hospital in order to be close by for follow-up appointments. The yellow on the path to the left reflected her desire to return to her college and her feeling that this would be the better path. The green leaves on the tree seem fairly balanced on both sides and she stated that she was able to see potential for growth in both options. The small green dot depicted her place on the path at the time the image was created. She seemed to have a sense of calm about the uncertainty and an acceptance of her lack of control over the outcome. Although the future contained many uncertainties she was able to begin to look toward it, to imaging possibilities and prepare herself for challenges ahead.

Mary completed the tree during her final chemotherapy infusion and we used the following session to revisit and reflect on her artwork created over the course of her treatment. After reviewing all of her artwork, Mary returned to the photo collage she had done in our earlier session; she remembered she had left it unfinished and chose to end the session by adding to the image with tissue collage (Figure 9.8, on website). She added blue around and between the outer images and a ring of yellow orange around the centre. She cut a small piece from each of the emotion pictures and pasted these around the centre, explaining that the emotions had been so difficult that she felt each had taken a piece of her. She acknowledged that she had gained insight but also that she had lost something along the way. The image at the top, which she described as her game face, was the only image that she did not cut a piece from. Mary described the completed image as representing her emotional cycle throughout her chemotherapy. At the bottom she wrote something the doctor had told her at the beginning of her treatment, 'We have to make you miserable in order to get you better.' She added her own words, 'The cycle of chemotherapy, half-way through feeling completely devastated and upside down, in the center a ring of hope.' It was interesting that she had begun this image about halfway through her treatment when she described feeling most upset. At the time, she had not intended the emotional images to represent any particular progression but, in looking back at them, she described how they grew more painful and intense toward the bottom of the circle and less so toward the top. She described her current feeling state as sort of numb and felt that the image to the left of the top image depicted this feeling. She seemed pleased with the image when it was complete and it seemed to offer a sense of closure and time to reflect on the overall experience of her treatment.

The collage Mary created using her photos was an example of a combination of active and passive phases of creation (Cane 1983). She began the piece midway through her treatment but then let it sit unfinished for a while, bringing it out to add to it and further reflect on its meaning when her chemotherapy was complete. Cattaneo and Malchiodi (1988) wrote about parallels and connections between the creative process and the therapeutic process. Mary's process related to the stages of encounter Cattaneo described; the initial encounter with the image and the deeper experience of encounter with the meaning of the image. The initial encounter with the image happened when Mary first created her collage but a deeper encounter with its meaning occurred when she returned to complete the piece and recognized the emotional cycle it represented.

Lachman-Chapin (1983) and Rubin (1982) both described how art therapists use their creative and artistic abilities in working with clients. I found that taking photographs of Mary allowed me to use my creativity to support her process and this helped to deepen our relationship. Creating photographs was a collaborative effort and allowed me to take a more active role in helping her to reflect on her identity. I believe the success of this intervention was influenced by my past experiences as a photographer, which allowed me to take on this role with confidence and sensitivity.

Additionally this work had an element of performance to it, which appealed to Mary's interest in drama and theatre. She had been a dancer and a drama major at college and had been active in these activities for a long time. McNiff (1992) has written about using performance art as a way to extend and deepen a dialogue with visual images. He wrote:

Performance art relates to images that have emerged from paintings and helps the actor to establish bonds to feelings and images that have been 'inwardly experienced.' The performance offers both the opportunity to reenter the feeling of the experience and to travel to yet another place . . . Performers describe how the enactment 'moves something' . . . they describe how it is the engagement of the body that deepens the work.

(McNiff 1992: 126–7)

For Mary, our photography session allowed her to create outward expressions of feeling states she experienced. Viewing the images she created, using body language and expression, helped her to reflect on her feeling states on a deeper level and to bring more of herself into her emotional imagery.

A note about post-treatment

My work with Mary continued for approximately four months immediately following her cancer treatment. At this time we continued to focus on her sense of self and integrating the treatment experience. She faced new challenges because she transferred to a new college and struggled with wanting to fit in but feeling very different from others as a result of her experiences. Artwork and photography again helped her to express her feelings of loneliness and isolation. By this time she was well-versed in using her artwork as tools of self-expression and even shared her pictures with some of her friends as a way to try to share with them what she had been through. At the time we ended treatment she seemed confident in her ability to use her art-making as a coping tool and shared that she intended to continue with her visual journalling.

Conclusion

My work with Mary, a late adolescent cancer patient, reflected her stage of development as well as how her illness impacted on her ability to achieve the tasks of this stage. The tasks of late adolescence involve separation from family, investment in a significant relationship and making plans for a career and future. Due to her illness and the need for chemotherapy treatment, Mary was forced to live at home and return to a status of being very dependent on her parents. At the same time she ended a significant relationship and felt a sense of loss and betrayal as she watched her ex-boyfriend move on to a new relationship while she was too ill to be out and meeting anyone. In the face of great uncertainty about her health, it was difficult to plan for or even imagine her future.

Estelle (1990) described how artistic expression could be especially helpful for adolescents who are feeling alienated from others. In the different phases of our relationship, Mary's work explored integrating new aspects of her identity as a cancer patient. Exploring and expressing relationships and emotions through her artwork helped her to move toward achieving a sense of identity and working through a second individuation process.

Mary's work in art therapy helped her to express and contain intense emotions related to her illness and treatment. When I first began seeing her,

her images were passive and she seemed depressed and without much hope. She and her mother had a close and conflicted relationship; Mary recognized that her mother contributed to her stress and frustration but at the same time she needed and depended on her mother to care for her. There was a conflict in her desire to break away from her parents but also her need for them to support her through her illness and treatment. Separated from her peer group, she struggled with issues related to identity and belonging. Art therapy helped Mary to symbolically act out and explore her emotions, giving her a safe place to respond to and reflect on her experience and relationships. Additionally, photography therapy interventions helped her to examine more directly her sense of self and how her identity was affected by her diagnosis and treatment. Once she was able to contain and symbolize her emotions and conflicts, Mary also began to be able to gain some sense of autonomy and to begin to explore and accept her new identity as a cancer patient. This was evidenced by Mary taking a more active role in managing her illness and treatment.

References

Cane, F. (1983) *The Artist in Each of Us* (revised edition). Craftsbury Common, VT: Art Therapy Publications.

Cattaneo, M.K. and Malchiodi, C.A. (1988) Creative process/therapeutic process: parallels and interfaces, *Art Therapy*, 5(2): 52–8.

Estelle, C.J. (1990) Contrasting creativity and alienation in adolescent experience, *The Arts in Psychotherapy*, 17: 101–7.

Ewald, W. (1998) All kinds of veils, *Double Take*, 4(3): 68–77.

Lachman-Chapin, M. (1983) The artist as clinician: an interactive technique in art therapy, *American Journal of Art Therapy*, 23: 13–25.

McNiff, S. (1992) *Art as Medicine: Creating a Therapy of the Imagination*. London, Boston, MA: Shambhala Publications.

Malchiodi, C.A. (2003) Psychoanalytic, analytic, and object relations approaches, in C.A. Malchiodi (ed.) *Handbook of Art Therapy*. New York: Guilford Press.

Meeks, J.E. and Bernet, W. (2001) *The Fragile Alliance: An Orientation to Psychotherapy of the Adolescent*, 5th edition. Malabar, FL: Krieger Publishing Company.

Minar, V. M. (1999) Art therapy and cancer: images of the hurter and healer, in C.A. Malchiodi (ed.) *Medical Art Therapy with Adults*. London: Jessica Kingsley.

Muuss, R.E. (1988) *Theories of Adolescence*, 5th edition. New York: McGraw-Hill.

Rubin, J. (1982) The search for formula, or how to use one's own creativity in art therapy, in A. DiMaria (ed.) *Art Therapy: Still Growing*, pp. 121–2. Alexandria, VA: AATA, Inc.

Wilson, L. (1985) Symbolism and art therapy, II. Symbolism's relationship to basic psychic functioning, *American Journal of Art Therapy*, 23: 129–33.

Winnicott, D. (1953) Transitional objects and transitional phenomena, *International Journal of Psychiatry*, 34: 89–97.

10 The Healing Journey: a ten-week group focusing on long-term healing processes

Elizabeth Goll Lerner

Introduction

The Healing Journey is a ten week programme developed to invite people to experience their illness and wellness from the perspective of the whole person, as an opportunity to emerge into a sense of balance, wholeness and integration. It is for people involved in long-term healing processes from illness or injury or who have been dealing with recurrence of similar symptoms or illness over a long period of time (such as cancer, diseases of the blood, chronic fatigue syndrome, chronic pain, pre-menstrual syndrome (PMS)). It is also appropriate for people who have survived a significant illness and are continuing to feel the effects of that experience. The group explores the life changes that occur because of illness or injury; the journey that takes place during the healing process; the spiritual aspect of the experience; the definition of wellness and the relationship between the physical discomfort or illness and the person going through it. The group includes discussion, work with art materials, selected readings, guided imagery and movement based on the ability of the participants. Techniques and topics are subject to change based on innovation and the group that has formed. The programme takes place in the Washington DC metropolitan area, which includes Maryland and Virginia.

Individuals with life-threatening and serious illness or injury often find themselves in the necessary world of hospitals, physicians, radiology technicians, practitioners of complementary medicine and support groups, to name only a few. Each contact with a healing professional, group event and instructional use of time is a necessary step in the educational and treatment process of an illness. Patients I had contact with in various settings were interested in exploring their experience through a different lens.

I experienced a long-term healing process and learned that exploring the dimensions of such a process in depth brings forth amazing possibility in the evolution of the individual. I created this programme so that others might have the opportunity to witness and be witnessed as they undergo profound changes in psyche, surroundings, relationships, and view of the world. I wanted others to receive acknowledgement and support in the decisions they make, understanding they may gain or losses they may find themselves sustaining.

This programme was created because the experience of long-term illness/healing is a profound and multi-layered one. People react in different ways to the shock of a serious illness and significant changes in their lives. Regardless of the method or manner, the introduction of a significant illness puts one in a different position on the earth. That position needs attention and exploration and integration with what has been before.

Another impetus in the creation of this programme was to allow individuals with serious illness or injury to expand the criteria with which they viewed and so manifested their experience of being in a medical treatment process. It can be cataclysmic when life as we know it changes forever, through no choice of our own. Inherent in the group process is the opportunity to explore the shocking impact of this realization. The programme provides participants with an opportunity to identify themselves partly, but not solely, as patients with a serious illness, while maintaining an active participation in their own healing process. The way we categorize ourselves has a profound impact on our journey through healing.

Effort is taken to create an environment that will encourage the individual to utilize the perspective of 'the journey' in healing. For example, participants are encouraged to ask the following questions: What is emerging as a result of the experience of illness? Where am I on the path of this journey? What choices am I making and what turns do I take? What is driving me to make the choices that I am making? What do I feel is contributing to my wellness? How do I locate the part of myself I need to use to guide me through his journey?

The Healing Journey is a psycho-educational programme, which involves looking at a variety of milestones/issues from the four perspectives outlined earlier: the physical; the emotional; the psychological; the spiritual. Each group session involves discussion of the assigned readings in conjunction with guided imagery/meditation involving personal responses, that session's topic, work with art materials and continued discussion. Movement and sacred circle dance is incorporated, based on the abilities of the group members. The goals of this programme are to help the participants to integrate these four aspects of being in relation to their illness, their relationship with their illness, their relationships (significant others, children, friends, doctors, care givers and so on), and the significance of the transition they are in. It is a programme in which the individual finds commonality not only with the group members, but also with the authors selected. Participants are invited to find a voice that relates to their essential experience and their authentic self.

A complete exploration of inner and outer experience takes place. For example, participants may discuss how they feel about their body in one session and the reaction of a family member to their illness in another. In both instances the focus is on tuning into or mobilizing aspects of the self in the service of the whole person and the creative and healing energy within the individual.

Participants are not only exploring their physical experience by identifying pain or concerns, changes in abilities or the healing of surgical wounds; they may also be tuning into the cells in their body through guided imagery or meditation and visualizing healing energy affecting all the cells of the body. Individuals may be exploring how their physical being is affecting their thoughts or feelings, or their connection to specific ideas about spirituality. Through this examination, individuals may move from being at war with, or let down by their body to being in conversation with, or even embracing their body. Identifying how one feels about one's body and various parts of it is critical to getting a clear view on all levels of the physical experience and how that experience is serving various aspects of the self.

When concentrating on the emotional experience of being in a long-term healing process, not only are feelings identified and addressed but also how they manifest or precipitate physical, emotional, psychological and spiritual changes in the individual.

Each topic involves a fleshing out of these considerations. Thus there is a focus on utilizing resources, which may support the healing process. Attention is paid to everyday life and transitions or transformations that occur during a long-term healing process. Selected readings are handed out and recommended (although not mandatory) for each session. Discussion, guided imagery/meditation and use of art materials are all significant aspects of the programme. Movement or meditative circle dance is sometimes added depending on the group which has gathered.

Once the group experience is complete there have been many opportunities to integrate essential aspects of the act of being in a healing journey and explore ways to optimize daily living within the complexity of this journey.

Issues that are key during the group process are:

- relationship with: self; significant others; children; caretakers; friends; doctors; other treatment providers; illness; wellness; outside world;
- control;
- fear/panic;
- loss;

- isolation;
- mourning;
- death;
- birth;
- wholeness;
- balance;
- emergence;
- Questions: Who am I becoming? How does that affect all the relationships listed above?
- How am I using or do I use the experience of my illness?
- How am I able to assess my next steps and the decisions I must make?
- Who are my partners in healing?

Benefits for participants:

- When individuals have a serious illness their world tends to revolve around the illness. It is as if the illness or the fact of the illness dictates life's every move. Participation in this group opens the lens and allows the individual to live life incorporating the necessities of living with an illness but not being controlled by it.
- They have the experience of commonality and exposure to others involved in the healing process.
- Through personal exploration, readings and group involvement they have the opportunity to gain some detachment from their illness and develop other methods of viewing life with an illness and a recovery process.
- They have an opportunity to be exposed to persons in all stages of recovery.
- They can evaluate their position in relation to their illness/recovery from a variety of perspectives. A brief explanation follows.

Physical perspective

Anything that relates to the body can be covered. Some examples are:

- the body and how it feels, significant physical problems such as pain, fatigue, numbness;
- remedies or treatments the individual has experienced;
- exercise;
- diet;
- how one moves through space;
- appointments with physicians and other related practitioners;
- sexuality;
- body image.

Emotional perspective

How do individuals or the group feel about what is occurring in their lives? What is the emotional relationship they have with their illness? What relationships are affected because the individual is in a long-term healing process?

Psychological perspective

What are the person's thoughts? How do thoughts about the illness/recovery affect their emotions and physical well-being? How does one interpret medical information? What is communication like with the practitioners involved? What is the quality of the relationship with the practitioners involved? What do individuals think about the readings? What do they think about the way relationships are going in their lives? What is the effect of their illness or injury on various aspects of their lives?

Spiritual perspective

What is it that individuals view as spiritual? How is that important or unimportant in their healing process or their lives? What have they noticed about faith or lack of it in relation to their illness/recovery? Is there a place for meditation or guided imagery? How do their thoughts about spirituality relate to the evolution of their healing process?

Programme description

Creating the environment

To establish an appropriate environment for this type of group one must think about what a 'holding' space or sacred space should consist of. Creating a sacred space is integral to the group's ability to think, breathe, exist out of a box and create an entity together, rich in continuous support and dialogue. In essence one must take the first step, creating the container within which to work.

A sacred space can be created anywhere. Discussion of the sacred in this context is not a discussion of religion or religious beliefs. It is a discussion of value and expansion; being held and flying out; complexity and simplicity. It is a paradox. Simply put, it is about setting apart a time and energetic space in which to honour one's own process and honour the process of each individual who sits with you in that space, in that time, for the duration of the ten-week process.

The agreement of a group of people, to make a time, a space, a meeting sacred takes only the agreement to do so. It is an agreement that within the prescribed purpose and chosen framework all will be honoured, all will be confidential and that the ears with which we hear and the leeway we allow ourselves to have is permitted to exist in the realm of possibility.

The definition of sacred is contextual. It is a setting apart from the rest of the world for a period of time during the group sessions to attend to an inner experience. It is the 'making special' by the group leader and the participants that sets this tone. The group leader must consciously and directly state that the time set for the group is a time to create a sacred or special environment in order to serve oneself and fellow group members embarking on this journey together.

A few flowers are also a good idea. The impact of flowers or other natural objects is more than aesthetic. It is extremely important to bring some quality of the natural world into the room. A flower, plant, rock or shell brings in life force energy, the premise being that there is energy all around us that we can tap into and utilize for our benefit. The natural world reminds us that there is something outside each of our bodies that has a life force, and that we can tap into that life force in whatever way is suitable for the individual. If this programme takes place in a hospital setting, or members have particular sensitivities or allergies, precautions will need to be taken. Individuals usually participate in this programme after hospitalization. However, aspects of it may be used at any stage of illness or healing in any setting.

Outline

This is the itinerary of this programme. *I use the word itinerary as I do in the introduction of the first group session. This is a journey.* I am listing the session topics by weeks 1–10.

1 Introduction
2 The physical nature of the experience
3 The physical nature of the experience in relation to emotion, thought and spirit
4 The emotional nature of the experience
5 The emotional nature in relation to physical process, thought process and spiritual process
6 The psychological nature of the experience
7 The psychological in relation to the physical process, emotional process and spiritual process
8 The spiritual process
9 The spiritual in relation to the physical process, emotional process and thought process
10 Final group session. Wrap up

Group members are invited to explore the topic prior to group sessions by doing the assigned reading and by noticing changes that have occurred or are occurring. This can be by remembering a book or article that had meaning, a place or a flower; noticing a thread that travels through the experience even if no words are present to define it; exploring relationships with oneself and others. Participants are informed that over time reflecting on the previous weeks will make the exploration richer.

Each group session involves discussion of the assigned readings, guided imagery/meditation involving that session's topic, work with art materials and continued discussion. Movement and sacred circle dance is incorporated based on the abilities of the group members.

The readings

The readings relate to the topic of the week. The choice may be based in part on discussion in the previous group session. Should a change be made based on group content it would be an add-on to the list handed out at the first group meeting. It might be something read aloud during the group in order to tie in the focus of the previous group or a theme, running through the group process, that was considered important to highlight at a given moment in the life of the group.

Group composition

It is important to note that the group composition in the Healing Journey is not restrictive regarding diagnosis. The criterion for admission is to have or have had an illness or injury that has a long-term healing process and is impacting, or has impacted on an individual's life in a complex and significant way.

In general the group composition often involves cancer patients but may be quite varied. Typically patients with a similar diagnosis are grouped together in support groups or groups related to illness. I have found it quite beneficial to group together individuals with a variety of diagnoses in the enrolment of the Healing Journey. One significant benefit has been a more expansive participant view of the definition of illness, wellness and health. While it is certainly important for patients to have the experience of being with others who are facing the same or similar diagnosis or diseases, for some there comes a time when having a broader scope is extremely valuable. It is important to step outside oneself and the ethnocentrism of one's own illness in order to view the process of healing from a variety of perspectives and evaluate the definition of wellness for oneself.

The screening process

Phone interviews are conducted for screening purposes. Individuals who may not be appropriate for this particular programme at the time of interview are referred elsewhere. Some individuals may be appropriate candidates for the programme later on in their recovery process.

People respond differently to various stages of illness. Some may want to be reflective and focused from day one; others may need to participate in a group of this nature farther down the treatment road. It is important to evaluate readiness, just as one would for any group. Participants come with a wide range of interests and needs. Some are interested in exploring the spiritual; some want to have an opportunity to discuss their physical and emotional experience in depth; some want to attend to how they see themselves in the world as a result of their illness. Others wish to explore the ramifications their illness has had on their lives and relationships and some simply want to be around people who have undergone significant life changes due to illness or injury. There is always discussion of issues about death, pain and treatment, and where the experience of being in the face of death or an altered existence has taken one on the journey.

The creative process

The Healing Journey programme is a creative process. Each aspect of the group invites participants to create or re-create new ways of thinking, feeling or positioning themselves in relation to the topic of the day.

The use of art materials in each session allows the participants a variety of opportunities. It allows each member time and space to have a private experience during the group session. Using the materials provided in relation to the theme creates a relationship with the topic that integrates the four aspects (physical, emotional, psychological, spiritual) of concentration. After a check-in with group members and discussion of the topic, a guided imagery is done to focus individuals in their own process. The guided imagery is focused on the day's topic and is always related in some way to the natural world. Participants are asked to draw or paint images after the guided imagery. Work with clay is also encouraged if the setting and group make-up allows. They are given a specific focus but always invited to pursue anything that has bubbled to the surface that is of significance to them at the time.

The integration of other modalities with the use of art materials tends to bring issues closer to consciousness and creates an integrated flow of energy with which to work when using the materials. It is often a challenge at the beginning. Many participants are unfamiliar with using art materials, but drawing or painting from the source of one's energy is different from creating a still life. Once people become comfortable with the knowledge that the focus of art in an art therapy setting is on the individual's expression or statement rather than the perfection of the artistic criteria, they are set free of previously taught judgements about their work. Of course these differing expectations are introduced in the description of the group and in the first group meeting. Although this group is a psycho-educational one, it is stated that it is therapeutic in nature. The introduction and explanation of art materials is done from the perspective of art therapy.

The discussion of the topic of the day in connection with the guided imagery and the art-making, and then the further discussion of the art productions, creates an extraordinary number of touchstones on a topic throughout the day's session and within the 10-week process as a whole. Each time a topic is touched on it is fleshed out more and more. Aspects that could not be discussed or tolerated earlier come around again and again in ways that are unobtrusive and part of the sea of the journey.

There is a parallel process taking place between the topics discussed, the revolving nature of how each topic is touched upon from each of the four focal points, and the return to guided imagery and the making and discussion of artwork in each session. The images created continue to give clues to the participants' symbolic language and feelings, thoughts or decisions about a wide range of topics from many different points of view. The work viewed over time shows a great deal about the ground the group member has traversed.

Participants are offered the opportunity after completing the programme to meet individually with me to do a picture review of the 10 weeks and discuss their art and personal experience of the process. That meeting is scheduled as a separate session.

The end result is that each individual on completion of the programme has had many opportunities to find the position on the earth he/she believes he/she is in and would like to choose. Participants have had a chance to evaluate and process their feelings and thoughts about a wide variety of experiences, people and wishes and have a better sense of where they truly want to be in the landscape of their lives.

Having a serious medical illness or injury changes the face of the world. It changes both the inner and outer view, the sense of intactness, the perception of time. I used to say it was like being on the moon while being on earth. The individual goes through a parallel process within our very midst. People in a relationship with the individual believe they understand what is happening, but it is very difficult to understand the separateness of the experience of illness when one is well or has never been seriously ill. There is a different evaluation process around physical choices, be it activities or energy shared with a friend. The health-filled human body once taken for granted is changed. The task is how, and at what point in the process, one discovers how to reintegrate into a life on earth and what new or distinct qualities that life might have.

A group composition

The group to which I will be referring consisted of five women. The composition of the group consisted of participants with two varieties of cancer, an ailment related to organ function and PMS.

The ideal number for this group is six to eight participants. The total number is often reduced by one or two participants, for various reasons. The programme can be run with one or two additional participants but the group length would need to be extended to accommodate the numbers. The programme runs for 10 weeks and each session lasts two hours.

I will track one woman's participation through the group, touching on various points in the group process while giving a context of the group discussion and highlighting some of the readings. A suggested list of books can be found at the end of the chapter.

The woman, whom I will call Jill, was in her mid-forties upon interviewing for the group. Her hope regarding the group was to make connections with others and learn to live better with her disease (breast cancer). Her hopes for herself were to feel better about her changed self and her decreased ability to contribute to her community. She also wanted to relieve herself of the burden she felt she was carrying and move on. She was married with two children. She had many concerns about death, physical symptoms, treatment decisions, her life and her self-image as a result of her illness.

Depending on the age and the responsibilities of the individual certain issues will have more weight than others. Members with adult children were more focused on their own paths than on the needs of a family.

In the first group all members were quite frank about a variety of issues and told their stories. I learned at the following group session that much was stirred up. People came in stating that they had been quite affected by the first session and found that certain issues highlighted themselves as areas that needed continued attention. The journey had begun.

As with all art therapy groups the first picture often introduces the template of issues or concerns on which the person is focused. In this instance, Jill's picture focused on her hair and the decisions that surrounded it throughout treatment as well as the symbolic aspects of the evolution of the treatment process and being given care (Figure 10.1, on wetsite, entitled 'Acceptance', 'Connections' or 'Belonging'). It is a discussion of three relationships. The upper left corner symbolizes a night nurse who cared for her in the hospital and helped her make important decisions by encouraging her to follow her heart. The nurse cared for her and brushed her hair when Jill was unable to do so. The centre represents a woman from the beauty shop who washed her hair and who hugged her when she was well enough to return. She found it a surprisingly warm gesture. The third relationship pictured was with her son who was very excited when her hair fell out because it meant that the medicine was working. He was a big part of her healing inspiration. Caretaking, caregiving and trusting herself continued to be important aspects of this woman's progress.

The relationships that promote care and healing and especially inspiration or partnership in healing are the gold nuggets of the healing journey. It may be a family member, it may be a stranger and it may be a practitioner. These people may change during the journey but each has a gift to give that leads to the next step.

The issue that arose between sessions one and two for Jill was not new and was significant: the split between body and mind; a tendency not to want to pay attention to the physical. The picture drawn in the second session, 'Physical nature of the experience', depicts a brick wall dividing her head from her body. There is a link with the symbol of a book because she stated that reading helps to make the connection from body to emotion to spirit. There are question marks throughout the body that ask, What is it that the body knows that I don't? Lightning bolts symbolize recurrent head-aches and a dog is a link to feeling connected to nature and to herself and represents another significant relationship.

Much of the group process involves making a connection between the mind and the body. How do we have a dialogue, keep the wavelength open, be tuned in? And what information or wisdom do we glean by cultivating that integration?

Next I will discuss session four, 'Emotional nature of the experience'. We did a beautiful dance from Romania called 'The Midwives' Dance'. It is said to have been danced by the women in the community when a woman was in labour. It highlights community support and the power of bringing someone or something new into the world. It was in this group that Jill found herself in perspective within the community and within our circle. She drew a light blue angel in the centre of the paper that she said symbolized a spiritual connection and, on the right hand side, the yellow flowers that were the centrepiece in the group circle that day. The flowers had great vitality. She discussed her family beach vacation and discussed how difficult it can be to have needs that take us away from the expectations of a family while simul-taneously knowing that we must respond to our own needs. She drew the peaceful aspect of the vacation on the lower left. (Figure 10.2, on website.)

By the next session, still involving the emotional process, she was draw-ing in a completely different way with a great deal of strength. One of the readings in that session was about forgiveness, for which she did not feel she had a great capacity. She drew a brown mound with a black dot out of which grows a yellow rose bush with very strong blossoms and stems. The yellow roses are surrounded by white and by tears, and the picture is entitled, 'If only I could' (Figure 10.3, on website). She stated that the white was to show that the rose image was not real yet but this is what it would look like if it were. The fact that she chose not to obscure the roses in any way suggests that she is certainly in the process of moving towards her goals. There is a change in her work at this point. Her pictures have a different strength from this point forward. This drawing suggests that she is farther along than she believes. She is well on her way in the process of finding a sturdier ground. The next work, made in the same session, is a spiral which she visualizes when she 'wants to find her centre', called 'Trusting myself'.

Session seven, 'The psychological in relation to the physical, emotional, spiritual' brought forth a large willow with long roots, entitled 'I want to be a tree' (Figure 10.4, on website). There is a small pool from which the roots drink. She stated that the blue represents both water and sky as if the picture were circular – taking in the universe. The picture is interesting because the willow is quite large in comparison to the pool and the roots are long and deep. The tree really needs the water but is flourishing with the minimal offering and lack of grounding. The suggestion is that Jill has begun to flourish herself, begun to see what she might take from the universe and her surroundings, and has roots with which to become grounded. Her needs have become more defined, conscious and available as she begins to explore certain issues more fully. She exhibits her connection to nature and the health she feels when communing with nature. There is ambivalence about being grounded in the earth but the beginning of feeling solid and complete.

This picture and other themes discussed in the group illustrate the difficulty of being taken out of one's life, finding various strengths once again as well as new strengths from which to draw, and re-emerging with consciousness. People will have different sets of circumstances, thoughts, feelings and decisions about what their needs are when it is time to participate in life more fully and what it is they need to support their health and wellbeing. There are stages of re-entry, which vary from person to person in length. There are often many questions. Sometimes there is great clarity. There is the unanimous feeling that life is now lived differently – in this group, more honestly and fully.

In session nine, Jill drew a picture of those aspects of her life that assist her in making spiritual connections (Figure 10.5, on website). She drew her dogs because she communes in nature with them daily. She also drew an element of a story that dealt with a child taking his teacher, a Shaman, to his resting place, and then going off on his own journey to find himself. The elements of death and birth, endings and beginnings are a paramount theme for all group members. There is also the critical need to strive to find the place, the way, the person with whom one can be totally oneself. There is no time not to heed the voice from within.

In the final session, 'Closure' Jill is asking, 'Where am I going?' This is the title of her picture, which shows the page tilted in a diamond shape (Figure 10.6, on website). Out of the dark blue form come multicoloured threads reaching to the top of the page, through a bridge and a rainbow to a circle which corresponds with a circle at the bottom in the blue. The circle signifies a thumb print. She stated that the fingerprint represented who she is which is what she was trying to find out. She ended the journey with a question and a work that illustrated the myriad of questions and the length of time it takes to find the place where one wants to stand.

The atmosphere of this particular group was one of deep nurturing and support for each other and deep introspection and nurturing of oneself. Each group member brought a view from his/her own perspective that made significant impact on the others. The reflection of this impact enabled group members to pursue their individual needs or calling. This group, as others have, chose to work together with me for some time afterwards in other psycho-educational programmes and programmes created specifically for the evolution of their group.

Conclusion

Some people are focused on continuing the changes in their lives or behaviour that came about because of their illness or injury. Others want to heal from the effects of their illness.

Sometimes this programme is enough. Sometimes it is a doorway to further exploration. Often a thorough examination of the experience of illness and healing may close a chapter and allow one to begin anew, and sometimes the progress through the illness and beyond assists in highlighting that which needs attention in one way or another and begins another path.

Further reading

Excerpts from the list of books which follows have been assigned or read aloud at one time or another in this programme. This is not a complete list of books.

Carlson, Richard and Shield, Benjamin (eds) (1989) *Healers on Healing*. Los Angeles, CA: Jeremy P. Tarcher.

Cousins, Norman (1979) *Anatomy of an Illness*.

Duff, Kate (1994) *The Alchemy of Illness*. New York: Bell Tower.

Frank, Arthur (1991) *At the Will of the Body: Reflections on Illness*. Boston, New York, London: Houghton Mifflin Company.

Lansdowne, Zachary, F. (1986) *The Chakras and Esoteric Healing*. York Beach, ME: Samuel Weiser.

Levine, Stephen (1987) *Healing into Life and Death*. New York, London: Anchor Books, Doubleday.

Levine, Stephen (1991) *Guided Meditations, Explorations and Healings*. New York, London: Anchor Books, Doubleday.

Ponder, Catherine ([1966] 1985) *The Dynamic Laws of Healing*. Marina del Rey, CA: DeVORSS and Company.

Siegel, Bernie (1990) *Love, Medicine and Miracles*. New York, London: Harper and Row.

Thich Nhat Hanh (1991) *Peace Is Every Step: The Path of Mindfulness in Everday Life*. New York, London: Bantam Books.

Wilber, Ken (1991) *Grace and Grit: Spirituality and Healing in the Life and Death of Treya Killam Wilber*. Boston and London: Shambahla.

11 Musing with death in group art therapy with cancer patients

Paola Luzzatto

Introduction

Life is precarious and unpredictable. This is a truth that nobody can deny. Nevertheless, this truth comes to most cancer patients as a shocking realization. The awareness of one's vulnerability and mortality and the fear of the ultimate loss, the loss of the self, may lead to anxious feelings and thoughts and to a depressed state of mind. Most psychotherapists would agree that to be able to accept death as part of life, intellectually and emotionally, is a form of maturity and wisdom that may decrease the anguish caused by an illness like cancer. In this chapter I am going to suggest that art therapy offers a unique way of increasing awareness of the existential connection between life and death. I will illustrate this aspect of the art therapy modality with some examples taken from a variety of art therapy groups that I have led at Memorial Sloan-Kettering Cancer Center, New York, with patients diagnosed with different types of cancer, and at different stages of their illness. This chapter does not focus on the use of individual art psychotherapy with cancer patients, which in my opinion activates different therapeutic factors and would merit a separate chapter.

Art therapy and the 'third way'

For a long time, and in many cultures, doctors and relatives used to hide the truth of their illness from cancer patients, in order to protect them from the distressing thought of death. Slowly, for a variety of cultural and socio-logical reasons, cancer patients are not only becoming entitled to know their diagnosis but also being helped to deal with the reality of their illness. In many cancer centres all over the world, support groups are becoming available, and patients are encouraged to talk about their fears, and also about their fear of death.

The reality is not as simple, and there is no clear-cut answer. Health professionals have learnt to accept that while some patients need to share their negative thoughts and anxious feelings in a group, other patients need to protect themselves from a self-revelation that could increase their distress, and their 'not-wanting-to-talk', or 'wanting to talk about something else' has to be respected.

Also in art therapy it is possible to move in two opposite directions:

1 some patients may need to make images clearly focused on 'the negative': anger, fear and death, as a form of catharsis;
2 other patients may reject the white page, complaining of poor imagination, or they may draw pictures clearly focused only on 'the positive': peace, beauty and love, as a form of self-soothing, or as a form of denial.

These two extreme forms of self-expression are important. The art therapist must understand when they are functional and when they become dysfunctional for the patient; they may be used for defence, but they may be used for personal development, too.

Between the need to 'get rid of the negative', and the wish to be 'reassured and supported', art therapy also offers a 'third way'. This third way is part of a process that Bion would call a process of 'thinking'. This chapter is about moments in time, in a group art therapy setting, when some of our cancer patients have allowed the 'thought' of death to emerge, without rejecting it and without being overwhelmed. The patients have often been surprised by their image, and they have spent some time looking at it afterwards, together with the art therapist and the other patients, as a form of reflection, almost as a source of meditation. This 'third way' has a lot to do with the ambiguity and complexity of the symbolic language; it is characterized by the presence of several levels of meaning, and by a variety of feelings, especially 'negative and positive' feelings at the same time.

When a patient refers 'symbolically' to death – and this is what this chapter is about – there is a special atmosphere in the room. The art therapist and the other patients half know and half do not know what the patient is referring to. The patient half knows and half does not know what kind of image has emerged, and how meaningful it is, or will become. The skill of the art therapist is to accept and respect the image, to help the patient and the group to stay at that symbolic level as long as possible, to encourage a meditative attitude, free association and symbolic elaboration (Jung 1968). Here I have called this experience, for want of a better phrase, 'musing about death'.

The setting

Adult cancer patients often feel intimidated by the white page, maybe more than other patients. I have asked myself why, and I think that the white page may be a symbol of the unknown, and for cancer patients the unknown may be particularly frightening. This fear may block the patient's feelings and the patient's imagination and it may prevent the patient from being helped by art therapy.

In order to deal with this problem, which is quite common and may be frustrating for many art therapists who work in cancer centres, a number of years ago I started to offer a series of ten weekly art therapy workshops, called the Creative Journey, in which patients are guided and encouraged to explore different art materials and different techniques (such as collage, the squiggle, touch painting, and so on), so that the 'white page' does not dominate their mind and does not block their imagination.

It is my experience that during the ten weeks of the Creative Journey the patients lose the fear of the white page, and start to listen freely to the images emerging from their deeper selves. At the end of the ten weeks they often wish to continue art therapy, in order to develop further their symbolic language. In this case they may join another ten-week group that we call the Creative Journey II. Here they start the session with a white page in front of them, and this time they are familiar with the use of the art materials and art therapy techniques that they have learnt during the Creative Journey.

The patients may also attend a third type of group: the Drop-in Art Therapy Open Studio that is open from morning to evening one day a week. They may drop in any time during the day, and stay as long as they like, especially when they come to the hospital for treatment or for medical appointments. The art therapist is available to facilitate image-making in case an individual patient feels stuck. One wall in the room is covered by pictures made by previous patients: these images may be inspiring and they may help the newcomers to understand what art therapy is about.

The material selected for this chapter is taken from these three types of group interventions: the Creative Journey I & II and the Drop-in Open Studio. The three groups share the same basic rules, which I summarize as follows:

1 At the beginning of each session, the patients are encouraged to spend a few minutes in silence, to move their mind away from the outside world and towards the inner self, and they are encouraged to respect any image that may emerge during the session.
2 'Visual sharing' is emphasized. The patients will work individually, will give a title to their work, and will place the finished picture on a board on the wall. All patients will spend some time looking at each other's images, and reading the titles.

3 'Verbal sharing' is optional: the patients know that they are entitled to remain silent. Nevertheless, they usually like to share some feelings and thoughts about their image (content and meaning).
4 'Verbal feedback': any patient who has made a picture may ask for a feedback from the group. The feedback is neither an aesthetic judgement nor a psychological interpretation: it is a personal response, often in the form of a free association.
5 'Visual feedback' is encouraged. A patient may feel intrigued, or inspired, or disturbed by an image made by another patient, and may respond with another image, on the same day or during one of the following sessions.

Images about death

I will try to convey to the reader the experience of being in a group where an 'image about death' may emerge from one of the patients. I have been able to distinguish three main ways in which 'thinking about death' has developed in art therapy groups. These three categories may be called images from dreams, the death of loved ones and images about one's vulnerability and mortality.

Images from dreams

The three images from dreams that I report here were all made during different groups: the first one was made during the Creative Journey, the second one during the Drop-In Open Studio, and the third one during the Creative Journey II. Using a dream is a fairly safe and very evocative way to think about death. The image about death may be made and denied at the same time: 'It was just a dream!' When a patient makes an image of death from a dream, it is possible that he or she intentionally wants to move from the unconscious level of the dream to the more conscious level. Making the image does transform the dream, and talking about it does transform it even further (Freud 1980). At the end of this process the patient often feels 'different': something has happened, for the patient, and for the group.

'The guardian'

A patient started to play with brush and tempera, then a strange creature appeared on the paper: it looked like an illustration from a mythology book. A title was given: 'The Guardian'. The patient said the image was connected to a dream she had had some time previously, and she reported the dream to the group:

I was on a small boat. In the dream I knew the boat was taking me across a river, and this was the river separating the world of the living from the world of the dead. I was not scared; I was in the middle of Nature, and it looked like a natural process: it had to be like this. When I reached the other side of the river, a creature like this one appeared, stopped the boat and said: 'This is not your time. You have to go back. You will come when it will be the right time for you.'

She continued to talk:

I woke up. I was pleased to be alive. This dream has been important to me, but making this image has made it more real . . . I now feel that the passage to the other side is not so terrible: my time will come and I hope I will be ready.

The level of 'existential awareness' in the group was intensified. Another patient mentioned the pleasure of reading myths and fairy tales, and how important it was for her to deal with themes of life and death through mythological symbols. Another patient said: 'It must be good to go when one is ready . . .'. A silence followed, and it felt comfortable.

'Peaceful'

A patient came to the Open Studio saying that she had had a strange dream during the previous week, and she wanted to paint it. She used soft pastels, and she worked on the painting for a long time. The scene was of a coffin, with five people standing behind the coffin, in a semicircle. The Star of David was up on the wall, above the coffin. The title was 'Peaceful'. She told the art therapist that she had dreamt that she was dead, and in the dream she could look at her coffin from outside herself:

I saw five people standing near my coffin, still, silent, not threatening, almost protective. They were very similar one to the other, like shadows, not real people: I did not recognize any of them.

She said it was not a bad experience to have that dream, but it was a bit scary. Instead, she was surprised that it became a very good experience for her to paint this scene from the dream. She liked her picture, and she felt peaceful when looking at such a calm scene. Her drawing was placed on the wall, and remained on the wall for many weeks, because it was obvious that many patients coming to the Open Studio found the picture quite intriguing and liked to look at it, asked questions about it, and felt inspired by it.

'The trumpet'

During the Creative Journey II a patient started a collage. She obviously had the dream in her mind when she came in, as she started to look at the magazines in a very purposeful way, searching for landscapes. She worked very intensely to represent the beauty of the clouds in the sky and their colours, through a sophisticated use of the collage technique. She said she saw in the dream 'a lot of clouds, colourful and beautiful, moving in the sky', and she said:

> In the dream I was part of nature, on earth. Suddenly I heard a trumpet, I looked at the sky and I saw it was God's trumpet. I am not sure I saw God, but I saw the trumpet, and I heard the sound of it: in the dream I knew it was calling some people to die and to move to the sky with Him. I was on the earth, and I felt very small and I kept looking at this magnificent scene.

She did not say whether in the dream she was called to die or not; it seemed as though she was only 'looking'. An image by Michelangelo, found in one of the magazines on the table, was used to represent God. The beauty of the collage mitigated the frightening power of 'God'. She asked for feedback, and one patient responded to the beauty of the clouds; another patient said she felt very moved by the little flower in the meadow below, which reminded her of her childhood.

The death of loved ones

I have seen many cancer patients painting an image about death, then saying they were thinking of the loss of a loved one: a friend; a grandmother, a mother ... It was always difficult to understand whether the aim was to overcome the loss, or to 'think about' death, or their own death. In this section I will report on an intense, mainly non-verbal, interaction within a ten-week group of the Creative Journey II, with eight patients. The process was triggered by one image, entitled 'Transition', made during the first session: it became a kind of thread, which lasted for ten weeks, until the end of the group. It did not become the main theme in the group, but certainly one of the main themes. During the ten weeks, every patient in the group made at least one image about death! I will try to describe the process, which was both verbal and non-verbal.

1 *Transition*. This was the first image about death in the group, made during the first session. It was an abstract composition, made of two separate watercolour cards, each quite small, and painted with vertical coloured stripes: one started with red and ended with black; the other one started with black and ended with yellow. The work was entitled: 'Transition'.

   The patient explained that she was thinking of a friend of hers, who had died during the previous week. The black line in the centre indicated the moment of death, which was at the same time an end and a beginning. It was a spiritual image: she expressed her conviction that there was 'life beyond death'. This picture was looked at in silence, with some patients getting up from the table to look at it from close and read the title. It was obviously giving the others food for thought. This became even more obvious during the following weeks.

2   *Do not go gently.* On the second week, a patient made what she called the 'atheist' modified version: her black vertical lines in the centre of the page were thick and jagged, instead of being fine and vertical, and contained the sentence 'Do not go gently' (a line from a poem she remembered), which became her title. She told the art therapist and the other patients that she was not a believer in the afterlife, and she had to express her own image of death, which was not peaceful.

3   *The death of a child.* On the third week, another patient painted a child – a little girl – from the back, lifting her arms towards a beautiful rainbow, and said: 'This is the death of a child'. She added: 'Death must be different for a child!'

4   *Death and life.* Fourth week: a patient drew the profile of her two hands on paper, and then enriched the image with beautiful leaves and thin delicate branches, which were connecting the two hands. She said she was thinking of the death of a friend of hers; she wanted to represent death and everlasting friendship at the same time.

5   *'Looking at the sky'.* During the fifth week, a patient represented her dead grandmother as a large circle in the sky, almost a sun – or a full moon – with a face and body inside the circle, and she represented herself as a little child inside a little circle, on earth, with a little arm pointing towards the sky.

6   *The centre of my being.* The following week a patient repeated the theme of the dead grandmother. She found in a magazine a picture of an old lady playing the piano, and she placed it in the centre of the white page: around it, she glued other pictures from magazines, representing herself in different moments of her life. She explained that the picture in the centre was her grandmother, who used to play the piano, and the music she heard as a child was still inside her . . . 'maybe in the centre of my being . . .'.

7   *Mother, where are you?* A patient found in a magazine a picture of an archaeological site, with two archaeologists looking at some bones, in the shape of a skeleton, obviously found during an excavation. She gave this a title: 'Mother, where are you? Are you listening to me?' (This patient later asked for some individual sessions, to deal with her early feelings of abandonment, which were affecting her reaction to the cancer diagnosis.)

8   *Death as mystery.* This non-verbal dialogue about death, which had lasted for nine weeks, was given an ending by the powerful intervention of another patient during the last session. She painted with thick brush and tempera an evocative black and white abstract pattern, and called it 'Death as mystery'. It looked as if she wanted to give the group a pause in the exploration about death. Mystery is beyond what is known and what

is unknown; beyond agreement and disagreement. The answer from the group was a moved and respectful silence. A patient asked to get a copy of her image. 'I would like to frame it and keep it in my bedroom.'

Images about one's vulnerability and mortality

Natural catastrophes, like lightning, eruptions and earthquakes, are common symbols for the cancer diagnosis. They usually mean: 'I suddenly felt I was dying.' From that moment on, the images of vulnerability and mortality may be very different for each patient. It is important to give patients a chance to find their own symbolic language. They need to express and experience in a supportive environment how this basic awareness affects them. I mention some of the most recurrent symbols:

- *A black cloud.* A black cloud may threaten the person's life centre. This may be expressed in an abstract way, but sometimes it is the image of a real person who fights against a surrounding cloud.
- *An object in a precarious position.* It may be a rock on top of a mountain, or a man who walks on a rope, to express the precariousness of life after cancer.
- *A danger hiding in the background.* It may be a tiger behind a tree, or a bomb that may explode at any time.
- *The clock.* Clocks, of any shape and size, are often added to a painting, or to a collage, to say how the personal experience of time has changed.
- *The body is not the same any more.* This is expressed in a variety of ways: the body is fragmented, the body is fragile, the body is fighting . . .

It is quite common that a patient draws a symbol of vulnerability and mortality, and in the same picture adds a symbol of strength and life. Here the power of art therapy is particularly effective: what is not possible in the verbal process is possible with symbolic imagery. The visual language of the images allows the contemporary presence of opposite feelings and thoughts. This is very comforting for the patient.

Conclusion

At the end of this chapter, I can confirm that a special meditative attitude about death and mortality, which I have called 'musing about death', has been possible, and has been useful, during a number of art therapy groups that I have led with cancer patients. Helping the patients to get rid of the fear of the white page has been important in this respect. The connection between the aesthetic, the emotional and the conceptual levels has also been important: it was left to each patient to move in from different angles. I have mentioned the respectful silence and the visual and verbal sharing and feed-back as important elements of the process: I need to add that smiles and laughter were also common, especially as a response to humorous symbols of vulnerability and mortality. I have asked myself whether any art therapy technique was most appropriate to facilitate the patient along the path of existential awareness. I have concluded that the techniques are the same ones that we may use with any other populations. During an art therapy session images may emerge in many different ways: some patients prefer to work with what is in their mind, some patients prefer to start playing with art materials, others are inspired by pictures made by the other participants in the group. Also the images about death emerged in these ways. The only difference, in medical art therapy and specifically in psycho-oncology, may be that these patients are often physically and emotionally so fatigued that maximum simplicity should be the rule. A small white page; one picture from a magazine; a squiggle: sometimes these are sufficient tools, and they may take the patient and the therapist a long way towards the mystery of death and of life.

Acknowledgements

I thank Jimmie Holland, MD, for giving me the opportunity to set up an art therapy service at Memorial Sloan-Kettering Cancer Center (MSKCC), New York. Bonnie Gabriel, who was my first art therapy intern at MSKCC, has helped me throughout the years to develop the Creative Journey: I thank her for her sensitivity and cooperation. I am grateful to the patients who partici-pated in the art therapy groups: their capacity to stay with the existential awareness of death without denying it and without feeling overwhelmed has been a source of strength for them: it has been for me a learning experience and a constant source of inspiration.

Further reading

Bertman, S. (1991) *Grief and the Healing Arts: Creativity as Therapy*. New York: Batwood Publishing Company.
Bregman, L. (1999) *Beyond Silence and Denial: Death and Dying Reconsidered*. Louisville, KY: Westminster John Knox Press.
Connell, C. (1998) Rites of passage, in C. Connell, *Something Understood: Art Therapy in Cancer Care*. London: Wrexham.
Freud, S. (1980) *The Interpretation of Dreams*. New York: Penguin Books.
Jung, C.G. (1968) Analytical psychology: its theory and practice, Tavistock Lecture No. 5. London: Routledge & Kegan Paul.
Stern, D.B. (1997) *Unformulated Experience: From Dissociation to Imagination in Psychoanalysis*. London: The Analytic Press.

12 Fear of annihilation: defensive strategies used within art therapy groups and organizations for cancer patients

Barry Falk

Introduction

The following chapter is a comparative study of two art therapy groups with cancer patients. Both are located within the south-east of England, one situated within a hospice and the other within a cancer treatment centre in a large hospital. The purpose is to look at the factors which determine how an art therapy group engages with or defends against the therapeutic task. Despite having similar issues each group has formed its own particular way of working within the therapeutic space. It is this difference between the groups that I shall focus on to gain a better understanding of why, when faced with the huge existential issues around death and dying, one group is more 'task-oriented' than the other. As well as looking at the internal factors, the issues pertinent to this client group, I shall also explore the external factors at play in the wider institutional setting to show how one influences the other. The aim is to understand better the complex interplay of group defences adopted against the overt death anxiety present within these groups and in the work settings.

The groups

The two groups chosen for this study are both art therapy groups set up to provide psychological support for cancer patients at the point of diagnosis, rediagnosis, whilst in treatment, after treatment or approaching death. One is set within a hospice and is a part of the day care service, the other takes place within a cancer treatment centre and is for outpatients attending the centre for chemotherapy or radiotherapy. Both groups are mixed in terms of gender and diagnosis. The former group is comprised of patients over 65, receiving palliative care, with generally low mobility; the latter is predominantly made up of fairly mobile younger patients receiving non-surgical cancer treatment. There is, however, a certain amount of overlap between the groups in terms of prognosis and states of health; those attending the hospice may be relatively stable in their illness and even be discharged due to good health, whereas some of the patients attending the cancer centre may have a very poor prognosis. Likewise there are similarities between the two groups in terms of the issues being addressed, such as fears connected with being diagnosed with a terminal illness, adjusting to changes in body image, the loss of a familiar/responsible role, issues of social isolation, the fear engendered in others by the cancer, the effects of ongoing treatment, frustration around loss of control and greater dependency on others.

The hospice art therapy group takes place within an art room. It has an available water source, good light, large table space and a busy, creative atmosphere. There is, however, a lot of 'clutter' in the room in the form of art materials, bric-a-brac, framed pictures, painted plates, special occasion cards and so on, which is strongly associated with arts and crafts; it is used on other days for this purpose. There is also dumping in the room in the form of a large, unstable, unhealthy table and a large, black, unusable relaxation chair. The art therapy group therefore feels as though it is borrowing the space, a space more readily associated with arts and crafts or as a storage room.

The cancer centre group is set within a conference room. The room needs to be adapted before each session to accommodate a circle of chairs and an art table. It is fairly large and thus allows for movement from one area to another. Conference presentation equipment and desks are set at one end of the room, there is grey carpet on the floor and no water source in the room. It is a safe, uninterrupted space but not an art room. It is also situated within, and therefore strongly associated with, the hospital.

Curative group factors

There is much written about the curative factors of group psychotherapy. Foulkes (1948) saw groups as essential to understanding the individual within the context of the wider situation, i.e. the family, society, and so on. Group analysis was perceived as offering the ideal milieu for therapeutic work with the aim of 'curing' a patient's neurosis and socially normalizing him/her. Yalom (1983) listed the main curative group psychotherapy factors as:

Instillation of hope, universality, imparting of information, altruism, the corrective recapitulation of the primary family group, the development of socializing techniques, imitative behaviour, inter-personal learning, group cohesiveness, catharsis and existential factors.

(Nitsun 1996: 10)

Waller (1993) similarly writes about the curative factors pertinent to interactive art psychotherapy groups, which include:

Greater atmosphere of trust in the group once the 'performance fear' of art-making has been confronted, art as an alternative to words and media for play, image-making resembling 'free association', and the artwork containing symbolic meaning as well as a reflection of the 'here-and-now' material of the group.

(Skaife and Huet 1998: 8)

Similarly the curative/healing factors intrinsic to art-making and creativity have been much written about. Zammit, working with a client suffering from a life-threatening illness, describes the art process as following a sequence:

1   an exploration into the nature of her illness;
2   expressions of inner change;
3   expressions of painful emotions and physical suffering;
4   expressions of resolution and celebration; and
5   expressions of a newfound spirituality.

(Zammit 2001: 27)

For Zammit, art-making is ultimately a self-healing activity which fits into a deep-rooted cultural belief in the healing power of creativity. Predeger also writes about the healing value of art as well as highlighting the need for a group support system for cancer patients, in this case a women's breast cancer support art group: 'Art became an opening to connect within the group and share in the human condition' (Pedeger 1996: 48). Likewise, Baron places emphasis upon the curative factors of the group for cancer patients, stating that it provided a place to 'reenergize themselves and com-bat feelings of isolation . . .' (Baron 1985: 23) as well as being a setting which challenges negative feelings and confronts individual denial through group reality testing.

Thus the art therapy group offers a place for group members to share and normalize their experience; to become aware of and challenge their use of denial; to offer and derive support from each other, thus partaking in social interaction when they are often feeling socially excluded; to express their grief and fear in a place where this is acceptable, understandable and in fact the common experience; and to take part in a creative activity which can act as a catharsis to expressing very difficult feelings, improve self-esteem, aid communication and socialization, and potentially even heal.

These curative factors are the incentive for art psychotherapy groups, but less frequently documented are the difficulties and anxieties inherent in group work, especially non-directive psychotherapy, and group resistance to engaging in the therapeutic task of dealing openly with the existential issues being addressed. Groups can often present a resistant, united front and utilize the art-making as a form of distraction and denial of the therapy process. To understand this better it is necessary to look more closely at group resistance.

Resistance within the group

'If one assumes, as Kubler Ross does, that death is inherently terrifying, then news that I have a terminal illness must be met with either outright fear or denial' (Walter 1994: 74). Within the hospice group, death hangs heavy; there have been many losses during the lifetime of the group and these are remembered and often commented upon in the form of recollection by the 'survivors'. In this sense the group is a microcosm of the hospice in general where bereavement is in the nature of the setting. Generally in psychotherapy the death anxiety is not explicit but is part of the underlying existential anxiety, whereas within cancer care/palliative care death is overt and openly discussed as an imminent issue. Reminders are seen in the clear deterioration of group members, confirming the fear and underlying assumption of all those attending the hospice that this is a place which you enter but do not leave. Hospice and death are thus intimately linked. Yet unexpected death, despite the hospice setting, has often shaken the group and significant losses continue to resonate and be remembered.

However, these issues of loss and dying, so apparent in the hospice, are broached only briefly within the session or not spoken about at all, and a feeling of bravado is often the presenting group face. The group has effectively rejected the art therapy materials that I offer and chosen instead to use the art and craft materials supplied by the hospice, often continuing projects, such as plate painting, already started on another day. Art activity tends, thus, to take the form of decorating and 'colouring in', which feels safe and distracting. As Pratt explains:

> Art therapy is sometimes confused with diversionary creative activities. Engaging with art materials can be extremely satisfying and thereby have a therapeutic effect. It distracts the patient from their daily concerns as they become absorbed with painting or claywork . . . But there is more to art therapy than this.
>
> (Pratt 1997: 48)

Art-making as a form of free association and subsequent key to under-standing is avoided within this group. The question is why does this group, which changes membership regularly, continue to present such a united and anti-psychotherapy front, whereas the cancer centre group, which also has a changing membership and faces similar issues, engages quickly and deeply with the psychotherapy process.

The obvious differences between the two groups are age, mobility and progression of illness. The hospice group is drawn from a generally older population; referrals to the hospice are often made when the illness is far progressed, when death is imminent and health is very poor. The con-sequence of this may be that they feel less in control and therefore more like recipients of treatment, thus agreeing to attend the art therapy sessions through group/staff pressure, not necessarily through choice. Psychotherapy too is not a common experience for this generation. The difference, there-fore, between myself and the group members is noticeable in terms of cul-tural perspective (the language of psychotherapy) and my relative youth and health (the enviable psychotherapist). Resistance may well be based upon a difference of perspective: 'A difference between an older generation that copes silently and stoically, and a younger generation that copes through talking and sharing' (Walter 1994: 74).

Death and absences have also been a difficult factor within the cancer centre group; losses are remembered and new group members are required to adjust to a group psychotherapy situation perhaps not experienced before. Yet issues around illness and dying are quickly and deeply engaged with, both verbally and within the art-making. Though there are defences, projections and basic assumption tactics these are the 'normal' regressive parts of the group process, not a rejection of it. Members of the group are mostly around my age and are drawn from a generally younger population group, therefore often sharing more cultural assumptions with me. This may be an important factor in the group's willingness to accept my role as therap-ist but I don't think it is a dominant factor; older people have participated in this group and relatively younger people have joined the hospice group, yet the culture of each group has remained the same.

Another important factor is the intention of the patients attending the therapy. At the cancer centre an appointment system is used; the group members attend at a set time for a set purpose and maintain strict con-fidentiality between group members outside the session time. The group is a slow-open one, that is, one which allows new members to join when a place becomes available, so that even though there are frequent absences and losses the group is aware of its membership. At the hospice, however, an open group system is adopted; group membership is more variable as I am often unaware of who will be attending week by week, in keeping with the quick referral system of the day care. Also, the group members continue to see each other outside the session time, thus blurring the boundaries and allowing the external hospice culture to influence the group. This creates a less stable base to the group. The hospice group also feels like a captive audience; they are encouraged to attend the art therapy though I feel they are often not fully aware of what is involved or what therapy, in this context, means. This is in part due to the way in which the nursing staff explain the service to them as well as perhaps a wider feeling of ambivalence about why they are attending the hospice: meeting the need for social contact but evoking fear about entering a place of dying and loss. The hospice group can therefore be seen as being less stable in terms of group membership, with greater ambivalence concerning the therapy and about the hospice, and greater merging as a defensive strategy, thus creating a more unified yet resistant group face.

The anti-group

Defence mechanisms are in themselves complex and multiple and include such unconscious behaviour as 'sublimation, substitution, displacement, perversion, condensation' (Foulkes 1948: 8). The term 'defence mechanism' was first conceived by Freud to describe the ego's defences against the 'id', initially referring to sexuality but later encompassing any anxiety-provoking situation (for instance the death instinct). Bion related these defence mechanisms to groups, using the term 'basic assumptions' to refer to the three types of defences usually adopted: dependency, fight or flight, and pairing. These he explained as regressive responses to the anxiety of being in a group. He saw two types of groups: the 'work group', whose members focused cooperatively upon the group's function/task, that is the therapy work, and the 'basic assumption group', which was resistant to the common purpose of the group. Categorized in this way the cancer centre group is an example of the 'task-oriented work group', whereas the hospice group is a 'basic assumption group'. One of the striking factors for me of running the hospice art therapy group is the way in which the group effectively avoids becoming too involved in the therapeutic process and resorts to regressive defence mechanisms:

> Bion (1961) gives the example of a markedly uncooperative group that was at the same time a very united group, the point being that its very negativity gave the group cohesion. This is an important aspect of the anti-group: the creation of a negative, sometimes destructive, counter-group unity that works against the therapeutic purpose.
>
> (Nitsun 1996: 110–11)

This is borne out in the hospice group. Though it accepts my role in setting up, holding and clearing away the room it rejects the type of therapy I am offering whilst still continuing to attend regularly. It effectively takes control of the space verbally and non-verbally but behind the heightened bravado is a strong denial and resistance to engaging in the therapeutic task of working through difficult feelings. Instead, these feelings are split off and projected out into exterior situations and places, for instance bemoaning bad nursing standards at the local hospital and offhand care from GPs, or galvanized around common enemies, for instance refugees who are blamed for taking up valuable health resources, or dangers such as new, untreatable hospital viruses (akin to their own illnesses!). Bion's fight or flight defences are relevant here: the group is behaving as if it were under attack and thus gathering together to fight often paranoid flights of fantasy.

Another basic assumption defence common to the group is the pairing of dominant males. This display of strength has been encouraged by the group. On a subconscious level this can be seen as a group wish to generate life, the 'messianic hope', in reaction to diminishing strength and impending death. It can also be seen as a way of undermining and wresting control away from me. In this way conversation is often used as a tool to silence me, not allowing me to get a word in edgeways!

> In basic assumption mentality . . . there is a collusive interdependence between the leader and the led, whereby the leader will be followed only as long as he or she fulfils the basic assumption task of the group . . . The leader who fails in these ways will be ignored, and eventually the group will turn to an alternative leader. Thus the basic assumption leader is essentially a creation or puppet of the group, who is manipulated to fulfil its wishes and to evade difficult realities.
>
> (Stokes 1994: 23)

The process of silencing the therapist is an interesting one and raises the question of which part of the communication is being silenced, an answer to which can be sought within the countertransference. As a consequence of the 'silencing', or blocking, I am often left feeling disempowered, angry and rejected. These, I surmise, are the unacknowledged feelings of the group projected into me. As Nitsun points out, such anti-group behaviour 'tends to evoke considerable despair and feelings of failure in the conductor . . . A sense of hopelessness in the conductor may in fact be an important signal of an anti-group at work' (Nitsun 1996: 56).

These anti-group tendencies are understandable given the destabilizing effects of the illness: the group feels as though it is clinging to a life raft trying to survive internal and external threats – a very real concern for the survival of the group. This anxiety is common to such groups where drop-outs, absences and losses are a feature; where illness, dying and death are the main issues. What is pertinent here is the way in which the hospice group merges to present such a strong anti-group front. The same anxieties are present within the cancer centre group but are used as a tool to spur exploration (anxiety being a necessary feature of a psychoanalytic group). 'The task of the therapist is to reduce anxiety to comfortable levels and then to use this existing anxiety to increase a patient's awareness and vitality' (Yalom 1980:

188); 'In work-group mentality ... members are able to mobilize their capacity for co-operation and to value the different contributions each can make' (Stokes 1994: 23). This is very much the way that the cancer centre group operates.

The unified, consistent anti-group face presented by the hospice group suggests that the underlying anxiety feels too threatening to be acknowledged and worked with. Thus the 'task' is not acknowledged, the 'therapy' rejected. Instead, the group is united around the task of denying the complex feelings evoked by illness, death, dying and loss. This unspoken denial is not, I feel, confined to the group but is also rooted within the hospice culture, and in fact forms an unconscious, collusive denial between staff and patients. Interestingly this seems to be borne out not only in the way that the strong anti-group tendency continues on beyond the fluctuation of group membership but also in the way in which the hospice culture reacts to the art therapy.

The wider setting therefore needs to be studied to try to understand further the way in which external institutional factors can influence the way a therapy group works: 'The in-patient group is not "free standing" but is always part of a larger therapeutic system' (Yalom 1983: 459).

Institutional anxiety

The hospice setting is one fraught with complication. It occupies a Victorian building roughly adapted to the requirements of the hospice. Space is an issue as rooms and corridors are not purpose-built for wheelchair users or for the professionals working within them. The art room has two offices attached, one for the lymphoedema nurse and the other for the aromatherapist, who both need access via the art room! The day care nurses' office is a cramped space boxed in by filing cabinets. Parts of the hospice have recently been closed for heath and safety reasons and staff have had to be relocated. Territories have thus been fought over: the purpose-built education room is now office space for the home care team, the dining room now the education space, the day-centre meals now eaten in the upstairs day room. As a consequence of this, firm therapy boundaries have been impossible to establish because of seemingly insurmountable and inflexible practical obstacles, such as the lymphoedema nurses requiring access via the therapy space during session times, late arrival of patients to the session due to late pick-ups, dumping of useless objects in the room, and the adopting of a space already loaded with its own type of art activity. Some of this behaviour may be viewed as 'sabotage' and it is a relevant factor to bear in mind that the art therapy/therapist may evoke envy in the staff as well as the patients. Within the hospice I am employed on a sessional basis and my role, perhaps, is perceived as a relatively easy one, whereas the nursing staff have a more time-consuming job to do dealing with the hands-on, messy, physical care of the patients. Also, when the group attends the therapy the day room is often left empty, leaving the nurses redundant, which may evoke resentment.

In theory the room at the hospice is an ideal space for art therapy: an art room with good light, a water source and a creative atmosphere, as opposed to the cancer centre where a conference room, without water supply, needs to be adapted for use. Yet the art room is loaded with associations and compromised by interruptions. It thus feels too unsafe for any deep inter- action or personal disclosure, whereas the conference room, for all its faults, maintains its strict therapy boundaries and thus creates a safe, consistent, boundaried therapeutic space. The open group structure of the hospice group is perhaps complicit with these looser boundaries, the art therapy merging with the rest of the day care programme, whereas at the cancer centre strict therapeutic boundaries have been easier to establish, partly because of the tighter group structure but also because the art therapy is kept distinct and private from the rest of the centre: the sessions take place upstairs (the chemo- and radiotherapy are downstairs) and are kept safe from interruption. This means that external institutional factors are not such an influence over the group's development, despite the presence of 'medical-looking' equipment within the room and the association with the cancer centre as a place for medical treatment. Group members only use the room for art therapy so there is the consistency of a safe, uninterrupted space. Though the centre is one which they attend for cancer treatment, the room is far enough removed for the therapy not to be compromised by this. Therefore the boundaries are much safer, the sessions treated as appointments and the intention of the clients clearer.

In order to understand how an institution can influence an art therapy group situated within it, it is therefore necessary to study the complex defence mechanisms at play.

> Like individuals, institutions develop defences against difficult emo- tions . . . central amongst these defences is denial, which involves pushing certain thoughts, feelings and experiences out of conscious awareness because they have become too anxiety provoking.
>
> (Halton 1994: 12)

These defence mechanisms operate within hospital culture/caring pro- fessions in general, so it is worth referring to Lyth's study of the nursing service in a general hospital to understand the possible anxieties and defence strategies adopted by the nursing profession: 'The nursing service . . . bears the full, immediate and concentrated impact of stresses arising from patient care . . .' (Lyth 1970: 46); '. . . the intense anxiety evoked by the nursing task . . . precipitated just such individual regression to primitive types of defence' (Lyth 1970: 62). Inevitably those involved in the intimate task of nursing the dying are deeply affected by the loss and pain that they witness. To cope with these unbearable feelings defence mechanisms are unconsciously used. According to Klein these are the primitive defence mechanisms that she refers to as the 'paranoid schizoid defences', such as splitting, projection and projective identification, in which unbearable feelings are projected out into a recipient/external situation. These defences are used by both patients and staff and recipients of these unspoken feelings can unconsciously take them on board as their own, thus further complicating the mixture of feelings evoked within both staff and patient. The interpersonal emotional interaction between nurse and patient is thus necessarily a very complicated one involving unconscious processes.

Within the organizations being studied here is the added factor of a deep-rooted, existential fear of self-annihilation.

> Melanie Klein takes as her starting point the fear of annihilation. This fear is of something that destroys from within. This 'something' is the inner workings of the death instinct, but it is experienced phobically. By that I mean that although the feared object is an element within, it is experienced as being outside.
>
> (Symington 1986: 257)

This 'phobic' response to death and dying, as something which cannot be acknowledged as within, must create huge ambivalence for staff/professionals working with this particular client group, an ambivalence in which denial of death is often employed as a coping mechanism. This denial can also be illustrated by the wider social fantasy in which

> The health service is unconsciously seen as a 'keep-death-at-bay service'; whilst the stated task is the treatment of illness, there is also an unconscious task of providing each member of society with the fantasy that death can be prevented.
>
> (Stokes 1994: 121–3)

Though both the hospice and the cancer centre deal overtly with death and dying I believe there is still this unstated anxiety about death. Additional to and as a consequence of this there is also, I surmise, a culture of hopelessness based upon the reality of the patient's condition. The role of the nursing staff to care and the pressure put upon them to be seen to cope with and sort out often insurmountable problems (such as dying!) compounds the underlying anxiety. Within the hospice, as compensation for the inherent failure of the staff to actually save the patient, an overly friendly attitude is often adopted. Speck writes: 'One of the dangers . . . is that of "chronic niceness", whereby the individual and the organisation collude to split off and deny the negative aspects of caring daily for the dying' (1994: 96). I am aware that this often bears out within the hospice. A pertinent example is the 'eating ritual' which has evolved during a younger persons' evening. The younger persons' day/evening is run for patients under the age of 65. Food is served around a long table halfway through the evening and consists of an extended three-course meal. The meal brings to mind images of the 'last supper'; there is something urgent and ritualistic to it, a gorging which feels ill-suited to the business of dying. This feeding frenzy brings to mind thoughts about bulimia and the stuffing down of emotions; within the countertransference there is an associated feeling of nausea. Despite discussions between myself and the daycare leader to rearrange the timing or have a more flexible cold buffet-style dinner, any change to the meal-time is strongly resisted. The result is that the mealtime cuts across the time available for a 90-minute group session and limits individual work. In this situation the culture of psychotherapy struggles against this more dominant culture in which feeding and socializing are the priority. I am aware that within the hospice being studied here the hierarchy of staff, from doctor to matron to day care leader to staff to patients, creates a power culture in which any challenge or disruption to the system is strongly resisted.

As a consequence of the unacknowledged fear evoked within the hospice I feel that there is huge unconscious anxiety which permeates into the art therapy group and creates a strong, collusive, anti-group culture; one in which art therapy is held as art activity, not psychotherapy, and where the main function of day care is to entertain and distract the patient. Because of the open group system and other contributory factors, such as compromised space, the therapy is loosely boundaried and subsequently less secure and more open to these external influences.

The collusive therapist

Within the anti-group culture I am often silenced, my viewpoints overridden and thoughts resisted, both by staff and patients. This silencing has a cumulative effect upon my role as therapist, in effect blocking my thinking. When I am no longer able to challenge or openly discuss issues I am then drawn into this culture, forced to be the group's puppet. By holding back on thoughts both within the session and outside I am in fact collusive with this group denial. Within the cancer centre, where I am operating in a complementary role to the consultants and nurses, I am allowed my autonomy to practise and am not drawn into the surrounding culture.

I am not advocating that the therapist remain separate from the surrounding team – far from it – but I am very aware of how a powerful culture of denial draws the therapist into a collusive role which undermines the type of therapy being offered. Within another hospice in which I run similar sessions there is none of this resistance. Instead there is a much less hierarchical culture in which I am included more in staff and multidisciplinary meetings and thus allowed a voice. Subsequently the sessions are rarely interrupted, understanding between myself and staff is much clearer and there is a clear distinction for the patients between the art activity being offered in the dayroom and the art therapy being offered in the conservatory.

Conclusion

The intention of this study is not to criticize the care offered by hospices. It is important therefore to note that hospices were set up with the aim of providing physical, psychological and spiritual care for the dying person, and that hospices in general are able to provide a higher level of care for the dying person than general hospitals by virtue of the higher ratio of staff to patient and the specialization of the staff team around issues of palliative care and symptom control. 'The setting up of hospices outside of the NHS was intended by Saunders to demonstrate a quality of care that would eventually change standards within the NHS' (Walter 1994: 143). On the whole this 'quality of care' is present within the hospice being studied here, yet the art therapy, I believe, highlights underlying psychological factors which need addressing.

Groups in general evoke anxiety and complex defence structures. With this client group in particular, however, and also within the staff team caring for them, including myself, there is also the very real threat of annihilation. It is worth remembering that hospice referrals are made once a patient is deemed to be beyond recovery and that the hospice itself is a place of dying, reiterating the hopelessness of the situation on the one hand and the wish to heal on the other. For the patients the ambivalence evoked by attending a hospice or cancer treatment centre is huge, centred around the need for social contact but evoking anxiety about loss and dying. As shown in this study, art psychotherapy groups do not necessarily lead to deep engagement with the therapeutic task but instead can lead to powerful group denial of the underlying issues, an anti-group culture in which regressive defence mechanisms are employed and with which the therapist is forced to be collusive.

Working within a hospice or hospital requires a 'flexible approach', due to the instability of patients' health and the priority of their needs. Within such an uncertain system art therapists may find it necessary, as I have, to offer an appropriate service such as an open group or more art activity-based therapy. But without a clear understanding of the way in which the art therapy is integrated into and affected by the surrounding culture, I have found that these therapy groups become too insecure to engage in deep therapeutic work, are open to influence from external institutional anxieties and undermine and sabotage the role of the therapist. As demonstrated, a collusive, often unconscious cultural resistance to deep therapy work can then be set up – a group and institutional denial which, rather than tackling the presenting psychological issues, seeks ways to avoid them.

References

Baron, P.H. (1985) Group work with cancer patients, *Pratt Institute and Creative Arts Therapy Review*, 6: 22–36.

Bion, W.R. (1989) *Experiences in Groups, and Other Papers*. London: Routledge.

Foulkes, S.H. (1948) *Introduction to Group-analytic Psychotherapy*. London: Maresfield.

Halton, W. (1994) Some unconscious aspects of organisational life – contributions from psychoanalysis, in A. Obholzer and Z. Roberts (eds) *The Unconscious at Work: Individual and Organizational Stress in the Human Services*. London, New York: Routledge.

Lyth, I.M. (1970) The functioning of social systems as a defence against anxiety, in I.M. Lyth, *Containing Anxiety in Institutions*. Tavistock, London.

Nitsun, M. (1996) *The Anti-group: Destructive Forces in Groups and their Creative Potential*. London, New York: Routledge.

Predeger, E. (1996) Womanspirit: a journey through art in breast cancer, *Advanced Nursing Science*, 18 (3): 48–58.

Pratt, M. (1997) The creative response, *Palliative Care Today*, 5 (4): 48–9.

Skaife, S. and Huet, V. (eds) (1998) *Art Psychotherapy Groups: Between Pictures and Words*. London: Routledge.

Speck, P. (1994) Working with dying people, in A. Obholzer and Z. Roberts (eds) *The Unconscious at Work: Individual and Organizational Stress in the Human Services*. London, New York: Routledge.

Stokes, J. (1994) Institutional chaos and personal stress, in A. Obholzer and Z. Roberts (eds) *The Unconscious at Work. Individual and Organizational Stress in the Human Services*. London, New York: Routledge.

Symington, N. (1986) *The Analytic Experience: Lectures from the Tavistock*. London: Free Association Press.

Waller, D. (1993) *Group Interactive Art Therapy*. London: Routledge.

Walter, T. (1994) *The Revival of Death*. London, New York: Routledge.

Yalom, I.D. (1980) *Existential Psychotherapy*. New York: Basic Books.

Yalom, I.D. (1983) *The Theory and Practice of Group Psychotherapy*. New York: Basic Books.

Zammit, C. (2001) The art of healing: a journey through cancer. Implications for art therapy, *Art Therapy: Journal of the American Art Therapy Association*, 18 (1): 27–36.

13 Creating through loss: how art therapists sustain their practice in palliative care

David Hardy

Introduction

In this chapter I will argue that therapists working in the field of palliative care should be more open to acknowledging their own needs and feelings of loss when clients die. I have come to this conclusion as a result of reviewing the art therapy literature written by practitioners working in palliative care, and I have noticed that there has been a reticence about looking at this feature of our work. I will try to examine why this has been so. The second part of my chapter will consider the arguments for and against working with transference and countertransference with this client group and I will draw upon my own experience to demonstrate the positive advantages that can be accrued by working in this way. A more active engagement with transference and countertransference issues can enhance practitioners' efforts in this field and enable us, as art therapists, to retain our own creativity and versatility and, by extension, to be truly attentive to our clients. Finally, I will try to demonstrate that being aware of transference issues is necessary not only for sustained good practice, but also for long-term 'survival' of the therapist as well. Since my thoughts on this matter arose from a review of the literature, I will present this by way of an introduction to my arguments.

A literature review

During the previous ten years there has been a proliferation of publications as art therapists working with the terminally ill have written about their work. Camilla Connell has been at the vanguard of this movement and like many of her colleagues she has stressed how the symbolic component of art can facilitate the expression of strong and sometimes conflicting feelings which may be considered too difficult to put into words (Connell 1998a). At a time of great vulnerability, when the patient may feel very dependent, this can be a considerable relief. As well as providing an immediate outlet for expression, several authors also describe how the symbolism in a picture can provide an important buffer between a patient and the very raw feelings which are sometimes exposed (Connell 1998a; Thomas and Kennedy 1995). Symbolism enables patients to readdress and interpret their feelings from a safer place, either in a session or at a later date. Connell (1998a) and Szepanski (1988) both emphasize that the symbolism in a picture can reson-ate and change in meaning over time, which not only enables the client to safely express difficult and powerful emotions but also facilitates the conflu-ence of competing thoughts as well. This feature of the process perhaps also reflects the ambivalence many clients feel as they come to the end of their lives (Szepanski 1988), and it is considered a specific attribute that art therapy can bring to this area of work (Connell 1998a; Wood 1998).

Thomas, amongst others, describes how art therapy can enable patients to achieve an insight into some of the psychological features that could be aggravating their physical pain (Thomas *et al.* 1998; Trauger-Querry and Haghighi 1999). She sees a direct causal link between the reduction of stress through these interventions and a diminishment of pain in her clients. By providing her patients with an opportunity to express pent-up and often overwhelming feelings of frustration, either in a cathartic manner or by a gradual process of working through, she enables patients to assume a greater feeling of control (Thomas and Kennedy 1995). The facility of art therapy to mobilize previously untapped resources by accessing the unconscious is described as invaluable in this regard (Connell 1998b).

The aesthetic feature of the art therapy process is addressed by Connell, who calls for resources for patients to be creative in a way which for them is novel and fresh. This is very important, she says, for increasing patient self-esteem. Emphasizing the healing process of art, Connell describes the pro-cess of making a picture, using the art materials and engaging in this way as bolstering patient morale and fulfilling a basic human need to be creative (Connell 1998a).

Most of the literature reviewed so far appears to focus primarily on the restorative qualities of making an image. It is my contention, though, that being supportive or providing the art materials is not always enough. As Luzzatto writes, the creative component of art therapy is not necessarily helpful for clients who may already feel blocked, empty or bereft (Luzzatto 1998). In reality, as she points out, they are a diverse client group who need to be responded to in a variety of ways. Some, overwhelmed by distress, may exhibit acute dysfunctional states. Other cancer patients may develop psy-chological conditions unrelated to their primary diagnosis, while, for a few, pre-existing mental health problems may return as a consequence of this turn of events (Luzatto 1998). Few of the authors I have reviewed have looked at or considered these issues at all. The need to assist patients to express their feelings about their illness appears to take precedence over nearly every other issue, including the need to think or work with the transference in the session (Coote 1998; Connell 1998a; Thomas 1998). As Brown and Peddler have observed in the field of palliative care, the focus on more humanistic approaches has placed a strong emphasis on the need to facilitate expression, perhaps over and above the need to always understand what the expression is about. As they characterize it, there has been a move away from talk to action (Brown and Pedder 1979). Ignoring or minimizing the role of transference is a mistake in my opinion, since any contact between a client and a therapist, with or without a picture, necessarily involves a degree of reciprocity, which in turn infers a transference interaction.

At this juncture I will continue my review of what has been written about this feature of our work in this area and then go on to discuss why it appears to have been so frequently overlooked.

Transference in palliative care in the art therapy literature

The glossary of *Art Therapy in Palliative Care* defines transference as a psychoanalytic concept whereby: 'the client displaces feelings arising from previous relationships (for example with parents) onto the therapist and/or the image in art therapy. Recognition of this process enables the therapist to identify and work with unresolved childhood conflicts' (Pratt and Wood 1998: 194).

The definition itself is not contentious. What is surprising, however, is how few art therapists working in palliative care refer to transference in their interactions, in this text or elsewhere. Val Beaver's description of her work is unusual therefore, because she does acknowledge that transference occurs in her interactions with a group of young prisoners with HIV and AIDS (Beaver 1998). In this setting, she says, she sometimes occupies the role of 'mother/therapist' and has to pay special attention to the role of sibling rivalry in the group (Beaver 1998). Paola Luzzatto (1998) more directly addresses the issue of transference when she frankly acknowledges the conflict she experiences when working with this client group. She is torn between offering 'art psychotherapy', with its attendant insights and focus on the internal world, and her wish to facilitate more 'supportive' interventions by fostering in her clients a creative relationship with their artwork. Such clients, Luzzatto states, warrant a range of interventions, including working with the transference (Luzzatto 1998). Her solution is to work with patients on a time-limited basis in a process she calls the 'Creative Journey'.

In this, her patients are encouraged to develop a personal imagery, through which their internal world is gradually reconnected to the external. Implicit is the idea that 'transformation' of meaning emanates from the patient through the medium of the picture. In this way, the transferences that do occur happen principally between patients and their pictures. Like Beaver, Luzzatto appears cautious about actively working with transference interactions that may take place between the therapist and the client. Possibly both authors feel that working more assiduously with the transference would be inappropriate in what is usually quite short-term work. The result is that the meaning, if any, of such dynamics remains largely unspoken.

There does seem to be a large but often unacknowledged anxiety about raising issues which clients may not have the energy or time to resolve (Skaife 1993). On this point the psychiatrist Jennifer Barraclough has argued that the brevity of therapy for clients in palliative care compromises and restricts practice in this sphere. There is insufficient time, she writes, for either party to establish a sufficiently trusting rapport (Barraclough 1994). Yalom (1980) characterizes this concern as 'why stir up a hornet's nest?' Why should therapists encourage patients to delve into the past when they should be preparing themselves for a sudden shortened future? (The inevitably heightened anxiety such an exploration entails, he argues, is usually intense but also short in duration.) He, and others, state that the proximity of death actually heightens patient responses to therapists and intensifies their work (Yalom 1980; Wood 1990; Schaverien 1998). Wood, too, illustrates that meaningful transference interactions can and do take place, even within the course of a single session (Wood 1990). Whether these should necessarily be brought out into the open remains for me an open question, which depends upon the context of the session and the nature of the interaction between the therapist and the client.

Significantly it is Joy Schaverien (1998), a therapist who does not routinely practise in palliative care, who addresses the issue of how transference can be used in this area of work. She describes her analytic work with a client who developed terminal cancer during the course of his therapy with her (Schaverien 1998). She addresses the very personal and caring feelings induced in her by these encounters and describes the series of dilemmas which necessitated her to re-evaluate her work. Over the course of two years, she is idealized and denigrated by this man, the subject of envy and attack, which she tries to addresses in an analytical way. On occasion this entailed challenging or contradicting her client. Only by holding onto her analytic framework, Schaverien emphasizes, was she able to stay therapeutically close to him until the end (Schaverien 1998).

In her interesting analysis of the art therapy literature on palliative care, Sally Skaife (1993) provides further insights into why practitioners appear to minimize their role in the therapeutic process. She alludes to the continuing influence of the 'hospital arts' movement on this branch of the profession, which has historically discouraged 'morbid introspection'. Its emphasis on patient diversion and self-improvement, she suggests, has implicitly discouraged any meaningful focus on the psychotherapeutic relationship between the therapist and the client in the hospital setting. Less than ideal working conditions and the expectation that the majority of this work is short-term has also compounded the reluctance of art therapists practising in palliative care to look at their practice in this way (Skaife 1993). On another level, Skaife points out that it is possible that therapists unconsciously avoid too close an attachment to their clients because they anticipate and fear that they themselves may become the object of an envious attack. The inevitable disparity in their respective positions, she points out, may cause the therapist to avoid any situation (such as making an interpretation) which could precipitate such an attack. Conversely, the failure of therapists to analyse their own feelings when working in this sphere, she cautions, can also lead to practitioners colluding or otherwise becoming over-attached to their clients (Skaife 1993).

As has been noted, art therapists working with the terminally ill seem generally hesitant to engage in this way. In this regard, Connell seems to sum up the prevailing feeling when she writes: 'The therapist's task is to attend, witness and wait. She provides the conditions through which the process can be given form and should not try to hinder it through inappropriate insertion of herself' (Connell 1998a: 90).

To her the therapist is an attendant, a facilitator or an ally (Connell 1998a). A more overt intervention, she argues, is an intrusion, a manifestation of our need to feel needed and as such a betrayal of the process, widening as it does the gap between the therapist and the client (Connell 1998a).

In the following part of this chapter I review how therapists have written about and worked with the difficult issue of countertransference.

Countertransference in palliative care in the art therapy literature

I recognize that interacting with patients in the manner just described, working with and thinking about transference and countertransference, is not appropriate for every situation. In reality, art therapists in palliative care need to respond to their clients in a variety of ways. Nevertheless, attachments are formed and alliances are made. Despite their best endeavours, I think art therapists do come to rely on seeing certain clients at a certain time. When these clients die their absence can be very keenly felt.

In their study of psychotherapy work with young people with AIDS, Cohen and Abramowitz demonstrated that therapists often required clients to mirror their own self object needs (Cohen and Abramowitz 1990). In these situations, therapists experienced narcissistic injury, fragmentation, depression, anxiety or burnout when their patients deteriorated or died (Cohen *et al.* 1990). I, for my part, have certainly found myself feeling very disturbed at a time when I thought a client I had worked with for a long period was going to die. Recently, while away on holiday, I was aware of a strong impulse to send another a postcard from abroad. I knew then that I had formed an attachment to this man and that I felt guilty about going away, because I feared that I would not see him again.

Although in her article 'Men who leave too soon' Schaverien is talking about the problem of premature closure in another sphere, I think her comments are also apposite to therapists working in palliative care (Schaverien 1997). Thus, using the language of sexual intercourse, she describes how in such cases the therapist is frequently frustrated. In this sense, fulfilment is prevented by premature termination and becomes a very significant depletion (something, I would suggest, that art therapists working in palliative care experience on a very regular basis). Harold Searles indeed thought that unconsciously patients provide a central meaning to therapists' lives. They validate and make real the therapist's own idealized self-image (Young 1995). Given these comments, it seems unwise to minimize the impact on a therapist of a client's death or deterioration.

How, then, do we as art therapists continue to cope and not just cope but continue to interact with our patients in a vigorous and creative way? How can we operate amongst all this loss without ourselves becoming defended? The truth is perhaps that, to some extent, we cannot. Thus, Sally Skaife has demonstrated that art therapists often unconsciously adopt a variety of defences to protect themselves from becoming overwhelmed by loss, including diminishing the distinction between themselves and their clients (Skaife 1993). By blurring the boundaries between the two parties in this way, she says, therapists appear unconsciously to try to negate the awful reality that one of the two is well and will survive and that one will not (Skaife 1993). This type of merger would appear to be defensive (as opposed to creative) and represents a form of denial in our work, which I would contend is more widespread than is generally acknowledged. (Interestingly it also represents a defence at the opposite end of the spectrum to that alluded to by Connell (1998a). She suggests that therapists unconsciously protect themselves from anticipated loss by being over-interpretative, thereby placing and then maintaining a distance between themselves and their client.)

Yalom is adamant that denial is both a ubiquitous and powerful defence. He states that it plays 'a central role in the therapist's selective inattention ... like an aura, it surrounds the affect associated with death whenever it appears' (Yalom 1980: 58). By its very nature, of course, denial is difficult to address. Even with the intervention of rigorous supervision it can pass by unnoticed, since it will influence the work that we choose to discuss. The client whose impending death may be causing us considerable unease, who re-evokes previous losses in our own lives, can thereby be ignored in supervision, simply through the process of omission. Yalom makes it clear that clients, relatives and health professionals involved in the care of the dying are all affected by denial. For the therapist, though, it can clearly cloud our judgement, lead to over-involvement and identification or, conversely, an estrangement from our clients as they approach the end of their lives (Yalom 1980).

At this juncture I would like to propose an alternative and, I hope, creative way of working with these powerful transference interactions. This will involve discussing the work of several theorists, who feel that therapists should accompany their clients in a more meaningful way than has been considered in the literature so far.

The therapist as a partner in the process

Michael Balint wrote of a stage in the development of the human psyche as resembling a *harmonious interpenetrating mix-up* (Balint 1966). In this stage the environment is perceived as having no sharp boundaries, enabling it and the individual to penetrate each other. He proposed that during certain stages of a therapeutic interaction, a similar fusion between the therapist and his/her client could and should be allowed to reoccur. Harold Searles echoed many of these thoughts when he wrote that deeply regressed symbiosis was the hallmark of the best type of analytic work (Young 1995). Thus, 'For the deepest levels of therapeutic interaction to be reached, both patient and therapist must experience a temporary breaching of the ego boundaries which demarcate each participant from the other' (Searles in Young 1995: 187).

These and similar ideas have also been explored by Rosemary Gordon in her seminal work *Dying and Creating: A Search for Meaning* (1978). Thus she describes a similar synergy as being crucial to the process of individuation and so to the process of creation. In her view, the merging of the therapist and the client replicates the earlier primary fusion between mother and child. In this re-equated dyad the client can oscillate between fusion and separation, symbolically experimenting with his/her creativity in the transitional or third space. Thus the patient gradually becomes confident enough in his/her own capacity to create and adapt to consider again (or maybe for the first time) the possibility of letting go or, as Gordon puts it, of accepting the inevitability of death. She describes this as a lifelong process, first approached in infanthood, thereafter intermittently through the course of one's life, and with renewed vigour at its end. It is my contention that such processes often occur when a therapist works with the terminally ill. Indeed, such an accompaniment of a patient is in my opinion crucial, if as therapists we are really serious in assisting patients to create new meaning. Intimacy,

Yalom makes clear, is fundamental to creativity and so to life and only the most self-possessed or truly original person can accomplish this completely on their own (Yalom 1980). Schaverien does not hesitate to write about her client on this aspect of her work: 'The love I felt for him . . . came to serve an additional purpose once his terminal illness was diagnosed . . . enabling me to accompany him in a way which might otherwise have proved more difficult' (Schaverien 1998: 58). To disavow her feelings of attachment to this man at this point, she states, would have been disingenuous and defensive, a distancing response, itself induced by her own overwhelming feelings of loss and unhelpful or even harmful in such a situation.

To illustrate some of the points that have been raised by the authors I have been reviewing, I will conclude this chapter by describing my work with two clients at a hospice.

Tina

Soon after I had started my job in the hospice, a young Asian woman called Tina was referred to me for individual art therapy. She had been diagnosed as HIV positive only a few months before and was thought by the staff looking after her to be having trouble coming to terms with her diagnosis. She was strikingly beautiful and clearly much younger than the other patients who were attending the centre at that time. Tina was also very aware that she was the only black patient attending the day centre and this seemed to exacerbate her strong sense of alienation. Her youth and her diagnosis also made her feel that she did not fit in. It was not surprising therefore that from our very first session she expressed strong feelings of being out of place. She felt strongly that she was an alien in a foreign land.

This sense of isolation and exclusion was portrayed in a series of images made at that time depicting a series of desolate islands, cut off from the mainland. Other images of barren mountains and foothills and deserted villages both confirmed Tina's sense of isolation and abandonment and the bleak reality of her homeland, which had been gravely depopulated by this terrible disease. None of the these images show any sign of life. All of them seem bereft.

In one of these images (made in our fourth session) the bow of a small boat appears on the side of the page. In front of it, and still some way off, an island emerges from the sea. It is battered by the waves and the six palm trees appear to be bent by the wind. Tina spoke in this session about what she imagined I thought about her and her disease. She had said before that she had contracted the illness through sexual contact and now she wondered if I thought she was promiscuous or had got what she had deserved. She went on to say, with some feeling, that she felt that no man would be interested in her sexually again (this feeling was perhaps reflected in the isolation and unapproachability of the islands in her pictures). An important part of her life, it seemed, had come to a close.

At the time I felt very sorry for this young woman and the predicament she found herself in. I tried to imagine what it would feel like to experience oneself as untouchable in the way that she appeared to. In retrospect I also wonder what role I played in that session for her in the transference. It is possible that maybe at some level she was thinking of the reaction of her father when she articulated her thoughts about her supposed promiscuity, since it soon transpired that she wanted to keep her diagnosis a secret not just from the other patients in the hospice but also from her family back in Asia as well. She feared their disapproval and possible rejection and vowed not to return to Asia until she really felt that she was dying. Tina seemed to me, though, to be penning herself into a dreadful corner. Her frequent protestations of homesickness indicated where she wanted to be, but to her mind this place had now become irrevocably associated with her eventual demise.

Prior to the commencement of our fifth session, Tina, I felt, manipulated a situation in the hospice which resulted in our being seated alone together to eat a Christmas meal. After this, when the session started, Tina referred to the forthcoming marriage of a near relative (an event she thought she would exclude herself from). She confessed to having fantasies about being married and of being 'normal' again. She then asked if she could have a cigarette. She appeared to me to be trying to challenge the boundaries of the session in various ways. Thereafter, she began to ask me about my private life, where I lived and with whom. It seemed that on some level she wished to join with me and, when I put this to her, Tina admitted that she looked at me and at other people in the street and felt envious of their lives. She repeated her fear that, as she had contracted the disease through sexual contact, no man (including myself) would find her attractive again. In the light of the developments in this session, I subsequently wondered whether the appearance of the boat on the edge of the picture made by Tina in the last session was more significant than I had at first realized. It seems possible, looking at it again, that her fantasy was that in some way I could sail in and rescue her.

Although Tina denied feeling rejected, she subsequently became very attacking. I could not know, she said, what it was like to realize you were going to die young. I often felt criticized and got the impression that Tina wanted me to feel as bad and as helpless as she did. Above all, she seemed frightened and this fear permeated our encounters over several months, until we at last reached a quieter place. Here, she became more reflective, but sadder as well.

The last picture Tina made in the art therapy session, she described as 'what if'. It shows an Asian woman in traditional dress, with her back to the viewer, supervising a small boy playing with a kite. On top of her head rests a luminous golden pot. The picture seems carefree but is also redolent with meaning. The 'what if', Tina explained, referred to her thoughts about how her life could have been had she not contracted HIV. It seemed a sad place to finish but it also encapsulated Tina's situation.

Tim

In my experience it is not uncommon for patients unconsciously to seek to live out their lives in those around them. It seems a basic human need to aspire to influence and shape events, and even people, and maybe particularly when people sense that they are coming to the end of their lives. Usually this aspiration is played out on siblings, partners and friends, but occasionally it is projected on to health practitioners as well. I felt that an elderly man called Tim, who was dying of myeloma, made these and other projections during our session time.

Many of Tim's pictures depict sometimes youthful but frequently elderly men, who always seem to be on their own. One picture shows a young man (Tim?), dressed in the fashion of the 1950s, casually playing with a ball against a wall (Figure 13.1, on website). Another picture depicts an older face which stares out bleakly from the page. Underneath Tim wrote 'What happens next?', (Figure 13.2, on website). Another depicts what was obviously a self-portrait encapsulated in a mirror resting on a chest. Underneath this Tim wrote 'On reflection, I cannot be sure.' (Figure 13.3, on website.) He seemed to delight in the pun and also enjoyed watching me try to decipher these often cryptic messages at the bottom of the page. They seemed in some way to match the persona of this enigmatic and deeply private man.

It was apparent from early on in our meetings that he took an interest in my life, about which I cautiously informed him. I felt that in this way Tim was briefly able to escape the confines of the ward (in which he had been for several months) to another place of potential, once occupied by him as he would see it, and now occupied by me. This enabled him to reflect on and re-evaluate his life, the lessons of which he was eager to pass on. There was an obvious identification between us (which I think probably flowed both ways) and the trust that this engendered facilitated changes in his artwork that enabled Tim to meaningfully address very painful issues surrounding his mother's death, as well as the dreadful feeling that life had passed him by.

In the transference, my role in these exchanges seems to me to be less clear. It is possible that I came to represent for this man an idealized and less damaged part of himself, but about this I can only speculate, since Tim forever remained cautious about revealing too much of himself to the prying eye. In the countertransference I certainly became aware of quite protective and almost paternalistic feelings towards him. These became stronger as he visibly declined.

At our last meeting he was too ill to do an image, but we were able to talk for a little while. He wanted to know about my recent holiday and was interested in the details of the trip. Although on this occasion feelings were not directly addressed, the regret in his voice when he said that he wished he had travelled more conveyed to me a perhaps deeper regret that he had possibly missed other opportunities in his life as well. He worried that he had not made an impact on the world. I was able to reply in all sincerity that that maybe he had, but in ways he had not ascertained. The meaning seemed to hang in the air, but I feel that he knew I was confirming I would miss him when he died. We both realized that our own particular journey was also coming to a close.

Discussion

I hope that it is clear from these examples of my work with patients in a hospice that transferences can and do take place. With Tina these seemed to change over time, as she became more used to me and the art therapy session. Sometimes I appeared to be equated with both the good and the bad objects in her life. Simultaneously, it seemed, I also came to represent both the means of her salvation and the focus for her envy. In this situation it seems clear to me that I did not (to paraphrase Connell) insert myself inappropriately into the sessions with Tina, since it was apparent that I was already involved!

On a different matter Luzzatto has written: 'Often patients interpret cancer in their body as a punishment, or an attack, or the sign of not being loved . . . they may need to change the meaning they have given to their illness or to change the response they have adopted to cope' (Luzzatto 1998: 748). Tina, I believe, thought about her illness in a similar way. As a consequence, she felt herself unloved and unlovable. Partly to rebut these awful feelings, I think at various levels, she aspired to join with me. Yalom has observed that this transference is not uncommon in such situations, the prevailing thought from the client appearing to be that 'as long as I am with the therapist, I will be safe' (Yalom 1980). In a situation like this, such a manoeuvre is primarily a defensive one and, as Skaife has illustrated, can equally well emanate from the therapist as well as the client (Skaife 1993). I would make a distinction between this dynamic, however, and what occurred during my interactions with Tim. To my mind the 'merger' that took place there was much more interactive and creative in feel. Thus, disclosing details about my private life to this man, such as where I was going on holiday, where I worked during the rest of the week and so on, while it may have transgressed the boundaries of the session in the strictly formal sense, in the context of these sessions actually helped to release something in this deeply private man. Harold Searles said that the client/therapist relationship had to be fully reciprocal in this way (Young 1995). Our mutual exchange, therefore, which to some extent this was, taking place as it did within the remit of therapeutic confines, actually facilitated this interaction and enabled Tim to engage in a way that I do not believe he would have done had I isolated myself within the confines of a therapeutic stance.

Both these clients evoked in me strong but very different responses. Although Tina may have initially been seductive, I soon experienced her as being very attacking indeed. Tim conversely praised the sessions and my role in them. It was sometimes difficult to detach myself from this to see what was not always so overt. Case, Dalley and Connell are therefore right to stress the importance of rigorous supervision, so that therapists may have the opportunity to understand their own responses properly (Case and Dalley 1992; Connell 1998a). Only in this way, I believe, will therapists retain their ability to effectively engage and disengage in the way that is so crucial for this area of work.

Conclusion

Traditionally, in working in the area of palliative care, there has been an emphasis on the cathartic role of the picture in the session to facilitate and contain. Writers like Connell show how effective this can be in promoting more adaptive and creative responses even in clients who are very close to death. However, failure to address transference issues is an omission, since it both underestimates the resources practitioners have to draw upon in order to 'survive' and potentially deprives them of a vital part of their practice. It is left to other writers (practitioners who do not generally work in this field) to usefully remind us of the importance of transference and countertransference in the therapy session. They show that, far from being a source for concern, such features can and should be treated as integral to the therapy interaction.

Practising in the area of palliative care is potentially fraught with problems as we continually work with people who subsequently die. As therapists we must remain aware of the effect this may be having on us as individuals, both in our professional lives and also away from work, if we are to endeavour to engage and disengage with the equanimity that our clients require. Above all, we must acknowledge that this work is difficult to sustain, for only by paying attention to our own needs can we more truly listen to those of our client. In the end I think Delmonte is right to caution that it is not necessarily the needs or motivations of the therapists who work in this area that are harmful, but their avoidance or denial (Delmonte 1996).

Note

Grateful thanks to the British Association of Art Therapists for allowing a substantial part of the paper 'Creating through loss' (2001) to be reproduced. It first appeared in *Inscape: Journal of Art Therapy*, 6(1): 23–31.

References

Balint, M. (1966) *The Basic Fault. Therapeutic Aspects of Regression*. London: Tavistock Publications.

Barraclough, J. (1994) *Cancer and Emotion*. Chichester: John Wiley and Sons.

Beaver, V. (1998) The butterfly garden: art therapy with HIV/AIDS prisoners, in M. Pratt and M.J.M. Wood (eds) *Art Therapy in Palliative Care: The Creative Response*. London: Routledge.

Becker, E. (1973) *The Denial of Death*. New York: Routledge.

Brown, D. and Peddler, P. (1979) *Introduction to Psychotherapy*. London: Routledge.

Case, C. and Dalley, T. (1992) *Handbook of Art Therapy*. London: Routledge.

Cohen, A. and Abramowitz, S. (1990) AIDS attacks the self: a self-psychological exploration of the psychodynamic consequences of AIDS, in A. Goldberg (ed.) *The Realities of Transference: Progress in Self Psychology*. London: Analytic Press.

Connell, C. (1992) Art therapy as part of a palliative care programme, *Palliative Medicine*, 6(1): 18.

Connell, C. (1998a) *Something Understood. Art Therapy in Cancer Care*. London: Wrexham Publications in association with Azimuth Editions.

Connell, C. (1998b) The search for a model which opens, in M. Pratt and M.J.M. Wood (eds) *Art Therapy in Palliative Care: The Creative Response*. London: Routledge.

Coote, J. (1998) Getting started: introducing the art therapy service and the individual's first experiences, in M. Pratt and M.J.M. Wood (eds) *Art Therapy in Palliative Care: The Creative Response*. London: Routledge.

Delmonte, H. (1996) Why work with the dying?, in C. Lee (ed.) *Still Waters*. Oxford: Sobell Publications.

Edwards, G.M. (1993) Art therapy with HIV-positive patients: hardness, creativity and meaning, *The Arts in Psychotherapy*, 20: 325–33.

Feldman, E. (1993) HIV dementia and countertransference, *The Arts in Psychotherapy*, 20: 317–23.

Gordon, R. (1978) *Dying and Creating: A Search for Meaning*. London: The Society of Analytical Psychology.

Halliday, D. (1988) My art healed me, *Inscape*, Spring: 18–23.

Holmes, J. (1973) *John Bowlby and Attachment Theory*. London, New York: Routledge.

Kearney, M. (1992) Image work in a case of intractable pain, *Palliative Medicine*, 6: 152–7.

Luzzatto, P. (1998) From psychiatry to psycho-oncology: personal reflections on the use of art therapy with cancer patients, in M. Pratt and M.J.M. Wood (eds) *Art Therapy in Palliative Care: The Creative Response*. London: Routledge.

Malitskie, G. (1988) Art therapy with kidney patients, *Inscape*, Spring: 14–18.

May, R. (1975) *The Courage to Create*. New York, London: Norton and Company.

Pratt, M. and Wood, M.J.M. (eds) (1998) *Art Therapy in Palliative Care. The Creative Response*. London, New York: Routledge.

Schaverien, J. (1997) Men who leave too soon, *British Journal of Psychotherapy*, 14(1).

Schaverien, J. (1998) Individuation, countertransference and the death of a client, *Inscape*, 3(2): 55–63.

Simon, R. (1981) Bereavement art, *American Journal of Art Therapy*, 20: 35–43.

Skaife, S. (1993) Sickness, health and the therapeutic relationship: thoughts arising from the literature on art therapy and physical illness, *Inscape*, Summer: 24–9.

Szepanski, M. (1988) Art therapy and multiple sclerosis, *Inscape*, Spring: 4–10.

Thomas, G. (1998) What lies within us: individuals in a Marie Curie Hospice, in M. Pratt and M.J.M. Wood (eds) *Art Therapy in Palliative Care: The Creative Response*. London, New York: Routledge.

Thomas, G. and Kennedy, J. (1995) Art therapy and practice in palliative care, *European Journal of Palliative Care*, 2(3): 120–3.

Trauger-Querry, B. and Ryan Haghighi, K. (1999) Balancing the focus: art and music therapy for pain control and symptom management in hospice care, *The Hospice Journal*, 14(1): 25–37.

Wood, M.J.M. (1990) Art therapy in one session: working with people with AIDS, *Inscape*, Winter: 27–33.

Wood, M.J.M. (1998) Art therapy in palliative care, in M. Pratt and M.J.M. Wood (eds) *Art Therapy in Palliative Care: The Creative Response*. London: Routledge.

Yalom, I. (1980) *Existentialist Psychotherapy*. New York: Basic Books.

Young, R.M. (1995) The vicissitudes of transference and countertransference: the world of Harold Searles, *Free Associations*, 5(2): 171–95.

14 Art therapy in the hospice: rewards and frustrations

Timothy Duesbury

Introduction

I began my career in palliative care as a final year art therapy trainee at a London hospice. Prior to this, I had a brief work placement in HIV through a degree course, and then, post degree, worked in a hospital with children living with cancer. Upon qualification, my trainee placement developed into a sessional post where, at the time of writing, I have been engaged for four years. During this time I also secured a second, part-time, palliative care art therapy post within the National Health Service in Guildford. In the hospice I used to run a group and to see clients individually. Now, partly due to lack of funding (but also as an adaptation to client needs), I only work individually with clients, my hours having been reduced to just three per week. In the NHS, I both run a group and see clients individually during one short day. Combining both of these positions, my client group includes cancer care, motor neurone disease, Parkinson's disease and distortion of body perception (as a life-changing condition).

Literature review

There follows a brief review of the literature, which considers some of the more problematic areas for staff working in palliative care. Themes include stress, institutional dynamics and professional isolation. The authors reviewed are mostly UK-based, as US and European work practices differ from those in Britain (see Skaife 1993). The exception is Belfiore, whose work seemed particularly relevant. Schaverien (2002) devotes a whole book to issues of psychotherapeutic work with one dying patient and takes the reader on quite a journey, looking in depth at many aspects of the therapeutic encounter. Later in the chapter there is a discussion of some of my own experiences (with reference to salient points from others writing before me) – the rewards and frustrations of palliative care work.

Alexander and Ritchie (1990) note that stressors of work in palliative care for nurses include patients below 40 years of age, patients in intractable pain, patients that are afraid to die, psychiatric symptoms, patients with young children and patients' relatives. Work with clients that are younger or of a similar age to oneself would seem to compound feelings of stress and anxiety. Alexander and Ritchie (1990) attribute this to an identification process. Wood (1998) cites Baker and Seager (1991) who comment on work with young people who die as stressful.

Belfiore (1994) looks at feelings that may be induced in palliative care workers. She considers that for some staff to be perceived as helpful implied for them competence and total availability. She used an art therapy group that enabled palliative care workers to become more aware of demands – both personal and those induced by the work place. She draws our attention to the notion of 'false self'. Rycroft (1995) attributes the concept of 'false self' to Winnicott (1958). Rycroft describes this notion as a defensive structure acting as an adaptation to an environment that has not met the needs of the child in the determining months of infancy. Belfiore (1994) describes these defensive structures for workers in palliative care as becoming their mode of interaction, as they oscillate between omnipotence and impotence. This may help to explain what Speck (1994) describes as 'chronic niceness' as palliative care workers strive to be seen as the perfect carers. Harris *et al.* (1990) discuss how regular contact with people who are dying forces one to consider one's own mortality, which increases one's fears about death. They go on to say how frequently forming a relationship with people who are going to die soon has been identified as stressful. Belfiore (1994) considers that palliative care staff may develop unhealthy defence mechanisms as a result of the demands of the work with patients and, we may surmise, because of the institutional demands that more work is done. Alexander and McLeod (1992) discuss organizations placing responsibility for staff dynamics firmly in their court. They feel that stressed staff need to be thought of in consideration to their working positions and that any problem may be institutional, and that institutions are to blame for pathologizing stressed staff as weak, whereas the true fault lies in the organizational structure. Alexander (1993) believes that palliative care workers are frequently over-optimistic as to what is achievable.

Alexander (1993) citing Weisman (1981), Alexander and McLeod (1992), and Finlay (1989) all comment on aspects of isolation of staff working in palliative care and, urging caution, advocate staff to find ways to offload their experiences for the sake of their own health. Edwards (1989) looks deeply at isolation for art therapists in general and understands it to have three aspects: recognition, integration and validation, and thinks about ways that these might be achieved. Sadly, many of the issues highlighted by Edwards are still prevalent fifteen years on and are much in evidence in my working environments. Writing in 1998, Wood considers that art therapists are well respected within teams. In my experience of palliative care work in two quite different situations, this holds true *within* the staff teams. However, institutional demands often seem to frustrate the support found within the team. This becomes apparent in demands for more clients to be seen (within existing contract times, when one's client list is full and there is a perception that administration and particularly processing time can be forfeited). With budgetary constraints and targets being ubiquitous the demand to treat more clients is probably a familiar pressure to all. Edwards (1989) cites Menzies 1977, who saw institutions creating defence mechanisms against anxiety when a different way of working challenges established procedures. This raised anxiety becomes a reminder of historical dynamics denied – reinforcing the anxiety but also the things avoided to date. Edwards sees validation of art therapy as key to its acceptance as a valued intervention. He questions whether 'empirical scientific knowledge' is as impartial as others may believe, but thinks that it still retains great influence in some work situations. Of course, this is not limited to palliative care art therapy and much of what is presented here will be applicable to art therapists working in other areas.

In hospice working, these pressures abound but are added to by an institutional response to counter the ultimate reduction in client interaction – death. This is, of course, a defence mechanism – denial. Yalom (1980) gives us a formula that may be useful in this regard: 'Awareness of Ultimate Concern–Anxiety–Defence Mechanism' (p. 10). The institution gets caught in a dynamic between expounding the reason for its very existence (to treat people who are living with a reduced life expectancy and who are near the end of their lives) and attempting to pretend that client lists are stable and full. Speck says:

> Just as I, in my role as chaplain, needed some space in order to regain my ability to think . . . so staff groups need space to understand what they are carrying psychologically as a result of the work that they do. The hospice or other care institution may then be able to re-engage with its primary task. It is the ability to tolerate ambivalence that can restore integration and the capacity to think, or, in Kleinian terms, move a group from the paranoid-schizoid to the depressive position . . .
>
> (Speck 1998: 100)

The root of this is institutional in its broadest sense, but influences others and so has echoes throughout, affecting teams and individuals. One's profession as an art therapist allows one to find a place to think – to process events in one's work and to understand and, therefore, to function more freely, more realistically, and more healthily.

In the palliative care institutions in which I work, it seems rare to hear of a person only completing their paid hours, with the norm being that most will stay to do something extra or finish a task for the following day. This includes ancillary, administrative, voluntary and professional staff alike. Feelings of needing to 'do more' can be understood as an existential response in the individual and in the institution as a fear of annihilation. This, combined with 'chronic niceness', produces a working environment where it is difficult to allow oneself to 'be' rather than responding to a denial-led ethos working towards ever-increasing targets. Kaye (1998) quotes Speck from 1994 as saying 'There is a collective fantasy that the staff are nice people, who are caring for nice dying people, who are going to have a nice death in a nice place' (p. 46). Higgins (2002) also notes 'hysterical merriment' affecting carers and patients alike. If the place where patients are to receive support colludes in this denial, how are they to find a voice to enable them to work through feelings? How are they to access and engage in therapy? When working in an environment which is in denial, partial or not, how is one to proceed? A familiar quandary is the theoretical approach that one adopts. Skaife (1993) highlights some interesting points. For instance, if a patient is physically unwell, it may be important to them that their mental health is not being called into question by a psychodynamic therapy. This is despite a form of psychotherapy being a useful intervention, she says (with reference to Kirby 1988), in order to explore issues of loss of power and other feelings brought about by a deterioration in health. She highlights practices that do not utilize the full rigour of a psychotherapeutic approach – not taking into account transference and countertransference, and suggests that this may be due to fear of envious attack on the 'well therapist' by the 'ill patient'. I feel that if the institution is less than supportive of psychotherapeutic work utilizing transference and countertransference then it can be difficult to employ such practices in one's work. Skaife notes that the context has to be right, with support from work places allowing space and time for an intervention to be useful to a client.

Psychodynamic work seems to challenge institutions. This can be partially understood in the light of defence mechanisms that we have acknowledged to be in place through an understanding of the literature discussed previously. If the institution is in denial of its shadow aspects – fear and anger about death and dying – then an attempt to expose and work with these feelings will obviously arouse a negative response. This may account for the frequently heard indicative 'to be more flexible' where perhaps the underlying message is 'please don't stir up and allow expression to those painful feelings'! A more humanistic approach, in which actualization emphasizes searching for more positive outcomes and empowerment (through identification of helpful attributes and utilizing them as strategies for future development), rather than explorative resolution, may be a more comfortable intervention for institutions in denial. This plea for flexibility has encouraged me to consider deeply my theoretical orientation. I have learnt to combine these approaches of exploration and development into one – where there is an interplay between explorations to help clients think about their motivations and how their past affects their present, and a process through which they feel empowered to develop new aspects to their lives and discover a future, even with a shortened life expectancy. Luzzatto and Gabriel (1998) advocate an integrative approach to art therapy. This includes promotion of insight and change in the inner world of the patient. Also, that their maladaptive behaviours be integrated with the use of transference and countertransference in the dynamic relationship between the client and the therapist. In my practice it has been a question of discovering what works – for the institution where the art therapy takes place, for me within those parameters and for my clients. It is a delicate balance to know when to delve and explore with a client and when to strive towards development. Connell (1992) notes that in psychology the use of art therapy as a diagnostic tool was previously a fashionable idea. She advocates a broader understanding of what art therapy can offer, saying that it can touch the psyche on different levels, using visual processes rather than logical ones. I feel that it has been useful for the clients for me to watch and wait, to see where they need to go at that moment, knowing that it may change as their needs fluctuate. This exploration has been, at various times, painful, disturbing and exhilarating. Schaverien comments that 'Physical illness does not stay within prescribed boundaries and inevitably the structure of the analytic frame has to be adapted to accommodate the deterioration of the patient's health' (2002: 10).

It is such an intimate journey, embarked upon by both client and therapist, that when it flows it is quite a heady ride. The therapy has to be understood as happening in the environment in which it takes place. Gestalt means 'wholeness'. Using the Gestalt Therapy notion of figure and ground, the institution, the multidisciplinary team (MDT), the space, etc., all form part of the (back) 'ground' and the interaction between my client and I are 'figure' (or what is focused on) – forming a Gestalt.

Rewards and frustrations

Just what are the pleasures – when things are so difficult? It seems a considerable challenge to describe to you how and why it is that I do my work in this area. It seems indulgent to say I feel humbled and privileged to be allowed to enter the emotional world of my clients at such a significant life stage. There is a joy that enables me to do just that and to return repeatedly even when it has been at its most painful. Recently, a group member

returned after a few weeks' absence to say goodbye. This person had experienced a dramatic downturn in health and looked very ill indeed, but had
been attending the group for a long time and had been highly committed to
it. It was deeply moving to us all in the group. A part of the joy in palliative
care work is the diversity and the immediacy of the interactions with clients.
A pleasure is in helping someone towards a method of discovery – a place
where they can begin to form understandings that may not be achievable
through any other means. As a facilitator one acts as a conduit. As a client
gains ability through increasing confidence as he/she experiences therapeutic
containment, the maternal holding shifts. A movement towards individuation occurs and one finds pride in the client's increasing abilities. Due to the
intense nature of the work, the rewards are as profound as the investment
has been high for both client and therapist. Schaverien (2002) says that 'The
experience of working with a dying patient is usually *engaging* . . .' (my
emphasis, p. 10). Beaver (1998) tells of feeling exhilarated, in awe and
humbled in her work, and that it was for her a privilege to work with her
client group. This has certainly also been the case for me in all of my palliative
care work.

The working environment can be very problematic. In 1998 Wood wrote:
'Art therapy should take place in an environment designated for that purpose' (p. 2). I have visited only a few hospices but recall, within this small
sample, art therapists being required to work in the main room of a day
centre and it would seem to be commonplace, at present, for art therapists to
have to share space and needing to pre-book rooms in which to work. This is
the case in one of my palliative care positions, where group work takes place
in what is normally the meetings room (it is carpeted and does not have a
sink) and individual work in a counselling room (again, it is carpeted and
has no sink). This, however, is preferable to the previously negotiated space
for individual work – a physiotherapy consulting room with sink and
linoleum but with a very clinical atmosphere. In all cases, furniture has to be
removed and other more appropriate furniture brought in. In another work
place, until recently I had to use the space that functions not only as the
dining area for patients attending the day centre but also as the general arts
and craft area. Therefore, the confusion between arts and craft and art
therapy for some patients (see Edwards 1989) who may attend both was
high (volunteers and some staff included). The feelings of clients who leave
art therapy during which they have experienced intense emotions, then
re-enter the same room for lunch thirty minutes later, must be difficult to
assimilate. In my conversations with other palliative care art therapists these
sorts of situations, sadly, do not seem to be rare. Simon Bell has commented
on this aspect of work, saying: 'Whilst meeting with Tom in a seemingly
secluded part of the day unit, we would often be disturbed by volunteers or
other staff who would unknowingly interrupt a session taking place' (Bell
1998: 92). Val Beaver adds to this, commenting:

To enable creativity and healing to take place there had to be a facilitating environment, a potential space where there was opportunity for reflection and reverie, and where the men could be protected from the harsh reality of prison routine, boredom and brutality – their own and others – at least for a while.

(Beaver 1998: 128–9)

It seems to me that art therapy in a prison must often be a harrowing experience, not least due to institutional dynamics. Not wishing to diminish this experience, art therapy in a hospice can also seem to be under threat from the 'providing' institution (invasion of space, lack of provision of space, impoverished contract hours and confusion between art therapy and creative therapy, and so on). It can often be a struggle to claim and establish a working space that starts to fulfil even minimum requirements of light, access to running water, privacy, etc. Wood (1998) discusses these points briefly and directs us to Case and Dalley (1992) for greater discussion. The National Institute for Clinical Excellence (NICE) guidelines produced by the National Health Service in 2004 comment upon appropriate facilities at points 5.14 (p. 77) and 5.37 (p. 81). A failure to recognize the benefits that properly resourced art therapy is able to give clients, and the knock-on benefits to the institution, clients' families and relationships and the systems in which they exist, limits what may truly be achieved. It is vital that these things are properly considered prior to introducing an art therapy service or its development. Working at bedsides on shared wards presents further dimensions that need acknowledgement when with a client. When there is only a flimsy curtain to pull around the client's bed, and while other patients may be attended to by staff, or have visitors, or domestic staff may be performing their duties, one is aware of the fragility of these boundaries. The therapeutic alliance, where one helps a client to develop a deep rapport and trust in the intervention on offer, becomes all the more important. In such situations, one tends to work in close proximity to clients and to lower one's voice. However, experience has shown me that trying to work with these factors can be beneficial. In one instance, I noted that I could overhear another patient's visitor and, remarking that it was like listening to the radio or to one's internal voices, wondered about my client communicating to himself. It opened up an unexplored avenue to our work. 'Whatever the practical constraints surrounding the location of art therapy sessions, the art therapist's task is to ensure that the surroundings allow enough privacy for a client to get on with their work . . .' (Wood 1998: 3). Not having a permanent space for art therapy has left me at times feeling 'homeless' and frequently at a loss about where to go in order to complete my work. Having the space to spend time to review clients' work is problematic, as is a quiet space for reflection whilst making process notes.

Professional isolation is a feature even though MDT working is common. It often seems hard for people from other disciplines to comprehend the true breadth and depth of what it entails to be an art therapist; it seems rare to work alongside someone else who is working psychotherapeutically.

However, being part of a small and compact MDT is often a reward of this area of work. When an art therapy referral is made, there is opportunity to discuss with colleagues their feelings about the potential client. Referrals may arrive from diverse sources, including nurses, healthcare assistants, physiotherapists or complementary therapists. Recently, an aromatherapist brought to my attention a man whom she felt was experiencing some difficulty due to the emotional impact his symptoms were causing him – ulcerated lymphoedema complicated by a cardiac condition. The referee felt that the medical team were somewhat at a loss as to how to support this man and she thought that art therapy might give him the chance to be heard and for problems to be acknowledged and confronted.

Without the good working relationships that I have fostered over the years, my sense of isolation would be much greater than it is. Alexander and Ritchie, writing in 1990, felt that developing work relationships for support was an area that needed attention.

Feelings of homelessness and isolation link to needing to find a place within the MDTs. If one is not able to do this, these feelings are compounded. In palliative care, it is frequent to be sessional and maybe only working in a team for a few hours per week. This can make linking and liaison with others profoundly difficult, if not impossible. It becomes yet another reason to feel the need to increase one's hours informally. Wood (1990) laments her lack of contact with teams due to her brief contracted hours as a palliative care art therapist. She regrets lack of contact with team members and notes: 'Unfortunately because I only work for eight hours a week I am unable to participate as a full member of the multidisciplinary team, and so do not attend the meetings where patients and new referrals are discussed' (p. 27).

Writing in 1993, Skaife notes the frequency of 'ad hoc' working positions at that time and how this made conditions for effective practice problematic. In one of my palliative care posts, I am employed for six-and-a-half hours per week and in the other for just three hours per week. In this position there is an immense pressure to want to develop the post – after all, how can one possibly begin to meet potential client demand? It is only potential demand, as it seems very like the proverbial chicken and egg – how can one generate demand if one is simply not there to meet it? So referrals remain low and the post remains impoverished. Coote, echoing my own experience, says:

> I am based in the day centre at the hospice, working with both day patients and in-patients on the wards. A limited budget allows only two and a half hours there a week. Considering the often brief time a

patient has at the hospice this inevitably limits the number of patients I will see.

(1998: 53)

Another palliative care art therapist once described to me a feeling that 'patients leave a "residue" as clients do not just bring with them cancer and death, but all aspects of their lives'. However, she also felt that this was partially ameliorated by the images containing many of the feelings. Sometimes one does not have regular clients and may have to wait for a new referral, either from a member of staff or a self-referral. For palliative care clients, time is often at a high premium. This increases the sense of urgency and the tension in having to sit with the waiting, desperately trying to 'be' rather than 'do'. Here, existential angst is hard at work, and living with the not knowing is hard for everyone, clients and therapists alike. The problem is, how can one sit in stillness and aloneness but also be ready to switch into a position where one is able to receive the extremes of emotion that the next person entering the room may bring with them? Anxiety is high. How should one hold this space? There is the possibility that someone, staff or volunteer, seeing me without a client, may enter the room even though they have been informed that this space needs to be kept for clients. If one begins an image, as a way of processing feelings, how would a client perceive this, and how to switch from artist to therapist in that instant that they pass the threshold? It has been described to me as like being in the trenches of the First World War: there are frequent long hours with no client and then suddenly all hell breaks loose as someone in crisis enters the room. When a client dies that one has been working with for a long time it is, of course, painful. Similarly it is also painful if a client who is at the end stage of their life somehow returns to therapy one last time; such is the depth of their engagement. One feels oneself 'hanging on' with them.

Supervision plays an essential part in this. It is a place of recognition – of one's role, of one's position (both in the work place and emotionally); a place of identity – where one can talk without the need to have to explain everything because one is understood professionally; and a place to chat and be human, basking in the light of being seen and accepted. Jones (1997) says that supervision allows time and space for many feelings to be processed concerning the work with people who are dying. Certainly, supervision enables me to continue to return to my work time and again.

It is not just their cancer or other life-threatening conditions that our clients bring but also other aspects of their lives; one finds oneself working within a holistic frame. It is not just the exceptionally intimate depth of work with someone close to the end of their lives but also the breadth, as we may consider past issues and family dynamics too, that makes this area of work so remarkably gratifying; we are working with past, present and future as an entirety. There is something profound in just 'being' with a client – whether or not they are making an image or talking. We may not have words at times in a session, my client or I, and this makes it difficult to describe the intensity, the beauty and the pleasure of the work between clients and myself. The engagement is equally deep on both our parts; it takes openness for the relationship to develop in this way. Therefore, I have to risk myself and commit myself to the therapeutic encounter in just the same way as my clients. Humanistic and existential models of therapy (forming a person centred approach) call for authenticity and positive regard. I feel that my clients deserve nothing less. Whatever the shortcomings of any place of work, the true pleasure comes from the engagement of clients and the journey that I feel humbled and privileged to embark upon with my clients. This is both the reward and the frustration of work in palliative care.

References

Alexander, D.A. (1993) Staff support groups: do they support and are they even groups?, *Palliative Medicine*, 7: 127–32.

Alexander, D.A. and MacLeod, M. (1992) Stress among palliative care matrons: a major problem for a minority group, *Palliative Medicine*, 6: 111–24.

Alexander, D.A. and Ritchie, E. (1990) Stressors and difficulties in dealing with the terminal patient, *Journal of Palliative Care*, 6(3): 28–33.

Baker, W.T. and Seager, R.T. (1991) A comparison of the psychosocial needs of hospice patients with AIDS and those with diagnoses, *The Hospice Journal*, 7(1/2): 61–9.

Beaver, V. (1998) The butterfly garden: art therapy with HIV/AIDS prisoners, in M. Pratt and M.J.M. Wood (eds) *Art Therapy in Palliative Care: The Creative Response*. London, New York: Routledge.

Belfiore, M. (1994) The group takes care of itself: art therapy to prevent burnout, *The Arts in Psychotherapy*, 21(2): 119–26.

Bell, S. (1998) Will the kitchen table do? Art therapy in the community, in M. Pratt and M.J.M. Wood (eds) *Art Therapy in Palliative Care: The Creative Response*. London, New York: Routledge.

Case, C. and Dalley, T. (1992) *Handbook of Art Therapy*. London: Routledge.

Connell, C. (1992) Art therapy as part of a palliative care programme, *Palliative Medicine*, 6: 18–25.

Coote, J. (1998) Getting started: introducing the art therapy service and the individual's first experiences, in M. Pratt and M.J.M. Wood (eds) *Art Therapy in Palliative Care: The Creative Response*. London, New York: Routledge.

Edwards, D. (1989) Five years on: further thoughts on the issue of surviving as an art therapist, in A. Gilroy and T. Dalley (eds) *Pictures at an Exhibition. Selected Essays on Art and Art Therapy*. London, New York: Tavistock/Routledge.

Finlay, I.G. (1989) Sources of stress in hospice medical directors and matrons, *Palliative Medicine*, 4: 5–9.

Harris, R.D. *et al.* (1990) Nursing stress and stress reduction in palliative care, *Palliative Medicine*, 4: 191–6.

Higgins, R. (2002) Foreword, in D. Waller (ed.) *Art Therapies and Progressive Illness: Nameless Dread*. Hove, New York: Brunner-Routledge.

Jones, A. (1997) Death, poetry, psychotherapy and clinical supervision (the contribution of psychodynamic psychotherapy to palliative care nursing), *Journal of Advanced Nursing*, 25: 238–44.

Kaye, P. (1998) Some images of illness: the place of art therapy in the palliative care team – a doctor's perspective, in M. Pratt and M.J.M. Wood (eds) *Art Therapy in Palliative Care: The Creative Response*. London, New York: Routledge.

Luzzatto, P. and Gabriel, B. (1998) Art psychotherapy, in J.C. Holland (ed.) *Psycho-oncology*. Oxford: Oxford University Press.

Menzies, I. (1977) *The Functioning of a Social System as a Defence against Anxiety*. London: Tavistock.

National Institute for Clinical Excellence (NICE) (2004) *Guidance on Cancer Services. Improving Supportive and Palliative Care for Adults with Cancer. The Manual*. London: NICE.

Rycroft, C. (1995) *A Critical Dictionary of Psychoanalysis*. London: Penguin.

Schaverien, J. (2002) *The Dying Patient in Psychotherapy. Desire, Dreams and Individuation*. Basingstoke, New York: Palgrave Macmillan.

Skaife, S. (1993) Sickness, health and the therapeutic relationship: thoughts arising from the literature on art therapy and physical illness, *Inscape*, Summer: 24–9.

Speck, P. (1994) Working with dying people. On being good enough, in A. Obholzer et al. (eds) *The Unconscious At Work: Individual and Organisational Stress in the Human Services*. (First published in 1994). London: Routledge.

Weisman, A.D. (1981) Understanding the cancer patient: the syndrome of caregivers' plight, *Psychology*, 44: 161–8.

Winnicott, D.W. (1958) *Collected Papers*. London: Tavistock.

Wood, M.J.M. (1990) Art therapy in one session. Working with people with AIDS, *Inscape*, Winter: 27–33.

Wood, M.J.M. (1998a) Art therapy in palliative care, in M. Pratt and M.J.M. Wood (eds) *Art Therapy in Palliative Care. The Creative Response*. London, New York: Routledge.

Wood, M.J.M. (1998b) The body as art: individual session with a man with AIDS, in M. Pratt and M.J.M. Wood (eds) *Art Therapy in Palliative Care. The Creative Response*. London, New York: Routledge.

Wood, M.J.M. (1998c) What is art therapy?, in M. Pratt and M.J.M. Wood (eds) *Art Therapy in Palliative Care. The Creative Response*. London, New York. Routledge.

Wood, M.J.M. (1998d) What is palliative care?, in M. Pratt and M.J.M. Wood (eds) *Art Therapy in Palliative Care. The Creative Response*. London, New York: Routledge.

Yalom, I.D. (1980) *Existential Psychotherapy*. New York: Basic Books.

15 A 'don't know' story: art therapy in an NHS medical oncology department

Maureen Bocking

Introduction

In this chapter, I will look at 'not knowing' as a feature of much of my art therapy practice with cancer patients at a London hospital. I will illustrate this with a case example of art therapy sessions over a period of two years until a patient's death in a hospice and some shorter casework. I will also reflect on the resonance of the theme of not knowing in my own life and choice of profession.

Giving patients as much appropriate information as possible is now part of normal hospital procedure and is assisted by the CancerBACUP organization. Understanding what is going to be done to them or what to expect relieves anxiety and stress and therefore assists recovery. Despite the best efforts of medical staff many questions inevitably remain unanswered or unasked. A diagnosis of cancer turns life upside down and changes everything. Uncertainty creeps in and new situations have to be faced. Dealing with practical matters may be easier than dealing with emotions. Much of the time we just get on with day-to-day activities and don't focus on feelings. Obviously, illness can undermine any aspect of life we take for granted, such as eating, sleeping, standing, walking, breathing, and put us in touch with primitive, childlike fears. These can threaten our sense of identity and the values that give meaning to life. The 'not knowing' I am thinking about is more to do with questions on a deeper level, about acceptance of uncertainty and willingness to explore something new. It is a challenge and art therapy opens a way to create our own meaning, of who we are and what is significant. Wondering is an openness to the unknown and makes it acceptable not to know.

Why art therapy?

Recently a patient asked me why I do art therapy and what I get out of it. I thought about it but it wasn't easy to answer. I felt a bit embarrassed to admit to getting anything out of it for myself, under the circumstances. All the literature and leaflets I hand out state that 'Art therapy is for patients to express themselves through the use of art materials in the presence of a qualified therapist . . .' and so on. I found myself questioning (yet again) my role as an art therapist and what it is like to hear so many stories, meet so many individuals for brief but crucial periods and not know where they have gone after they leave hospital. My role is to temporarily 'hold a safe space' for them to explore life and death issues. I am often left to deal with what this arouses in me. Also, am I allowed to find satisfaction in this work?

When I was asked to write this chapter I found myself going back to basics and taking a questioning position. For instance, what do I (as a person) bring to the session? How do I (with all my life experiences) meet the patients/persons/clients, with all of theirs? How does the therapeutic relationship happen? And how do the patients really experience me? Do we, as art therapists, look at the reasons we choose to do the kind of work we do? Why did I choose to work in a hospital environment with cancer patients?

When I reflected on the last question the answer was not difficult to find. I lost my father when I was 9 years old. At that time children were usually excluded from knowing about painful events like dying, funerals and feelings. I'd never seen my mother or father shed a tear. I believed men never cried. Nobody mentioned cancer. My father disappeared one day while I was at school and that was it. I went to the hospital with my mother to visit him but children weren't allowed in. I stood at the end of a long ward and wanted to know what was going on behind the drawn curtains. I was curious and sad but I comforted myself with the thought that one day I would find out.

Some years later I trained to become a nurse and at the back of my mind was the same curiosity and determination to know what goes on – behind the screens. At the time nurses were not supposed to waste time talking to patients 'unnecessarily'. I left nursing knowing about bodies but wanting to know more about that which was not spoken about: feelings, emotions and the human condition.

A lifetime of experience later, with a degree in fine art and a deep interest in people, I found my way to a personal inner landscape through art therapy training. Now I see my role as an art therapist as going into these inner places with other people who struggle with the state of not knowing. I aim to 'hold the ground' and offer a place of safety in which to explore the uncertainty of having a diagnosis of a life-threatening illness.

Meeting people as patients in a hospital setting

On a practical level, not knowing is a weekly occurrence for me. For instance, who I will meet that day? Will patients who I met the previous week have gone home? Will people who wanted to see me for art therapy actually feel well enough when the time comes? Will their visitors turn up unexpectedly or medical treatment clash with an arranged session?

Neither the patient or I know for certain for how many hours, days or weeks they will be coming to the hospital and whether a first meeting will be a 'one-off'. For this reason, patients are seen one-to-one and groups are not possible. In the ward patients need patience and waiting adds to uncertainty. They wait for ward rounds, treatment procedures, medication or chemotherapy, appointments in other departments, transport, meals or visitors. They don't know which bed they will have, who will be near them, when the doctor will come, what tests will show, what will happen next, when they will go home, and so on. People can be very busy as patients in hospital and hardly have time to rest.

As yet another person disturbing a patient's need for privacy, I have to respect their feelings and be sensitive to the body language or avoidance of eye contact that tells me just to 'go away'! I have learned to recognize polite excuses when someone finds it hard to say 'no' to the offer of art therapy. Members of the medical team or I might think a patient would benefit from art therapy but they choose to decline. Sleep can be more important, or the whole idea too unfamiliar and strange.

On the other hand I have also realized that it is important not to pass by someone who looks unlikely to respond to me, as sometimes such a person has indeed taken up the offer and used art therapy in a surprising and very worthwhile way. As I enter wards and meet the patients I have to accept my own uncertainty and the discomfort of 'not knowing'.

Being adaptable and flexible as a hospital art therapist

A moment of meeting between two people is a fundamental adventure. Who are you? An affirmation of identity, a split second appraisal of like or dislike, a friendly face in a strange place, or just someone to talk to? Bald heads, tubes and dangling bags of urine, body fluids in recycled cardboard kidney dishes, drips and monitors. Coughs, smells, lumps and bandages, cards, flowers, fruit bowls. Vulnerability and suffering. I walk into people's personal spaces with my box of paper and art materials and our eyes meet. Is what I am offering appropriate just now? It is a yes or no moment?

I have sometimes seen the process of meeting and establishing art therapy sessions as a series of hurdles to pass over. After making contact and agreeing to meet for an art therapy session, finding a suitable time can be quite tricky. The next step is deciding where the session will take place. Is the patient physically mobile and do they have use of their arm or hand, when attached to an IV infusion? Have they left their glasses at home? Can they sit up? Will the session take place at the bedside? How long will it last? Will it be the only time we meet or the start of a therapeutic relationship?

I tend to be a travelling therapist, carrying my box of materials with me and making use of quiet rooms or spaces by the beds. I also have use of one of the doctors' consulting rooms, with cupboards where art materials and artwork are stored. This provides a private place away from the wards where patients who are able can attend for art sessions and conversation. It is mostly free of intrusion, interruption and noise and it is a base for me to return to and to feel grounded in an otherwise 'free-floating' role.

Many patients want simply to talk to someone who will listen or, for various reasons, have only a single session of art therapy. Nonetheless, these can be very valuable experiences for them. In the following section I will give examples of 'one-off' sessions and the significance of the materials that are used. I will also describe examples of longer periods of art therapy work and the differing ways the theme of not knowing manifests itself.

Single sessions and the art materials

Art therapy is often a strange concept to people who have never heard of it before. Drawing and painting can be equally unfamiliar. Many people say 'I can't draw a straight line!' Others imagine it is an art class. I take with me brief, introductory leaflets to help explain that it is not about being good at art. The leaflet outlines the idea of expressing feelings through using art materials, in the presence of a qualified art therapist who will be there to listen and facilitate the process. I try to demystify the idea of therapy and talk about experimenting with the paint or whatever they choose. As long as someone wants to try it, I encourage them to do so and see where it may take us.

Making a start can be daunting. I keep a selection of picture postcards for people to look through for inspiration. Even if someone tries to copy a picture it soon becomes their own interpretation which will have a special meaning to that individual. I keep the usual range of pencils, crayons, paints, paper, collage materials and self-hardening modelling clay. I also have available a sand tray with a box of stones, shells and scraps of interesting-shaped wood. These can be used to create three-dimensional pictures in the sand. It includes a poetry book and miniature Japanese garden tools with a tiny rake for drawing. It is a wonderful way to create symbolic landscapes or to trace out imaginary life journeys. The sand pictures can be easily changed or smoothed away and sand provides extra tactile qualities to play with.

Sand was useful in another situation. A young girl who had lost her sight from a brain tumour came for art therapy sessions and painted pictures from memory. Although she enjoyed the feeling of using a paintbrush and moving thick paint around on paper, it seemed sad that she could not see what she had done. I helped her sprinkle sand onto wet acrylic paint and after it dried she could feel the textures and shapes she had made. It made the experience of painting more meaningful for her and helped build up her confidence.

I have found silk paints a particularly useful addition to the box I carry when working in the wards. They are easy to manage for bed-bound patients as the silk is held taut in a lightweight embroidery hoop. Although the inks have similar qualities to watercolour paints, there seems to be less anxiety and expectation about the finished result. The colours are vivid and tend to run very freely so the way the paintings turn out never fails to be a surprise. The silk fabric can be aesthetically pleasing and can create associations of preciousness. It can be an unconscious reminder that lives are precious and that the patient is special.

One elderly lady I was asked to see was anxious and withdrawn because she was about to be transferred to a hospice. She used silk paint and began by remembering how she was taught art at school. She tried to draw yellow roses and struggled to be accurate. As she gradually accepted the inevitable inaccuracies of her drawing, which was done with the outliner, Gutta, she relaxed and enjoyed herself. She began adding little pictures at the side to show me how she used to draw people. Then boats were added, which led her to tell me recollections of her father, who was a sailor, and her own memories of the sea. Telling her story enabled her to get more in touch with her sense of identity after a long stay in hospital. The choice of silk paint was important because it released her from the fear of 'making mistakes' and let her be herself.

A young man who used watercolour paints discovered that visualization through art could set his mind free from the feeling of being trapped by illness, at least for a while. I was asked to see him for art therapy because he was depressed. He told me he could not bear to see the sunshine outside the window because he could not go out and live his normal life. He closed the curtains and went to sleep in his darkened room to shut out everything he could not face.

As he told me sadly about all the events leading up to his admission to hospital, he doodled with paints, letting the colours bleed into each other as he worked his way down the paper. After a while he was surprised to notice that he had used rainbow colours and the centre was almost white. As we looked at it together and thought about what he'd been saying, he realized he had created a kind of space where his mind could 'fly'. I left the paints with him for a week and on my return he showed me several paintings he'd done on his own. He had enjoyed painting skies and mountain ranges. The particular qualities of watercolour paper helped him get in touch with flowing, fluid feelings. Pale sky or sea colours on damp paper can work almost magically to produce impressions of distant horizons. Like music or poetry, imagery can transport one to a different place. The rainbow often appears as a symbol of change and hope. Many patients use painting in that way, to catch hold of memories of happy times or places.

When I am asked to see someone for art therapy, I do not know if it will be a single session or the first of many. Patients attend hospital as in-patients or outpatients during a course of treatment. I may meet them at any stage of their illness. The following examples of casework are from longer periods of art therapy. The first is from work that took place over about six months and the second lasted over two years, until the patient's death in a hospice.

My first art therapy session with Jill

Jill (a pseudonym) made contact with me via the secretary of my immediate boss, the consultant who initiated art therapy in the medical oncology department. This is another of the ways in which referrals are made. As Jill was an outpatient our first contact was by telephone and we arranged for her to attend for an appointment with me so that we could discuss what art therapy was about and whether it would suit her.

Jill arrived with several bags of papers and books to show me, which she emptied out on the desk. She had collected articles from the *Guardian* on cancer, had all her own pathology reports and pictures of tumours from the internet, and she'd talked to doctors and her consultant who had tried to draw diagrams for her to explain the surgery she'd had. She wanted to get hold of slides of sections of tumour cells so she could see a cross-section of breast cancer cells, preferably her own.

Jill had been diagnosed fairly recently and had three lumps removed from her left breast. She'd had the lumps for over six months but been told they were benign and definitely not cancer. She was angry and articulate. She talked for an hour about her cancer which she wanted to understand in a surprisingly head-on way. She had been told hers was rare and slow-growing and her prognosis was good but did not believe it. She'd drawn her own visualization of the lymph glands and nodes and made a Christmas card cartoon of her breast in a sketchbook she brought to show me. It was a cross-section of her breast with all the alveoli looking like holly leaves coming to a point where her nipple was a little Father Christmas on top. She thought it would be a laugh to send it to her surgeon.

I could not help saying that I thought her need to understand intellectually was a way to try to control her situation and I wondered about feelings that might be underlying the busy preoccupation with gathering information.

We had a very lively conversation. I was almost overwhelmed by the amount of talk and 'stuff' flowing from her. She said she hated all doctors and nurses and all hospital procedures to a point where fear almost stopped her going ahead with her operation. She was concerned about her appearance and what had been done to her breast as well as losing the last chance to have a baby.

In this first session no art was done although Jill had brought with her two sketchbooks of line drawings like a visual diary. During the time she'd talked I tried to let her know that to some extent I would be with her in the exploration of what was going on inside her body, and emotionally too. I felt that she needed to recognize the part of herself that felt like a frightened vulnerable child in an out-of-control situation. Also, that having had things done to her which were painful but that she'd survived meant that she could do so again. She said she felt utterly alone and without inner resources, having no faith or religion and, unfortunately, no faith in the medical profession either.

My reflections on this session

Jill was being forced to go through a process of change for which she was unprepared. It seemed that she felt she could, by reducing it to a microscopic slide, 'freeze the moment' and be in control again.

I wanted to give her a sense of being accepted and held by me in a symbolic way. If we could assemble and hold her pictures we were also enabling her to tolerate her feelings. So far she had 'poured out' her story to me and my role was to listen and contain it.

Many of the metaphors that came to mind as I thought about the session with Jill were 'fluid', which reinforced the impression that art therapy could provide a form of container for her to 'spill out'. One of my aims would be to facilitate the discovery of inner resources Jill felt she was lacking.

For myself this was also the beginning of a process and my contact with the patient had an emotional impact on me. One way I could hold and reflect on what happened between us was to write down what I felt. This would also include all I could remember of what was said in the session.

Patrick Casement has written about the technique of 'self-supervision' in his book *On Learning from the Patient* (1985). Taking an objective view enables one to monitor the unconscious communication going on in the therapeutic relationship.

Ongoing sessions with Jill

In our second session Jill didn't know what to do but was ready to try new materials. I thought it might be useful for her if she could express herself on a large scale. She struggled all the time with physical tension that came out in her 'tight' voice and anger towards various people and institutions who she felt had treated her badly. She felt she was not being really heard or her complaints taken seriously.

I mentioned the possibility of making an outline of the human body into which shapes or colours can be placed as symbols of physical sensation or pain. This is an exercise used by Paola Luzzatto (1998). It may take the form of cathartic expression (taking negative feelings out on the paper, making a mess, throwing out the paper, etc.).

Jill liked the idea and her first painting was on a large piece of brown paper pinned up on the wall. On it she made an outline of her own body. She focused on the breasts and in particular on the scars made by surgery. Getting the colour exactly right was important and the detail of the breast sizes, as one was now bigger than the other. Other parts of the body were almost ignored and were definitely an afterthought. Once the figure was established another one was added. It was a smaller male figure and he was being attacked by the woman. She loomed up with outstretched arms flailing against him. He appeared to be falling backwards and was definitely the victim.

I commented to Jill that within the painting she could control everything that was going on. She could alter or change things. The image could be used to mediate between how she felt things to be and how she would like them to be. Jill's response was to add scalpels and bullets to her painting. They were being fired out of her breasts, like six-shooters in a Western, at the man who she said was her surgeon. She found it immensely amusing to attack him in that way and thoroughly enjoyed her power. She thought she would make it a gift to him at her next appointment. It was a straightforward expression of Jill's anger that appeared to be cathartic, but nothing like I had expected. Her diagnosis of cancer had brought many underlying issues to the surface, many of which would be discussed in future sessions.

Jill attended art therapy sessions every week for the next few months and her breasts were the central and ongoing theme of her artwork. Other painful issues to do with fertility, relationships, restorative surgery and her future life were discussed. One of the most controversial was whether it would be better to die rather than have more surgery if cancer reoccurred. My aim was to facilitate Jill's discovery of her own inner resources and a part of herself that would help her cope if she did have to face it again.

Summary of the work

In the weeks after our first meeting, Jill was still attending outpatient clinics for radiotherapy and for post-operative follow-up treatment. This was a period when feelings were raw. Her physical condition dominated her artwork. Her weeping wounds needed dressings to absorb them. The feelings that spilled out needed containment.

Jill chose to use pastels, crayons and coloured pencils which allowed maximum control of the drawn lines. Making the drawings of breasts was an opportunity for her to be in control – of the shapes and lines of her own body. She was able to express complex, often negative emotions to do with her perceived deformity. On one occasion she used modelling clay and made 3D images of herself 'as a piece of meat in the microwave'. It was like a replay in which she could take care of herself, symbolically, as she lay under the uncomfortable, dehumanizing radiotherapy equipment with felt pen crosses on her chest to guide the beam.

Jill's sense of humour has always been one of her strongest assets. It was the therapist's ally, in that it was her way of observing and being objective at the same time as experiencing intense emotion. It seemed to help her view her fellow-patients with compassion and to acknowledge the good intentions of the doctors in spite of her distrust of them. During the months we were meeting she stopped going round in circles quite so much, as she struggled with her ambivalent feelings. She could tell me about her inner 'primal scream' and create a collage to express and hold it at the same time. The main work of the therapy was to hold the space for Jill to explore the issues which were most important to her at that time; choice and personal control of her body and her destiny.

It is not possible for me to know if Jill's insights and subtle personal changes will sustain her in the long term. Only time will tell. In Jill's case I can admit to feeling satisfaction in seeing someone gain a stronger sense of their artistic creativity and potential. She has now returned to work and continues to see me for art therapy sessions once a month. She has left all her art therapy work with me for the present, so I am still holding her to some extent.

Longer term and more in-depth art therapy

A second example of art therapy was with a man in his early thirties who I will call James. A major theme in this casework is 'facing death'. As a doctor himself, James was totally aware of his prognosis and the processes his body would be going through as he approached his death. He knew about dying but he could not know about death.

James had been undergoing treatment for cancer over many years and when I met him he was having a course of radiotherapy into his spine. He planned to come to art therapy sessions as an outpatient after being discharged home. He was able to drive himself to the hospital and valued having the chance to do something for himself while not being able to carry on with his professional work.

James, like my previous patient Jill, had a great deal to say as well as having a lot of enthusiasm towards experimenting with art materials. He filled his time with me as if driven by tremendous urgency. While at first it was difficult for him to accept the awkwardness of his painting and the childlike imagery he produced, he was open to the idea of discovering meanings in his 'accidental' shapes, like pictures in clouds.

The way James used his sessions was to delight in letting himself play. He was willing to take risks and be spontaneous with mark-making. He enjoyed the sensual qualities of art materials and the unexpected mingling of colours and lines. The way he would proceed with the objective of mastering technique counterbalanced times when he could accept formlessness and mystery in his work. This characteristic reflected his personality and ability to live in the present moment and enjoy it while knowing he was facing a relentless deterioration in his health. In his earliest painting individual symbolic shapes without apparent purpose merged together in a chaotic mass with a dismembered male torso just visible in the centre.

While busy painting, James talked at length about his past and present situation. The art therapy sessions appeared to be deeply needed opportunities to tell his story and think about where it was going. Talking about his childhood, school, home, family relationships, bereavements, places he loved and his achievements, he was telling all that was 'known' and in a way this was safe, solid ground. From this position he could venture into the mystery of the unknown.

In the early weeks of our art therapy relationship, James did some drawings at home and brought them to show me. He copied a Dali painting of Christ on the Cross looking down at earth stretching out below him. He added words such as 'Why?' These paintings were shared with me but James's most personal thoughts about his religion and faith were too sensitive to put into words. However, they were profound and significant in his spiritual life. He let me know how his relationship with God influenced his feelings about his own death.

James's cancer spreads

About a year after James started seeing me for art therapy his cancer spread further into his spine and he could no longer walk. His wife brought him to the hospital by car and he came to my room in his wheelchair. Over the previous year he had produced many paintings that represented aspects of his personal journey. For instance, he brought memories to recreate such as places in which he had spent happy childhood holidays by the seaside, and one was a scene he visualized from a book he'd enjoyed. The scene was viewed from above, looking down at different places along the shore; some were rocky, some had thick forest and by a small sandy beach was a hut to shelter in. Two little sailing boats were out on the lake heading towards an island.

Although the landscape could have represented difficulties James needed to negotiate in his daily life, another way for this to be understood is as a representation of 'transference'. The two boats on water could represent the therapeutic relationship, and the island the therapy space.

Another painting James had planned in advance but needed to work out in the session was called 'Lifeline'. He imagined a structure like an egg timer with sands of time flowing down through it. He drew himself suspended above the hole and held up only by a 'web' that was his wife's love. The painting was fairly explicit in its reference to his sense of time slipping away beneath his feet. He wanted to put down on paper the stark reality of his situation, which we were then able to talk about.

Love also featured in a painting he called 'Transformation'. His wife was at the top of the paper undressed and being pulled in different directions by their two little children, while her tears were cascading down to him. He was dressed all in black with feet rooted into the ground. Her pale blue tears came to a point between them where they were transformed into pale blue heart shapes as they touched him. Beside him he painted a wheelchair and two golden gates. The gates were closed but pale blue light beamed over the top. It was a powerful image which contained both positive and negative feelings.

The art therapy sessions had become a place where James brought negative feelings when family relationships were going through stressful times. The image of his wife undressed and 'out of reach' above him could have been a portrayal of his sexual unavailability since becoming paralysed. He was unable, or perhaps chose not, to voice his feelings about that very painful area of his life.

Well-meaning friends added to the strain with their kindness and comments about wanting James to get better and 'back' to his old self. He found it hard to talk to them and felt isolated and lonely in the place he now inhabited. They could not know what it was like to be there and he could not explain.

Gateways – a visual metaphor for transitional states

Over a period of weeks the theme of 'gateways' appeared often in James's artwork. His gates varied in size but were always central and usually in the foreground of a landscape without people. They were closed gates but could be seen through. We talked about what the landscapes and gates might mean to James. He recognized how his feelings about the future resonated within the pale horizons and blocked pathways. There was poetry present in his idea of a piece of earth subjected to harsh cycles of change but never losing the potential of new life.

One day after James and I had been talking about the image of a closed gate he painted one that was open. There was also a figure for the first time. It was running towards a gap in the doorway. The most startling thing about the painting was that the figure was surrounded by flames and running towards green grass outside the gate. I imagined that the figure was trying to escape from fire and flames towards the safety of a peaceful scene. His explanation was quite the opposite. Paradoxically, the heat and pain represented being alive and the doorway opened into the 'unknown'.

I continued seeing James after he was moved to a hospice. He had been preparing himself for the end for a long time but when he could no longer be cared for at home it still came as a shock. He told me he was not ready and had not expected it to happen so soon. Some of his last drawings expressed anger and frustration and again it was useful for him to have somewhere to put negative feelings that he did not feel were a complaint towards loved ones. James also drew with crayons, a final 'gate' picture, completed with huge effort. It was a landscape with sheep grazing in fields beside water. Across the centre was an old stone wall with a gate standing open. The horizon line was between sky and glittering water. As he worked on his picture, he slipped in and out of dozing sleep because of his medication. He gradually disengaged from the outside world and in our final session he wanted me to help him with goodbye letters to his daughters.

James made full use of his creativity during his last two years of life. His wife wrote a letter to tell me how important art therapy was to him. At his funeral and memorial service James's paintings were displayed with pride and were valued by his family. Unlike the artwork produced in most other art therapy situations, which is not necessarily meant to be shared or displayed outside the therapeutic setting, in palliative care the artwork is often invested with special meaning and it may become a gift to others. James left his work with me until his last weeks in the hospice when he wanted to look through it with his wife. She chose paintings to keep and what was not wanted was returned to me to dispose of. He was pleased to give me permission to include his work in a folder of patients' paintings kept at the hospital for teaching purposes.

Conclusion

Although I am well aware of the definition of art therapy and my job description is clear enough, my perception of my role as an art therapist is not so clear. This prompted my basic self-questioning at the outset of this piece of writing and, partly, the choice of title. Malcolm Learmonth (2002) mentioned an (unrealized) ambition of his to be able to describe on the back of an envelope why art therapy works. He pointed out the challenge for art therapists to be able to describe the theory behind what they do and why, in language that is understandable and concise. I tried to do so but the depth of issues involved in the lives of the patients referred to here can only be briefly touched on.

I realized that my own uncertainty in my work is closely related to the patients' experience of 'not knowing' and could be understood as a form of unconscious communication going on between us. One patient I talked to poured out his frustration in the following words:

> I hate that sensation of wait and see. You're in limbo, waiting. It's the worse thing, nothing to go on, up in the air, no conclusions, no achievement, no dateline to stick to, don't know when it ends, nothing to tell people. You feel awkward; they don't know what to say to you, give clichés of comfort. It's easier to say 'I'm OK'; they can't do anything, that's just the way it is.

Art therapists would want to offer such a patient art materials through which to channel the intense emotion but in this case he was too wound up and refused them. It was an uncomfortable experience for him not to know what was happening to him physically and on a practical level. I stayed with him and with his not knowing for an hour. He wanted me to know that he was stuck with it hour after hour and day after day. It was almost unbearable.

In other examples of casework I hoped to demonstrate what I do and how I try to understand what goes on within the therapeutic relationship. It is necessarily a flexible approach in which I respond to patients' needs across a spectrum of 'therapeutic intervention'. At one end of the spectrum are patients who use art therapy in a way that could be called 'art psychotherapy' because it follows a psychodynamic model. For instance, we look at patients' childhood experiences that influenced their personality and coping strategies and perhaps explore possibilities for change. Work with a patient whom I saw for about six months was used to illustrate mid-length art therapy of a fairly psychodynamic nature. At the other end of the spectrum I may be more like a technical assistant and the art is about enjoyment rather than exploration of feelings. In between the two extremes are a diverse range of needs. I touched on some of the deeper issues brought by a patient who attended art therapy until the last weeks of his life. Being with someone who was using imagery to communicate and explore the experience of approaching death was deeply moving. It was the ultimate 'not knowing' which, for me, stirred up deep philosophical and spiritual questions that I continue to ask, but to which I know there are no certain answers.

References

Casement, P. (1985) *On Learning From the Patient*. London: Tavistock.

Learmouth, M. (2002) Painting ourselves out of a corner, *Newsbriefing, Newsletter of British Association of Art Therapists*, June: 2–5.

Luzzatto, P. (1998) The encounter with the body, in M. Pratt and M.J.M. Wood (eds) *Art Therapy in Palliative Care: The Creative Response*. London: Routledge.

16 An art therapist's experience of having cancer: living and dying with the tiger

Caryl Sibbett

> Back and forth autoethnographers gaze, first through an ethnographic wide-angle lens, focusing outward on social and cultural aspects of their personal experience; then, they look inward, exposing a vulnerable self . . .
>
> (Ellis and Bochner 2000: 739)

Introduction

Whilst Chapters 2 and 4 focused on the socio-cultural dimension of art therapy in cancer care, this chapter will focus more on the 'vulnerable self': my own experience of liminality as a cancer patient and art therapist. As outlined in Chapter 2, this is based on research undertaken for my PhD as a form of 'arts-based autoethnography' (Slattery 2001) and 'auto/biography' (Stanley 1992).[1]

First, I will explore my own experience of having leiomyosarcoma, a rare form of soft tissue cancer, and my related art-making. To develop the discussion from Chapters 2 and 4 this exploration will be done from an anthropological perspective, paralleling my experience with a rites of passage transition (Van Gennep 1960), associated ritual and particularly the state of liminality (Turner 1995).

Secondly, I will explore the impact on myself as an art therapist working with people diagnosed with cancer. I had been practising in cancer care for some years before my diagnosis and then stopped working in this area until my supervisor and I felt I was ready to commence again. It will be suggested that when working with those in liminal states we can experience what might be termed *secondary liminality*. The discussion will also refer to issues such as countertransference, restimulation, working with the dying and self-care.

Wounded storyteller

This story is an illustrated 'auto/biography' (Stanley 1992), or 'autopatho-graphy' (Couser 1991), as, in my role of 'wounded storyteller' (Frank 1997), I narrate my own experience both as a cancer patient and as an art therapist working with those affected by cancer. The research includes my own personal and professional voices and therefore this will not be an 'author-evacuated text' (Geertz 1988: 9). This will be made explicit by writing in the first person and by the inclusion of biographical and personally reflective material and artwork. The research explored the concept and experience of liminality – how I felt being in a liminal, transitional or 'betwixt and between' space (Turner 1995: 95), living and practising at the threshold between life and death. The story encompasses my attempts to make sense, through words and art-making, of having cancer and fluctuating between states of 'acute liminality' – heightened risk and reduced control – and 'sustained liminality' – less risk and more perceived control (Little *et al.* 1998: 1490), a fluctuation which may last for the rest of my life.

Congruent with literature on the structuring of autobiographies, my self-study is organized around 'turning points' or 'epiphanies' in my experience (Denzin 1989). This includes times that I regarded as a 'nodal moment' or 'point of crisis at which time ... lives underwent a wrenching' (Graham 1989: 98–9). However, my personal story is also an interpersonal one and so at times I include references to 'mentors who evoked' me (Palmer 1998: 21) by interweaving a number of voices with my own, such as those of some of my doctors and clients whose stories particularly resonated with mine.

Personal liminality

In trying to understand my own cancer experience I found the concept of liminality and its characteristics (Turner 1995) congruent with my experi-ence and thus to be 'a major category of the experience of cancer illness' (Little *et al.* 1998). Key characteristics of liminality – *limbo, power/powerlessness, playing, communitas* and *embodied experience* – all seemed relevant to both my cancer experience and art-making and I will now reflect on each of these.

Limbo

One characteristic of liminality is a sense of limbo, ambiguity, being 'betwixt and between' and 'out of time' (Turner 1988: 24–5, 1995: 95).

In the early summer of 1998 things were going well for a change. I had just successfully completed my first year of a Masters course at university and, with confidence growing, had decided to try to move from sessional therapy practice and teaching to pursue a more full-time career in these areas. However, I had also first noticed the lump on my arm. Although I didn't realize it at first, I was beginning slowly but inexorably to move into the realm of liminality and limbo.

After some time, when the lump did not disappear, I went to my medical practice several times between that summer and the next year. Each time I was given a probable diagnosis of a sebaceous cyst. However, because it continued to grow and be increasingly painful, I requested action and was referred for minor surgery. This was done in August 1999 by my GP who realized during the surgery that it was not a cyst and thus the nature of the lump was unknown. However, things took a turn for the worse because I later discovered that the removed tissue was not sent for histological analysis but was disposed of, meaning that I did not get a diagnosis. The lump had not been completely removed and so it continued to grow in size and painfulness and therefore I requested a hospital referral.

An additional difficulty was that the GP involved stated that it was not routine practice in that surgery to send such tissue for histological analysis, whereas I was informed by medical colleagues that guidance on minor surgery in general practice stipulates that 'All tissue removed by minor surgery should be sent for histological examination' (General Medical Services Committee and the Royal College of General Practitioners 1996: 5) and, referring to histology policy in basic surgical technique, it simply recommends 'SEND EVERYTHING!' I had various communications with the GP to try to ensure that practice would be changed to become congruent with this guidance, but this resulted in my having no confidence that such change would occur. Therefore I proceeded with a complaint that was subsequently upheld by an Independent Review Panel of the local Health and Social Services Board. This Panel also deemed the tissue disposal to be a 'grave error' with 'life-threatening consequences'.

Back at the time of the minor surgery, my lack of a diagnosis also meant that I was not rated as urgent and so the first available hospital appointment was in January. At this appointment I saw a specialist registrar who arranged for me to see the consultant surgeon. By this time my teaching and therapy practice had started again after the Christmas and New Year break. However, three days before the consultation with the surgeon I received a hospital letter telling me the appointment was cancelled and rescheduled for four months later. My sense that something was wrong urged me to refer myself privately to the surgeon whom I then first saw in late February 2000. Clearly he too felt that it was important to get a diagnosis because he scheduled day procedure surgery for six days later and a further appointment eight days after that to receive the results. This was one year and eight months after my first presentation to a doctor.

Surprisingly, looking back, I don't think I suspected consciously that I had cancer, even when the surgeon arranged surgery so promptly. Perhaps it was literally unthinkable. Certainly my family and I were not talking in terms of this, but rather I was caught up in just getting action. Even on the day I got the results I was alone and drove myself to the private clinic and was planning to teach that afternoon.

However, some part of me knew at some level that something was wrong. This awareness seemed to be a form of 'unthought known' (Bollas 1987: 282) based in the 'somatic unconscious' (Wyman-McGinty 1998). This urged me on to continue to seek medical attention despite several misdiagnoses, failure to get a histological examination and resulting lack of a rediagnosis, and hospital delays. The awareness perhaps manifested in some of my dreams and in artwork during those several years and urged me to action.

Prodromal symbols

A 'prodrome' (Gr. *prodromos*: 'running before') is an early symptom, occurring prior to and indicating the onset of a disease (MHI 2002). It has been suggested that drawings and dreams can have a 'prospective' element (Furth 1988: 23), for instance prodromal dreams of cancer (Hersh 1995). It has been further suggested that during cancer images can be a 'messenger' like prodromal dreams (Malchiodi 1998: 165–94) that can, even pre-diagnosis, indicate a pre-conscious knowledge of the illness and its outcome (Bach 1990; Bertoia 1993: 3), prognosis (Achterberg 1985) or dying (Mango 1992).

I first noticed the lump in early 1998, but my oncologist informed me that cancer had probably begun two years prior to being noticeable, i.e. around 1996. For several years before I discovered in 2000 that I had cancer, a number of artworks and dreams had been disconcerting and, at the time as recorded in my journals, had heightened my sense of being in danger and of my death. I had never had such dreams before this.

I found an unremembered drawing from 1996 depicting me with a skull-like face and a damaged left arm showing a mark highlighted on my upper left arm. The tumour site was in my upper left arm. In October 1997 I dreamt my right foot was painful and that there was something below the skin like a piece of bone. In the dream I worked it out through the skin and it was an inch long oval piece that was sent for analysis and proved to be a piece of shell. However, in the dream I knew a part remained inside my foot and this was not good. When I awoke I realized there was nothing in my foot but I was left with a sense of anxiety. In January 1998 I dreamt I was dancing with my own death certificate, but on waking was annoyed that I had missed the opportunity to look at the date on it. In April 1998 I dreamt I was in a stationary car being trampled over by a huge horse, then an ox and then my heart sank as I knew a herd of cows would follow and nothing could stop them and I would not survive. In 1998 I dreamt I was patting a tiger on the head and although it was large and powerful, it was letting me do this. It was life-threatening, yet a companion.

In October 1998 I made a 'self-collage' (Figure 16.1, on website, and front cover) in which the left side depicted threatening vulnerable aspects of myself and the right side depicted nurturing positive aspects. All the meanings below were recorded at the time of making the image. The image features a central tree and at its base are shells and horns and in its trunk is a metal DNA helix or caduceus. The () shapes between the helix are mandorla (almond-like) shapes that were recurring through my art during this period. On the left is 'dead wood', a 'petrified forest', that evoked feelings of death and terror. On the right is the Green Man, a figure that has been important for me since first appearing in my art in August 1996. He symbolizes an animate form of the tree thus representing life and contrasting with the death of the petrified forest. I also associate this figure with Mercurius (or Hermes) whom Jung (1981: para. 243) describes as the 'numen of the tree, its *spiritus vegetativus*' and as 'the life principle of the tree . . . The tree would then be the outwards and visible realization of the self.' Perry (1997: 149) describes Mercurius as 'he who abides at the threshold (of change)' and Mercurius is also known as Hermes, regarded by Stein (1983) as the guide of souls through liminality or threshold situations. On the left of the image, there are fragmented symbols featuring mother-of-pearl and a quaternity, whilst on the right are similar yet integrated symbols.

Regarding the mandorla shapes, in 2000 the specialist registrar indicated the area on my arm where the surgeon would operate by drawing such a shape horizontally on my arm and it was to become the shape of the surgery wound.

The week after making the collage I dreamt that two large lions chased me upstairs in my house. I was terrified because there was no way to escape from them although I woke up just as they were about to eat me. Was this a rising of danger toward consciousness?

In January/February 1999 I had two powerful death/reincarnation dreams. In the first I was travelling in a car and was being shown images, flashed to the front left, of places on the journey ahead. Then they began flashing rapidly and became distorted, surreal and terrifying and I was 'told' that these were now images of the journey ahead *after* my death. Later in the dream, after my death, I was in a huge covered area with crowds of people milling about. People were getting on large train-like vehicles and I knew I had to get on one. Although we did not know exactly where they were going, I knew they were taking us to the next life. At the time, I noted in my journal that Bertoia (1993: 124) suggests that rebirth 'refers to some form of transcending death, of being reborn into some new frame of existence' and it also applies to 'the development of some form of tolerance for the dying process and for what happens after this body dies'. Jung (1960: 410) suggests rebirth symbols of change, such as journeys and changes of locality, can be associated with changes in psychological condition and with approaching death. The next night I had another dream where I was in a corridor or room with many doorways to other rooms. I knew that each room was another life.

In February 1999 I made a 'self-box'; its front was open and I recorded at the time that the threshold seemed important. I hung strips of black crêpe on either side of the opening and this was very disconcerting at the time because I felt strongly that they related to my own death.

Looking back, this all seems curious yet could be unconnected to the fact that I had cancer developing throughout that period. However, the heightened death awareness these symbols brought was part of what prompted me to seek medical attention even though I was not consciously aware of cancer. Perhaps what might be termed *prodromal symbols* can occur in dreams and artwork during the early stages of disease such as cancer, thus communicating an 'unthought known' (Bollas 1987: 282) perhaps known by one's body.

Diagnosis

In late February 2000 my surgeon removed the lump by excising down to the muscle, commenting that I must be alarmed by how much tissue he had removed. Eight days later I returned for the results, alone. As I entered his room he told me that he had got the results earlier in the week but had wanted to see me in person. My alarm bells rang. As he told me the diagnosis, in an instant my world changed, time altered and I plunged into acute liminality. Some part of me was reeling whilst another part listened intently. He was saying I had a rare malignant soft tissue cancer. He was introducing me to my new 'companion' but, as often happens with introductions, I did not quite catch its name at the beginning. Later I checked its name and knew it to be leiomyosarcoma and then, as our relationship grew closer, I could sometimes call it by its contraction, LMS.

The surgeon was telling me he had 'smelled a rat', i.e. suspected cancer, before operating and now this was confirmed by histology. However, he also cautioned that he had been unable to get clear margins underneath the tumour despite exposing the muscle. I was being referred to an oncologist while they determined whether to operate again or not. Leaving the clinic I was alone and in shock and as I drove on the motorway to teach that afternoon, I was thinking: 'Put it away . . . don't get emotional . . . put it away somewhere; I have to put it away somewhere very secure. In a box, a box . . . heavily wrapped up and sealed. Wrap it up, wrap it up again, tie it up, sealed, packaged.' I was also wishing I didn't have to tell anyone so that they wouldn't have to be upset.

When leiomyosarcoma was confirmed I entered a limbo state on the threshold between life and death where both became simultaneously sharply real and surreal. I was experiencing liminality, which I later learned Little *et al.* (1998) describe as a major category of the cancer experience. Liminality stems from the Latin word *limen* meaning threshold (Turner 1982: 24). I was plunged into a 'betwixt and between' (Turner 1995: 95) space of risk, suspense and timelessness with a heightened emotional engagement with death and, paradoxically, life.

Over a period of time the doctors debated whether to perform more surgery but instead decided on radiotherapy. The sense was that the horse could already have bolted due to the delay in getting to hospital and the disruption of the tumour during the earlier minor surgery. The diagnosis also began what was to become an ongoing process of tests, CT scans and so on. There were seemingly endless hours of waiting – waiting for appointments, waiting for scan results, waiting for the sword to fall, or not. A visual metaphor emerged of having a 'sword of Damocles' (Cicero 2001) suspended over my head. I later discovered this metaphor had been used in the literature on cancer experience (Muzzin *et al.* 1994; Riskó *et al.* 1998; Self 1999).

Another metaphor that emerged was that when I got the diagnosis a tiger had appeared beside me. It had attacked me and left its scars. The 'wait and see' game began as the tiger would accompany me for the rest of my life, however long that was. What sort of relationship would this be? Would he be a meaningful companion or would he be a carnivore about to devour me, or both? The metaphor of cancer 'eating' can appear in patients' narratives (Skott 2002). The tiger was powerful, but I had no power over him. Later I remembered my earlier dream of patting a large and powerful tiger. The tiger represented many things including death, cancer, and my own body matter turning against me. I was later interested to discover that etymologically 'tiger' (*steig-*) links to sharp, prick, stab, stitch, tattoo, stigma (Pickett *et al.* 2000), and is thus symbolically relevant to my surgery, stitches and scars. I also later discovered that Feneron (1997) had used the metaphor of a tiger in a poem relating to her experience of breast cancer. The tiger could represent the liminal for, as Cooper (1995: 172–3) notes, it is 'Ambivalent as both solar and lunar, creator and destroyer.'

Some time afterwards I read the book *Life of Pi* and it resonated with my experience as the main character Pi survived a ship sinking only to find himself on board a lifeboat for many months with a Bengal tiger. Pi describes his fear:

> . . . fear, real fear, such as shakes you to your foundation, such as you feel when you are brought face to face with your mortal end, nestles in your memory like a gangrene: it seeks to rot everything, even the words with which to speak of it. So you must fight hard to express it.
>
> (Martel 2003: 216)

My artwork was a valuable form of expression, for example one piece entitled 'Limbo' (Figure 16.2, on website) expressed liminality and fear. In it, I depicted myself waiting in a limbo environment, motionless with fear yet expressionless. My head is wounded and bleeding. The shape of my head is visible through my hair and this seems to indicate fear of potential hair loss through future chemotherapy. I seem transfixed with shock.

The figure is tied up with string and this seems to represent my powerlessness.

Power/powerlessness

A second characteristic of liminality is a sense of powerlessness, submissiveness and silence (Turner 1975, 1995). My cancer diagnosis heralded a new phase of life in which I became a patient. During acute liminality lack of control was pervasive (Cunningham *et al.* 1991: 71; Little *et al.* 1998: 1485). My usual routines gave way as, often willingly, I had to surrender power and control to the medical routines. My life was in the hands of the doctors or fate or chance. My surgeon wrote to my GP: 'I shall be seeking the advice of my oncological colleague ... and hopefully we can formulate the most appropriate strategy ... she may well require wider removal +/– radiotherapy' (Consultant surgeon 2000). I was passive in my obedience during this liminal time (Turner 1995).

I felt caught up in the conventions of the medical culture where authority could at times be based more on title and uniform than on trust and entitlement (Philip 2002). However, the issue of power in healthcare is complex (Canter 2001), and I experienced it too as somewhat liminal in its ambiguity. Whilst I might wish to have had more control over my situation I could simultaneously be happy to trust in the fiduciary relationship with my therapist and some of my doctors based on my perception of their 'legitimate', 'expert' and 'referent' power (French and Raven 1959).

The artwork entitled 'Limbo' (Figure 16.2) also depicts my sense of powerlessness and silence. I am tied or 'stitched' up. It also depicts the overwhelming fatigue by which I was enveloped throughout the experience and particularly after the radiotherapy. My mouth and eyes are pinned shut with real pins, symbolizing the taboo aspect. It was difficult to feel or speak about my terror and I wanted to protect others and myself from distress. The issue of the failure to send my tissue for analysis was also difficult to speak about. Penson *et al.* (2001) assert that medical errors can have 'a disastrous effect on patients, staff, and institutions' and will 'always be a taboo subject'.

Another aspect of powerlessness related to my experience of the medical error and my attempts to ensure that medical practice changed as a result of my complaint against my GP. In the meeting of the Independent Review Panel of the local Health and Social Services Board I was told that its report would recommend changes in the practice's medical procedures. I asked the Chair of the Panel what power the Panel had to ensure any such recommendations would be complied with. I was concerned to be told I had asked a difficult question and that the Panel had no such power and indeed there could sometimes be a shortfall between what was recommended and what subsequently happened.

Paradoxically, as well as a sense of structural inferiority, liminality is also associated with 'ritual powers' (Turner 1995: 100) and heightened awareness of 'cosmological systems' as important (Turner 1982: 26–7). I felt empowered through some of the art-making. For instance, in my journal for the week beginning 29 October 1998 I recorded that I displayed the image 'self-collage' (Figure 16.1) and looked at it regularly as I felt it was very significant, perhaps an 'embodied image' or 'talisman' (Schaverien 1992). I recorded that this felt ritualistic and that I was reminded how 'One must observe the proper rites . . . They are what makes one day different from other days, one hour from other hours' (Saint-Exupéry 1971: 84) and how Waller (1983: 188) notes that 'The patient may use the object in a ritual.'

In the self-collage on the right is a quaternity containing a bejewelled web. This linked to an increased awareness of concepts such as interconnectedness, new physics and the Buddhist concept of Indra's Net, symbolizing our interwovenness and interdependence in the cosmos (Capra 1991: 151).

Playing

A third characteristic of liminality relates to 'varieties of playful experience' (Turner 1988: 124–5). Caillois' (1962) theories were useful in helping me understand my cancer and art-making experiences.

As a patient, I felt as though I was caught up in Caillois' (1962: 20) first type of play relating to *role play*, disguise, imitating or 'playing a part' (*mimicry*). I could hide from myself, denying or suppressing uncomfortable emotions and thoughts. Sometimes I was playing the role of a courageous patient, yet hiding the terror and responding to 'How are you?' with the expected 'I'm OK.' In this way I was operating at Berne's (1968: 163–4) interactional behaviour level of 'rituals' which involves stereotyped, implicitly agreed-to responses rather than 'intimacy' which would be spontaneous, game-free, congruent and open to vulnerability. Perhaps the former is ritual bound by *ludus* or convention and the latter can be ritual characterized by *paidia* or spontaneity.

I also identified with Caillois' (1962: 17–18) second type of play relating to *chance* or *fate* (*alea*). At times I felt I was a piece of meat being played with by fate, God, doctors, or the tiger. My future was conceived in terms of survival probability – the roll of the dice. A consultant oncologist/medical–legal expert reported: 'Ms Sibbett's chances of a five-year disease-free survival are of the order of 60 per cent. The ten-year survival figures are probably 30 to 40 per cent' (Medical–legal expert 2001). Chance could also be conceived as an either/or situation, not a spectrum. My own oncologist said: 'Survival probability figures are one thing, but actually for you it will either be 0 per cent or 100 per cent!'

Caillois' (1962: 14) third type of play relates to *competition* or *contest* (*agôn*) and sometimes I felt I was locked in a battle or struggle with cancer that I would either win or lose. This was a battle to the death. Yet it wasn't some externally caused wound or infection. In a sense I was battling with my own body, represented by the tiger. This heightened a sense of splitting from my body, for instance sometimes I felt as though my body had let me down by getting cancer, whilst at other times I felt as though I had let my body down by getting cancer. When I feared I might lose my arm I thought: 'Well, rather it than me.' However, the scars I now have seem special. Rather than being concerned about cosmetic impact as my surgeon feared, I regard them as marks of survival – the tiger bit but didn't win, not that time anyway. *Agôn* also has etymological links to agony and I experienced such pain in mind and body.

Caillois' (1962: 23) fourth type of play related to *vertigo* (*ilinx*) also seemed relevant as my senses reeled as I wavered on the precipice of suffering and death and I experienced the 'voluptuous panic' which can paralyse the mind. The sense of terror and desperation this evoked is depicted in the artwork 'Living Bone?' (Figure 16.3, on website), in which I am portrayed in a foetal position and scraping my face in despair.

I found art-making valuable in expressing the various types of play but also in counteracting the loss of control and power as it provided an opportunity for spontaneous improvizational play (*paidia*) which helped in the movement toward sustained liminality.

Communitas

A fourth characteristic of liminality relates to communitas which is a type of communion, equality and a 'liberation of human capacities of cognition, affect, volition, creativity, etc., from the normative constraints incumbent upon occupying a sequence of social statuses' (Turner 1982: 44). I experienced this most in cancer care charities such as in a patient action group or support groups for cancer patients. These could offer a sense of belonging and acceptance and permission to share. One difficulty within such communitas was that my cancer was rare and there was no specific support group and indeed at times I could feel a sense of being neglected whilst other more common cancers were privileged. Another factor was that the communitas with other cancer patients could give rise to a feeling that a person who had not experienced cancer would not understand. This was exacerbated or perhaps realized when such a person might respond to my expressions of having a heightened death awareness by saying: 'Well, we all know we're going to die some time.' Little and Sayers (2004) describe the heightened death awareness, or 'death salience', that cancer patients have: 'We all know that we will die, but there is a greater vividness and proximity in that knowledge for someone who has been through mortal extreme experience.' Having been bitten by the tiger, perceived its fearsome size, felt its hot breath, heard its claws and been locked in its gaze, is qualitatively different from knowing that there are tigers who will kill, yet not having personally encountered one.

Embodied experience

A fifth characteristic of liminality relates to 'embodied' experience and, for me, this was of fundamental significance in my cancer experience and related art-making. Indeed, art-making helped me to express and contain my embodied experience, as detailed below, and also to work on it, helping me to move toward sustained liminality and come to terms with the fluctuations between it and acute liminality.

The physicality of having cancer, and being treated for it, primarily featured pain, suffering, fatigue, various ordeals and multi-sensory aspects. My experience also featured issues of body/self image, cultural embodiment, and impact on sexual embodiment. It also involved expression of 'ideas', 'acts' and 'works of art' (Turner 1982: 12–15) which helped me portray and communicate some of the above, all of which are components of embodied liminality (Turner 1982, 1995).

I found it important to use art-making to express and record aspects of the impact of cancer and the treatment. Internal aspects, pain, fatigue, wounding and compromised sexuality are indicated in all of my artworks shown (Figures 16.1–16.4), which I regarded as 'embodied images' – ones in which feeling states are experienced and embodied (Schaverien 1992).

The image I created, entitled 'Living Bone?' (Figure 16.3), portrayed the embodied nature of my cancer experience. I felt ongoing pain and fatigue throughout my body, involving a loss of physical power (Glaus *et al.* 1996) which was also emotionally draining, indicated in the lines across the head and red lines down the back.

Aspects of my experience related to how the cancer came through to the skin, the burning of my skin in radiotherapy, and the pain felt in my skin and throughout the body. I resonated with Anzieu's (1989: 108) concept of an 'assaulting, destroying' function of the skin ego and the bodily skin in which he suggests that self-anger and self-destructiveness emanating from the id can be transported and 'become encysted in the surface layer which is the Skin Ego' so that 'The imaginary skin which covers the Ego thus becomes a poisoned tunic, suffocating, burning, disintegrating. We might therefore speak in this case of a toxic function of the Skin Ego.'

At one stage, after another surgery in hospital, a nosocomial or 'hospital-acquired' wound infection developed. Mine persisted for some time but I was aware of other patients whose infections became chronic, a condition which Gardner (1998) suggests is characterized by an embodied state of liminality as such people can live an indeterminate existence in between health and illness.

Another artwork, 'Clay Female' (Figure 16.4, on website), was a clay figure of myself and this also portrayed the importance of my body's experience. The figure was scored with lines of pain, stooped with fatigue, and the core of her body was missing in the shape of my cancer surgery wound. Her hands and feet were merged into the body so that she would be unable to protect herself and she had no mouth with which to speak or scream. The fatigue and the taboo aspects in Figure 16.4 reminded me of Beckett's (1959: 418) lines '. . . it will be the silence, where I am, I don't know, I'll never know, in the silence you don't know, you must go on, I can't go on, I'll go on.' Souter (2002) compares the experience Beckett describes with Bion's (1993: 116) concept of 'nameless dread' and notes that Beckett had psychotherapy with Bion.

As I faced the prospect of cancer foreshortening my life I experienced despair relating to actual and potential effects of the cancer and its treatment. My body/self image was compromised, I feared future chemotherapy and hair loss and, worst of all, probably now I could not consider having children. I experienced the gender identity chaos that is an aspect of liminality (Turner 1967: 98) and artwork was important in dealing with some of these loss issues.

I discovered that W. H Auden (1994) had written a poem entitled 'Miss Gee' about a woman with cancer and I sought out his *Collected Poems* in a bookshop one day to read the poem for the first time. It had a humorous rhythm and began 'Let me tell you a little story About Miss Edith Gee.' The poem continues with Miss Gee bicycling to the doctor to tell him she has a pain. He examines her and later tells his wife that Miss Gee has cancer. He adds that 'Childless women get it . . . It's as if there had to be some outlet for their foiled creative fire.' I found it emotional to read this as it resonated with my own fears and self-blame. More emotion was to come as the doctor relates his fear that Miss Gee is 'a goner'. Then Miss Gee gets taken to the hospital and the surgeon, on cutting into her, turns to his students and says: 'We seldom see a sarcoma as far advanced as this.' Standing in the bookshop I was stunned because I had not anticipated it mentioning sarcoma. Sarcoma is rare enough to be mentioned only sporadically even in the medical literature. The juxtaposition of childlessness, death and sarcoma was almost too much.

During one time of extreme despair in December 2003 I went into my bathroom and created a three-dimensional life-sized foetus out of flesh-coloured paper and some of my menstrual blood. It related to myself as a baby and to my situation of not having children. As I was creating it on the floor of the bathroom I realized it seemed like a miscarriage and thus represented the loss. I also tied up this baby figure with string and this seemed to echo Figure 16.2 and feelings of powerlessness.

On another occasion I painted a nude figure of myself and in the womb area I depicted a foetus. In the image, my body was pierced with real screws and there was a sense of the pun of 'I'm screwed', also meaning I'm going to die and perhaps relating to the medical error. I realized that in the painting I looked female, compared to earlier more androgynous representations of myself. I also laid out the painting as if it was myself after death lying flat. This was very emotional but seemed to bring some acceptance of my femininity – yet also that it was compromised, and acceptance of my future death – yet also of my terror of dying.

I empathized with the person diagnosed with cancer potrayed by Ellis and Bochner (2000: 756), who wished to use autoethnography and who describes her own experience as being initially optimistic, then pretending to be upbeat and

> a warrior who has learned from her experiences. But what I had to face as I wrote my story is that I'm scared all the time that the cancer will come back . . . I'm sorry, but cancer has not improved my life and I can't make it into a gift.

It is important to emphasize that, whilst some cancer patients can glean some positive aspects from their cancer experience, such as regarding confronting mortality as a 'turning point' that stimulates a life review and a profound search for wholeness (LeShan 1996), getting cancer in itself is 'not a positive and enviable experience' and indeed can be experienced as an 'abomination' (Ehrenreich 2001: 53).

I have found that having cancer is a complex, shifting experience filled with multiple meanings and lack of meaning. Perhaps like the tiger, it has appeared to me in different ways at different times. Yet fundamentally it is a carnivore. I waver in liminality, living or dying with the tiger.

Managing acute and sustained liminality

Throughout the fluctuation between acute and sustained states of liminality (Little *et al.* 1998: 1493) my own artwork gave me a means of expressing aspects of my cancer experience relating to various types of play: role play, chance or fate-driven, competitive and frightening (Caillois 1962), thus better enabling me to face the existential and physical fact of my *boundedness* or finiteness (Little *et al.* 1998: 1491). Art-making provided a therapeutic liminal space for improvizational play, thus enabling me to project difficult issues into the art, then own them since they had become visible, touchable, thinkable and emotion-able. Art therapy-related rituals and symbols enabled me to metaphorize my body and thus express my body's story of the physicality, structural inferiority/power, and sexual embodiment inherent in my cancer experience. Thus, paradoxically, art-making also helped me to accept and reduce stigma relating to my bodily *unboundedness* (Lawton 1998). It has also helped me develop a more constructive self and body 'I–Thou' rather than 'I–It' relationship (Buber 1970), which Turner (1975, 1982: 46, 1995) regards as an aspect of communitas.

Therapeutic liminality and containment promoted developmental oscillation between the paranoid–schizoid (separation) and depressive (reincorporation) positions (Klein 1946, 1975, 1988; Bion 1959) and thus helped me to deal with the 'shifting perspectives' dynamic of cancer experience (Paterson 2001; Thorne *et al.* 2002: 449).

All these aspects, along with processes such as supervision and personal therapy, helped me to monitor and manage the 'oscillating trajectory' and fluctuations between acute and sustained liminality (Little *et al.* 1998: 1493) and my heightened 'death salience' (Little and Sayers 2004). They helped me move to a position of beginning to practise again with such issues, whilst being aware that a significant movement toward acute liminality would render me unfit to practise again.

Arman and Rehnsfeldt (2003: 512) suggest that breast cancer nurses can find it difficult to speak about the suffering they encounter because 'both suffering and death challenge a person's individual view of the meaning of life and uncover one's own vulnerability'. Art-making helped me express my vulnerability and often voice otherwise unspeakable fears.

Thorne's (1991: 73–81) suggestion that the person-centred quality of 'tenderness' involves both one's vulnerability and one's ability for compassion provided a bridge between the personal and professional. Processing my own vulnerability was important for me as both patient and art therapist. This links to Coulehan's (1995) assertion that imaginative attention to the emotional life is vital in the therapeutic relationship which is 'at its heart an emotional connection'. He argues that practitioners need to 'unite tenderness with steadiness', that is, reason and fortitude with compassion, thus fostering their 'emotional resilience' (Coulehan 1995: 223–4).

Professional liminality

Before my own diagnosis, part of my art therapy practice was in institutions, charities and a hospital context, working with people who had been affected by cancer. Following consultations with my supervisor, some of this recommenced after my treatment was finished and I was fit enough to practise with such issues again. Both before and after my diagnosis I found it imperative to reflect on the reciprocal influence between myself and clients (Jung 1995:

57) and thus on countertransference, transference and projections. After my diagnosis it was particularly important to reflect on the relevance of my own cancer status to my practice.

Countertransference

The term countertransference is used here in a broad sense to mean what Case and Dalley (1997: 62–63) describe as 'the therapist's own feeling response to the client and the image in a therapy situation'. Schore (1999) suggests that it is a means 'by which the unconscious mind of one communicates with the unconscious mind of another'. I found it to be 'a highly important organ of information' (Jung 1995: 57). I needed to be aware that it could involve what Jung (1929: para. 365), quoted by Perry (1997: 141), described as 'unconscious infection' and 'the illness being transferred to the doctor'.

Similarly, I needed awareness that it could involve projective identification (Sedgwick 1995: 11; Perry 1997). Such projective identification 'breaks through the borders' of people present (Riskó 2001), and thus as an art therapist I could experience such projections. The therapist, acting as container, can identify with projections as if they were his/her own, thus perhaps going beyond the boundaries of empathy which Rogers (1957: 99) describes as the ability 'to sense the client's private world as if it were your own, but without ever losing the "as if" quality . . .'. Waller (2002: 7) suggests that staff working in dementia care are 'subject to massive projective identification which can be dangerous both for the staff and the patients'. Riskó *et al.* (1996) argue that oncology staff members can become the 'container' of cancer patients' 'bad objects' and 'hidden emotions' such as 'guilt, anguish, fear of death, anger and tension' and therefore staff 'frequently try to minimize patient contact (verbal and non-verbal), because these patients may have a significant effect on their emotional and psychosomatic stability'. Conversely, I needed to acknowledge my capacity to use defence mechanisms such as projection of my fears into clients, or a hypochondria-related flight into my own feared future ills to avoid being present with the client's actual current and future suffering.

Therefore, especially when working with those in liminal situations, it was vital for me, and indeed any healthcare professional, to be aware of such countertransference and projective identification dynamics and be trained and supported to contain them because otherwise patients can 'experience not the fear of dying made bearable, but a nameless dread' (Bion 1993: 116). I needed to draw on how my own art-making helped me to tolerate my own fear of dying. Clinical supervision was also an essential support in the management of my countertransference to clients and their artwork (Case and Dalley 1997).

Embodied countertransference

The embodied nature of liminality meant that 'bodily-based countertrans-ference' (Schore 1999) to clients and to 'embodied images' (Schaverien 1992) was particularly relevant in my practice. Ross (2000) suggests that therapy sessions impact on the corporeality of the psychotherapist as in 'somatic countertransference', which can be an aspect of the 'unthought known' (Bollas 1987: 282). Somatic countertransference can manifest as a physical sensation or 'felt sense' (Gendlin 1981) in the art therapist or researcher's body. Examples I experienced included feeling fear in the pit of the stomach, nausea or shame. Schaverien (2002: 136) suggests that bodily counter-transference is 'particularly difficult when working with a life-threatening illness'. She adds (2002: 141): 'When a patient is seriously ill, contamination may be an unconscious fear.' Thus it was important for me to keep working on any distortions of my own body ego as these 'must not trespass into the client's therapeutic experience' (Henley 2000: 76), and I found claywork particularly helpful in reflecting on this.

As a researcher, it was also important that I examine my own embodiment as 'an embodied, sensing, acting, socially situated participant' (Turner 2000: 53), and indeed Braud (1998: 216) suggests that consulting the wisdom of the body is part of ensuring an expanded form of validity. Inclusion of embodied awareness was congruent with my autoethnographic research approach which includes the researcher's body as a source of awareness (Ellis and Bochner 2000: 742; Spry 2001). Shaw (2001) advocates that psy-chotherapy process research should incorporate data from the researcher's embodied experience. Embodied awareness was another way of experiencing liminality for, as Spry (2001: 727) notes, autoethnographers can experience 'embodied liminality'.

Restimulation

At the potentially raw interface of tenderness and compassion (Thorne 1991) I was also vulnerable to restimulation of my own unresolved issues. Hospice contexts can evoke death anxiety (Bene and Foxall 1991) and I experienced this when visiting an ex-client, the same age as me, for the last time before her death. I had heard she was in a hospice (see Figure 4.4) and after visiting her, as we embraced and said goodbye at the door, she turned and walked away from me down the corridor. As well as all my feelings for her, I also wondered if one day my cancer would recur and I could be in the same hospice, facing my death. Another example was when I attended the funeral service of a male client in his thirties. As well as experiencing grief at the client's death, I also momentarily experienced the thought that I too could be in this crematorium after dying from cancer. I reflected that such examples of restimulation could also be attempts at self-protection through a retreat into my own sustained liminal state rather than staying present with the reality of the client's acute liminality or actual death. If such restimulation occurred when working with a client it could block my presence, thus impeding therapy. I have found personal therapy and clinical supervision vital in monitoring and trying to minimize such restimulation when with clients, yet also important in not denying my own death.

I needed to face my own death and engage in 'personal death awareness' work (Worden 2000: 133–6). Cohen (1983) suggests that psychotherapists can avoid making professional preparations in the event of their death because of the inherent anxiety involved. It was vital that I faced this and made professional plans in the event of my death.

It was also important that I be aware of and minimize the danger of aspects of my practice inappropriately restimulating my clients. For example, I tried to avoid using aprons that might restimulate their memories of hospital or theatre gowns. I was also aware of how relaxation audio tapes or directed visualizations featuring things like tunnels, sometimes used by staff in cancer care organizations, could restimulate memories of claustrophobia during MRI scans. I needed to take care with language which in other contexts could be neutral but in this context could have difficult meanings; for example, phrases like 'recurring symbol' or 'personal growth' could resonate with recurrence or tumour.

Secondary liminality

Even before my own diagnosis, my awareness of liminality was increased through practising art therapy with those in liminal situations such as those affected by cancer and in a 'betwixt and between' (Turner 1995: 95) state. This might evoke in staff and carers an experience of what might be termed 'secondary liminality', vicarious exposure to the liminality of those in liminal situations. This may be a relative of secondary traumatic stress (Stamm 1995) or the raised awareness of one's own 'actual and feared losses and existential anxiety', which those involved in grief therapy experience (Worden 2000: 134). Secondary traumatic stress can occur in art therapy (Malchiodi and Good 1998; Sweig et al. 1998) and in working with life-threatening illnesses such as cancer (Turner and Kelly 2000). Secondary liminality might differ in that it particularly relates to acute and sustained states of limbo, uncertainty, heightened fear, power and powerlessness dynamics, manifestations of play, communitas and embodied experience (Turner 1982, 1995).

Pearson (1999) researched dreams of caregivers of the dying and suggests that 'being with the dying is a liminal experience' because, like the dying, carers too are 'drawn to the border between life and death'. She quotes one minister as saying: 'Sometimes I don't know if I am with people here or there. Sometimes I feel like I've gone to the other side with them. Sometimes it's hard to come back.' Clinical oncology staff can experience repeated losses and are therefore faced with the collective impact of death as an existential fact and the cumulative grief associated with the deaths of clients (Mount 1986).

A metaphor that emerged from my experience of the cumulative impact of being a companion to the dying was that of Hermes who acted as the guide of souls (psychopomp) to Charon who then ferried the dead across the river Styx to the Underworld and who is described as 'a warden of the crossing' (Virgil 1966: 156). Interestingly, Turner (1986: 35) notes that the etymology of the word 'experience' links to meanings of 'to fear' and 'to ferry'. Stein (1983) regards Hermes as the guide of souls through liminality or threshold situations. However, what is the impact on humans taking on such a role?

It is important that art therapists and other healthcare staff acknowledge the impact of such repeating and cumulative experience. It is vital that self-care processes are normalized and encouraged in the realm of liminality, for instance communitas (Turner 1982) such as team support (Mount 1986) and 'survival bonding' (Wade and Simon 1993). A ludic (Turner 1982: 27) defence mechanism such as humour or black humour can help practitioners face yet manage liminality. Indeed, in traumatic work it can be liminal itself, for as Moran and Massam (1997) quote Janoff (1974: 303), 'Black humor cannot be described as being pessimistic or simply lacking an affirmative moral voice. Rather, it lives outside these limits in a terrain of terrifying candor concerning the most extreme situations.'

It would be important for healthcare staff dealing with liminality, and therefore susceptible to secondary liminality, to have particular training and support in managing acute, sustained and secondary liminality and its associated characteristics.

Conclusion

In reflecting on my story I found that liminality and its key characteristics were a relevant lens through which to explore my cancer experience. As Bolen (1998: 15) notes: 'When life is lived at the edge – in the border realm between life and death – it is a *liminal* time and place.' To be told one has a 'deadly disease' like cancer is to 'enter a liminal state fraught with perils that go well beyond the disease itself' (Ehrenreich 2001: 50).

Reflection on my art helped me express and process the 'oscillating trajectory' of my experience between acute and sustained liminal states (Little *et al.* 1998: 1493). Such art-making and associated rituals helped me both personally and professionally to tolerate my fear of dying and manage countertransference. Working with 'multivocal symbols' (Turner 1982: 27) and experiencing 'flow' (Turner 1982: 55–8; Csikszentmihalyi 2002) helped me process my vulnerability and 'tenderness', thus potentially fostering 'emotional resilience' (Coulehan 1995: 223–4). Similarly playing with and expanding my perception of open and fluid metaphors promoted the recontextualization of emotion and the 'generation of new meaning' contributing to 'resilience to trauma' (Modell 1997: 111).

I was also aware that my attempts to find meaning or stability needed to be viewed in the context of how humans experience the 'terror of death' (Becker 1973: 11). Terror management theory (Greenberg et al. 1986; Solomon et al. 1991) suggests that people who experience reminders of their mortality may need to 'affirm their threatened world view or self-worth' and thus self-reports of growth or benefits may 'represent self or world view protective strategies' which may be attempts to assert the belief that their life has meaning (Davis and McKearney 2001: 5–6).

Many types of illness narrative can co-exist and emerge and recede perhaps between perceived agentic and victimic poles (Polkinghorne 1996), such as those featuring curative 'restitution', unending 'chaos' and transformatory 'quest' (Frank 1997). This is dynamic, for, as Thomas-MacLean (2004) notes, the empowering nature of the 'quest' narrative can be dissolved by the chaos of recurrence; 'restitution' may not be possible in the face of incurable cancer. It is added that the term 'reconstruction narratives' may be more apt, and interestingly this inadvertently uses breast cancer terminology.

The literature and my own personal and professional experience suggests that a fluctuating state of heightened own-death/life awareness, potentially negative and positive, exists once the cancer experience is begun. Liminality 'is both more creative and more destructive than the structural norm' (Turner 1982: 47). Muzzin et al. (1994) suggest that having cancer is a 'living–dying' experience in which individuals are faced with the intolerable incompatibility of life and death.

The creative potential of liminality is that it offers a 'potential space' (Winnicott 1996: 41) in which artwork, acting as transitional objects, ritual and art-making, giving an inherent interplay of creation and destruction, helps to bridge between life and death (Gordon 2000). It can help to manage paradox, uncertainty and limbo as it develops what Keats called 'negative capability' (Rollins 1958). Thus perhaps art therapy can foster the creative potential in liminality whilst expressing and managing the destructive dynamics also inherent in liminality.

Turner (1982: 44) reminds us that liminality is 'an instant of pure potentiality when everything, as it were, trembles in the balance'. I wrote earlier that I was living or dying with cancer – the tiger. Rather then, I waver in liminality, living *and* dying with the tiger.

Note

1   My research motivation and methodology were outlined in Chapter 2. In brief, however, the auto/biographical art-based autoethnographic study was stimulated by my experiences of liminality in art-making and after cancer diagnosis. The research systematically investigated the relationship between key aspects of liminality and art therapy and my cancer experience and that of participating clients.

References

Achterberg, J. (1985) *Imagery in Healing*. Boston, MA: Shambhala.

Anzieu, D. (1989) *The Skin Ego*. New Haven, CT: Yale University Press.

Arman, M. and Rehnsfeldt, A. (2003) The hidden suffering among breast cancer patients: a qualitative metasynthesis, *Qualitative Health Research*, 13(4): 510–27.

Auden, W.H. (1994) *Collected Poems*. London: Faber and Faber.

Bach, S. (1990) *Life Paints Its Own Span*. Einziedeln, Switzerland: Daimon Verlag.

Becker, E. (1973) *The Denial of Death*. New York: Free Press.

Beckett, S. (1959) *Trilogy: Molloy, Malone Dies, The Unnamable*. London: John Calder.

Bene, B. and Foxall, M.J. (1991) Death anxiety and job stress in hospice and medical-surgical nurses, *The Hospice Journal*, 7(3): 25–41.

Berne, E. (1968) *Games People Play*. London: Penguin Books.

Bertoia, J. (1993) *Drawings from a Dying Child*. London: Routledge.

Bion, W.R. (1959) Attacks on linking, *International Journal of Psychoanalysis*, XL: 308–15.

Bion, W.R. (1993) *Second Thoughts: Selected Papers on Psychoanalysis*. London: Maresfield Library.

Bolen, J.S. (1998) *Close to the Bone: Life-Threatening Illness and the Search for Meaning*. New York: Touchstone/Simon & Schuster.

Bollas, C. (1987) *The Shadow of the Object: Psychoanalysis of the Unthought Known*. London: Free Association Books.

Braud, W. (1998) An expanded view of validity, in R. Anderson and W. Braud (eds) *Transpersonal Research Methods in the Social Sciences: Honoring Human Experience*. London: Sage Publications.

Buber, M. (1970) *I and Thou*. New York: Charles Scribner.

Caillois, R. (1962) *Man, Play and Games*. London: Thames and Hudson.

Canter, R. (2001) Patients and medical power, *British Medical Journal*, 323: 414, http://bmj.bmjjournals.com/cgi/content/full/323/7310/414 (accessed 2 August 2004).

Capra, F. (1991) *The Tao of Physics*. London: Flamingo.

Case, C. and Dalley, T. (1997) *The Handbook of Art Therapy*. London: Routledge.

Cicero, M.T. (2001) *On the Good Life* (Trans. Michael Grant). London: Penguin.

Cohen, J. (1983) Psychotherapists preparing for death: denial and action, *American Journal of Psychotherapy*, 37(2): 222–6.

Consultant surgeon (2000) Letter to GP. Unpublished personal medical records of C. Sibbett.

Cooper, J.C. (1995) *An Illustrated Encyclopaedia of Traditional Symbols*. London: Thames & Hudson.

Coulehan, J.L. (1995) Tenderness and steadiness: emotions in medical practice, *Literature and Medicine*, 14(2): 222–36.

Couser, G.T. (1991) Autopathography: women, illness, and lifewriting, *A/B: Auto/ biography Studies*, 6(1): 65–75.

Csikszentmihalyi, M. (2002) *Flow*. London: Rider.

Cunningham, A. *et al.* (1991) A relationship between perceived self-efficacy and quality of life in cancer patients, *Patient Education and Counseling*, 17: 71–8.

Davis, C.G. and McKearney, J.M. (2001) Post-traumatic growth from the perspective of terror management theory, *Running Head: Growth and Terror Management*, http://www.meaning.ca/pdf/2000proceedings/christopher_davis.pdf (accessed 13 August 2004).

Denzin, N. (1989) *Interpretive Biography*, Vol. 17. London: Sage Publications.

Ehrenreich, B. (2001) Welcome to Cancerland: a mammogram leads to a cult of pink kitsch, *Harper's Magazine*, November: 43–53. Breast Cancer Action website, http://www.bcaction.org/PDF/Harpers.pdf (accessed 13 August 2004).

Ellis, C. and Bochner, P.A. (2000) Autoethnography, personal narrative, reflexivity: researcher as subject, in N.K. Denzin and Y.S. Lincoln (eds) *Handbook of Qualitative Research*. Thousand Oaks, CA: Sage Publications.

Feneron, H. (1997) *Tiger in My Breast*. Los Altos, CA: Six Cats Press.

Frank, A.W. (1997) *The Wounded Storyteller: Body, Illness, and Ethics*. Chicago, IL: University of Chicago Press.

French, J.R.P. and Raven, B. (1959) The bases of social power, in D. Cartwright (ed.) *Studies in Social Power*. Ann Arbor, MI: Institute for Social Research.

Furth, G.M. (1988) *The Secret World of Drawings*. Boston, MA: Sigo Press.

Gardner, G. (1998) The human dimension of nosocomial wound infection: a study in liminality, *Nursing Inquiry*, 5(4): 212–19.

Geertz, C. (1988) *Works and Lives: The Anthropologist as Author*. Stanford, CA: Stanford University Press.

Gendlin, E.T. (1981) *Focusing*. New York: Bantam.

General Medical Services Committee and the Royal College of General Practitioners (1996) *Minor Surgery in General Practice: Guidance*. From the GMSC and RCGP in collaboration with Royal College of Surgeons of England, Royal College of Surgeons of Edinburgh, British Society for Dermatological Surgery, Joint Committee on Postgraduate Training for General Practice. London: GMSC and RCGP.

Glaus, A., Crow, R. and Hammond, S. (1996) A qualitative study to explore the concept of fatigue/tiredness in cancer patients and in healthy individuals, *European Journal of Cancer Care*, 5(2 Suppl.): 8–23.

Gordon, R. (2000) *Dying and Creating: A Search for Meaning*. London: H. Karnac (Books) Ltd.

Graham, R.J. (1989) Autobiography and education, *Journal of Educational Thought*, 23(2): 98–9.

Greenberg, J., Pyszczynski, T. and Solomon, S. (1986) The causes and consequences of the need for self-esteem: a terror management theory, in R.F. Baumeister (ed.) *Public Self and Private Self*. New York: Springer-Verlag.

Henley, D. (2002) *Clayworks in Art Therapy*. London: Jessica Kingsley.

Hersh, T.R. (1995) How might we explain the parallels between Freud's 1895 Irma dream and his 1923 cancer?, *Dreaming: Journal of the Association for the Study of Dreams*, 5(4): 267–87.

Janoff, B. (1974) Black humor, existentialism and absurdity: a generic confusion, *Arizona Quarterly*, 30(4): 293–304.

Jung, C.G. (1929) Problems of modern psychotherapy, in C.G. Jung, *The Practice of Psychotherapy*, Collected Works 16. London: Routledge and Kegan Paul.

Jung, C.G. (1960) *The Structure and Dynamics of the Psyche*, Collected Works 8. London: Routledge and Kegan Paul.

Jung, C.G. (1981) *Alchemical Studies*, Collected Works 13. London: Routledge and Kegan Paul.

Jung, C.G. (1995) *Modern Man in Search of a Soul*. London: Routledge.

Klein, M. (1946) Notes on some schizoid mechanisms, *International Journal of Psycho-Analysis*, 27: 99–110.

Klein, M. (1975) Infantile anxiety-situations reflected in a work of art and in the creative impulse, *The Writings of Melanie Klein*, Vol.1: *Love, Guilt and Reparation and Other Works*. London: Hogarth Press/Institute of Psychoanalysis.

Klein, M. (1988) *Envy and Gratitude and Other Works, 1946–1963*. London: Virago Press.

Lawton, J. (1998) Contemporary hospice care: the sequestration of the unbounded body and 'dirty dying', *Sociology of Health & Illness*, 20(2): 121–43.

LeShan, L. (1996) *Cancer as a Turning Point*. Bath: Gateway Books.

Little, M. and Sayers, E. (2004) While there's life . . .: hope and the experience of cancer, *Social Science & Medicine*, 59(6): 1329–37.

Little, M., Jordens, C.F., Paul, K., Montgomery, K. and Philipson, B. (1998) Liminality: a major category of the experience of cancer illness, *Social Science & Medicine*, 47(10): 1492–3.

Malchiodi, C.A. (1998) *The Art Therapy Sourcebook*. Los Angeles, CA: Lowell House.

Malchiodi, C.A. and Good, D. (1998) Secondary traumatic stress: self-care, self-empowerment, and authenticity. Paper presented at the 1998 American Art Therapy Association (AATA) Conference, Portland, November 1998. Audiotape No. 34. Denver, CO: National Audio Video Inc.

Mango, C. (1992) Emma: art therapy illustrating personal and universal images of loss, *Omega: Journal of Death and Dying*, 25(4): 259–69.

Martel, Y. (2003) *Life of Pi*. Edinburgh: Canongate Books Ltd.

Medical–legal expert (2001) Medical–legal report. Consultant clinical oncologist/expert witness. Unpublished personal medical–legal records of C. Sibbett.

MHI (2002) Medical glossary, *Med Help International*, http://www.medhelp.org/ (accessed 13 August 2004).

Modell, A.H. (1997) The synergy of memory, affects and metaphor, *The Journal of Analytical Psychology*, 42(1): 105–17.

Moran, C. and Massam, M. (1997) An evaluation of humour in emergency work, *The Australasian Journal of Disaster and Trauma Studies*, 1997–3, http://www.massey.ac.nz/~trauma/issues/1997–3/moran1.htm (accessed 13 August 2004).

Mount, B.M. (1986) Dealing with our losses, *Journal of Clinical Oncology*, 4: 1127–34.

Muzzin, L.J. *et al.* (1994) The experience of cancer, *Social Science & Medicine*, 38(9): 1201–8.

Palmer, P.L. (1998) *The Courage to Teach: Exploring the Inner Landscape of a Teacher's Life*. San Francisco, CA: Jossey-Bass.

Paterson, B.L. (2001) The shifting perspectives model of chronic illness, *Image: Journal of Nursing Scholarship*, 33(1): 21–6.

Pearson, C. (1999) Dreaming in a liminal time. Paper presented at the Annual Conference of the Association for the Study of Dreams, University of California at Santa Cruz, July 7, http://nauticom.net/www/pstubbs/pcdream.html (accessed 2 August 2004).

Penson, R.T. *et al.* (2001) Medical mistakes: a workshop on personal perspectives, *The Oncologist*, 6(1): 92–99, http://theoncologist.alphamedpress.org/cgi/content/full/6/1/92 (accessed 13 August 2004).

Perry, C. (1997) Transference and countertransference, in P. Young-Eisendrath and T. Dawson (eds) *The Cambridge Companion to Jung*. Cambridge: Cambridge University Press.

Philip, C.P.C. (2002) The white coat ceremony: turning trust into entitlement, *Teaching and Learning in Medicine*, 14(1): 56–59.

Pickett, J.P. *et al.* (eds) (2000) 'steig-', *The American Heritage Dictionary of the English Language*. Boston: Houghton Mifflin Company, http://www.bartleby.com/61/roots/IE498.html (accessed 2 August 2004).

Polkinghorne, D. (1996) Transformative narratives: from victimic to agentic life plots, *American Journal of Occupational Therapy*, 50(4): 299–305.

Riskó, Á. (2001) Close to the body. Lost Childhood International Conference, Ferenczi Sándor Society, Budapest, 23–25 February. *Onkopszichológia Online*, http://www.oncol.hu/psicho/index.html (accessed 13 August 2004).

Riskó, Á., Deák, B., Molnár, Z., Schneider, T., Várady, E. and Rosta, A. (1998) Individual, psychoanalytically oriented psychotherapy during oncological treatment with adolescents suffering from malignant lymphoma. 4th International Congress of Psycho-Oncology, Hamburg, Germany, 3–6 September. *Onkopszichológia Online*, http://www.oncol.hu/psicho/index.html (accessed 13 August 2004).

Riskó, Á., Fleischmann, T., Molnár, Z., Schneider, T. and Várady, E. (1996) Influence of the pathological psychological state of cancer patients on their decisions, *Supportive Care In Cancer*, 4(1): 51–5, *Onkopszichológia Online*, http://www.oncol.hu/psicho/index.html (accessed 13 August 2004).

Rogers, C. (1957) The necessary and sufficient conditions of therapeutic personality change, *Journal of Counselling Psychology*, 21: 95–103.

Rollins, H.E. (ed.) (1958) Letter to George and Tom Keats, 21 December 1817, in *The Letters of J. Keats: 1814–1821*. Cambridge: Cambridge University Press.

Ross, M. (2000) Body talk: somatic countertransference, *Psychodynamic Counselling*, 6(4): 451–67.

Saint-Exupéry, Antoine de (1971) *The Little Prince*. New York: Harvest/Harcourt Brace & Co.

Schaverien, J. (1992) *The Revealing Image: Analytical Art Psychotherapy in Theory and Practice*. London: Routledge.

Schaverien, J. (2002) *The Dying Patient in Psychotherapy*. Basingstoke: Palgrave Macmillan.

Schore, A.N. (1999) The right brain, the right mind, and psychoanalysis, *Neuro-Psychoanalysis*, 1(1): 49–54, Commentary. University of California at Los Angeles School of Medicine. Included in Schore, A.N. (2003) *Affect Regulation and the Repair of the Self*. New York: W. W. Norton & Company, http://www.neuro-psa.com/schore.htm (accessed 13 August 2004).

Sedgwick, D. (1995) *The Wounded Healer: Countertransference from a Jungian Perspective*. London: Routledge.

Self, M. (1999) The sharp edge of Damocles, *Student BMJ*, March, 7: 85, http://www.studentbmj.com/back_issues/0399/data/0399pv1.htm (accessed 27 July 2004).

Shaw, R. (2001) The embodied psychotherapist: an exploration of the therapist's somatic phenomena within the therapeutic encounter. Paper presented at BACP Research Conference, Bristol, 18–19 May.

Skott, C. (2002) Expressive metaphors in cancer narratives, *Cancer Nursing*, 25(3): 230–5.

Slattery, P. (2001) The educational researcher as artist working within, *Qualitative Inquiry*, 20 June, 7(3): 370–98, http://www.coe.tamu.edu/~pslattery/documents/QualitativeInquiry.pdf (accessed 2 August 2004).

Solomon, S., Greenberg, J. and Pyszczynski, T. (1991) A terror management theory of social behavior: the psychological function of self-esteem and cultural world views, in M. Zanna (ed.) *Advances in Experimental Social Psychology*, 24. San Diego, CA: Academic Press.

Souter, K.T. (2002) Medical technology and the clinical encounter, *Psychoanalysis Downunder*, 2 (April), http://www.psychoanalysisdownunder.com/PADPapers/medical_technol_kts.htm (accessed 13 August 2004).

Spry, T. (2001) Performing autoethnography: an embodied methodological praxis, *Qualitative Inquiry*, 7(6): 706–32.

Stamm, B.H. (ed.) (1995) *Secondary Traumatic Stress: Self-care Issues for Clinicians, Researchers, and Educators*. Lutherville, MD: Sidran Press.

Stanley, L. (1992) *The Auto/Biographical I*. Manchester: Manchester University Press.

Stein, M. (1983) *In MidLife: A Jungian Perspective*. Dallas, TX: Spring Publications.

Sweig, T.L., O'Rourke, R., Sarnoff, J.R. and Ursprung, W.A. (1998) Vicarious traumatization and the creative therapist: personal perspectives on the clinical underworld. Panel at the American Art Therapy Association (AATA) Conference, Portland, November. Audiotape No. 36. Denver, CO: National Audio Video Inc.

Thomas-MacLean, R. (2004) Understanding breast cancer stories via Frank's narrative types, *Social Science & Medicine*, 58(9): 1647–57.

Thorne, B. (1991) The quality of tenderness, in B. Thorne (ed.) *Person-Centred Counselling: Therapeutic and Spiritual Dimensions*. London: Whurr Publishers.

Thorne, S. *et al.* (2002) Chronic illness experience: insights from a metastudy, *Qualitative Health Research*, 12(4): 437–52.

Turner, A. (2000) Embodied ethnography: doing culture, *Social Anthropology*, 8(1): 51–60.

Turner, J. and Kelly, B. (2000) The concept of debriefing and its application to staff dealing with life-threatening illnesses such as cancer, AIDS and other conditions, in B. Raphael and J. Wilson (eds) *Psychological Debriefing: Theory, Practice and Evidence*. Cambridge: Cambridge University Press.

Turner, V.W. (1967) *The Forest of Symbols: Aspects of Ndembu Ritual*. Ithaca, NY: Cornell University Press.

Turner, V.W. (1975) *Dramas, Fields, and Metaphors: Symbolic Action in Human Society*. Ithaca, NY: Cornell University Press.

Turner, V.W. (1982) *From Ritual to Theatre: The Human Seriouness of Play*. New York: Performing Arts Journal Publications.

Turner, V.W. (1986) Dewey, Dilthey, and drama: an essay in the anthropology of experience, in V. Turner and E. Bruner (eds) *The Anthropology of Experience*. Champaign, IL: University of Illinois Press.

Turner, V.W. (1988) *The Anthropology of Performance*. New York: Performing Arts Journal Publications.

Turner, V.W. (1995) *The Ritual Process: Structure and Anti-Structure*. New York: Aldine de Gruyter.

van Gennep, A. (1960) *The Rites of Passage*. London: Routledge & Kegan Paul.

Virgil (1966) *The Aeneid*. Harmondsworth: Penguin.

Wade, K. and Simon, E.P. (1993) Survival bonding: a response to stress and work with AIDS, *Social Work Health Care*, 19(1): 77–89.

Waller, D. (1983) Art therapy as a creative therapy, *Self and Society, European Journal of Humanistic Psychology*, XI (4): 187–91.

Waller, D. (ed.) (2002) *Arts Therapies and Progressive Illness: Nameless Dread*. Hove: Brunner-Routledge.

Winnicott, D.W. (1996) *Playing and Reality*. London: Routledge.

Worden, W. (2000) *Grief Counselling and Grief Therapy*. London: Routledge.

Wyman-McGinty, W. (1998) The body in analysis: authentic movement and witnessing in analytic practice, *Journal of Analytical Psychology*, 43(2): 239–61.

Index

Page numbers in *italics* refer to figures and tables; *passim* indicates numerous scattered references within page range.

abstract designs 140
Achterberg, J. *et al.* 15
acute and sustained liminality 235–6
adaptability of therapists 212–13
adolescence
    case study 139–48
    identity development theories
        137–9
advertising/media 43–4, 46
agôn (competition/contest) 25–6,
    232
alea (fate/chance) 24–5, 231–2
anger
    in adolescence 139, 140, 142
    expression of 106, 107, 108–9,
        114, 142, 143, 217, 221
    'negative behaviours' 123–4
    towards medical staff 215–16,
        217
anti-group defence mechanism
    177–9, 182
anxiety
    death 175, 181, 238
    institutional 179–82
    see also stress
Anzieu, D. 233
aprons 22, 239
art materials 213–15
art therapists
    adaptability 212–13

and artists 83–4, 85
    frustrations 204–7
    isolation 200–1, 206
    motivations 211
    personal experience of cancer
        223–41
    rewards 203–4, 207–8, 211
    stresses 200–1, 207
    uncertainty 212, 221–2
    see also therapeutic relationship;
        therapists
arts and healthcare 83–5
Asian client, case study 192–4
Athern, J. and Madill, A. 27
Auden, W.H. 234
autoethnographic studies 12–13,
    223

Bakhtin, M.M. 20–1, 55, 65, 67
Balint, M. 191
Beaver, V. 187, 204, 204–5
Beckett, S. 234
Belfiore, M. 199, 200
Bell, S. 204
Bion, W.R. 27, 67, 68, 164, 177,
    178, 234, 236, 237
blood and womanhood 105, 106
body image 43, 55–7, 104–5
body outline exercise 217

body/ies
  inscribed 59–60
  modification 45–7
  objectification 8–9, 43–7
  souls and identity 48–9
  visible 43–4
  see also entries beginning
    embodied
Bolen, J.S. 13, 19, 25, 70, 240
Bolton, G. 84
bone marrow aspiration (BMA)
  120, 121–2
bone marrow transplant (BMT)
  125
Borgmann, E. 51
Bourdieu, P. 60–2
breast cancer, case studies 102–18,
  215–18
brief psychodynamic
  psychotherapy 129
British Association of Art
  Therapists 90

Caillois, R. 22–3, 24–5, 27, 69,
  231, 232, 235
capitalism 41, 42
Case, C. 129
  and Dalley, T. 17, 196, 237
Casement, P. 216
childlessness 234–5
child(ren)
  benefits of art therapy 120–1
  death of (image) 169
  pain control 121–4
  terminal phase 124–6
  see also parent–child
    relationships
chronotope (time space) 20–1, 55
clay
  breast 103, 105, 218
  female figure 104–5, 234
  foot 53
  pain relief 53, 104
clinical governance 93–4, 96–7
collage 141, 145–6, 167–8, 218
  'self-collage' 227, 231
colours 26
communitas 15, 28–30, 232–3

Connell, C. 21, 91, 93, 128–9,
  129–30, 185–6, 189, 190, 195,
  196, 203
consciousness 8, 9, 48, 49, 60
consent see permission
constructive liminality 69
containment
  artwork as 27–8, 67–8
  and bodily 'unboundedness'
    57–9, 69, 236
Coote, J. 85, 129, 187, 206–7
countertransference 189–91,
  237–9
  see also transference–
    countertransference
Csikszentmihalyi, M. 19, 28, 240
cultural defence mechanisms 69
cultural embodiment 60–2
Cunningham, A. et al. 21, 230
cure
  of children 120
  group factors 173–5

dance 155, 159
death
  anxiety 175, 181, 238
  awareness/'death salience'
    232–3, 236, 239
  confronting 114
  and dying 1–11
  group work (images) 166–70
defence mechanisms
  anti-group 177–9, 182
  body image, case study 104–5
  'compass of shame' model 66,
    67
  cultural 69
  denial 181, 190–1, 201, 202–3
  institutional 180–1, 200, 201,
    202–3, 240
  resistance 39, 42, 48, 175–7
denial 181, 190–1, 201, 202–3
Department of Health (DoH)
  86–90
depressive position 68, 236
diagnosis
  art therapist's personal
    experience 228–30

missed 225–6, 230–1
psychotherapeutic theory of
    response 67–8, 69
see also embodied liminality;
    liminal(ity)
disengagement 4–5
doll, use of 122–3
Douglas, M. 55, 57–8, 65
drawings (case studies)
    Jill 158, 159–61
    Mary 141–2, 144
    Mrs Verdier 114–15
    single session 130–1, 132,
        133–4
dreams 64, 166–8, 226, 227–8
    of caregivers 239
Dreifuss-Kattan, E. 20, 25
Dyer, A.R. 15, 17

Edwards, D. 200–1
ego defences see defence
    mechanisms
Ellis, C. and Bochner, P.A. 12–13,
    223, 235, 238
embodied boundaries 57–9
embodied countertransference
    237–8
embodied experience 16, 51,
    233–5
embodied liminality
    expression 52, 55, 64–7
    physicality 51, 52–5
    sexual embodiment 52,
        62–4
    structural inferiority and power
        52, 55–62
emotional perspective, group
    work 153
empowerment through art therapy
    22, 231
enactment through gestures
    109
endings, importance of 97
energizing effect of art therapy
    53–4
engagement 6
evaluation and research
    by therapist 93, 96–7

literature review 85–91,
    128–30, 185–7, 199–208
expression 52, 55, 64–7
    of anger 106, 107, 108–9, 114,
        142, 143, 217, 221
    of grief 105

'false self' 200
family 220, 221
    responses to illness 3–5
    see also specific family
        relationships
father–daughter relationship, case
    study 106–7, 108, 110–13,
        114, 115, 116
fatigue 53–4
Favara-Scacco, C. et al.
    121–2
fear of annihilation see anxiety;
    defence mechanisms
female figures 104–5, 234, 235
femininity 63
    blood and 105, 106
    see also breast cancer, case studies
flow 19, 20, 28
flowers 132, 154, 159
Foucault, M. 18, 19, 20, 55, 56,
    58, 67
freedom 44–5, 47
Freud, S. 8, 56, 104, 166, 177
friends/peers
    in adolescence 138, 139, 140,
        143, 144, 145
    responses to illness 3–5
frustrations of therapists 204–7

gateways, visual metaphor
    220–1
Geertz, C. 60, 224
Gestalt Therapy 203
gestures, enactment through 109
Goffman, E. 29, 38, 56
Gordon, R. 191
grief, expression of 105
group work themes
    fear of annihilation 172–84
    Healing Journey 149–62
    musings about death 163–71

group(s)
  benefits 152, 173–5
  composition 155, 158–61,
    172–3, 176–7
  creative process 156–7
  defence mechanisms 175–9, 182
  images about death 166–70
  institutional anxiety 179–82
  key issues 151–2
  perspectives 152–3
  programme 149, 150–1,
    153–61
  readings 155
  rules 165–6
  screening process 156
  settings 153–4, 165, 173,
    179–80
  therapist's role 182–3
'Growth, positive, expanding'
    image 144–5
guided imagery 156, 157

habitas/hexis 60–2
hair loss 63–4, 122–3, 158,
    234
Halton, W. 180
Halvorson-Boyd, G. and Hunter,
    L.K. 16, 25
Hardy, D. 129
Healing Journey, group work
    149–62
healthcare, arts and 83–5
heterotopias 18, 19, 20, 58
HIV, case study 192–4
hospices
  Marie Curie Hospice, London
    91–7
  see also institutional issues

identity 7–8, 43, 48–9
  development theories 137–9
  social construction of 39–42
  see also independence;
    individualism
ilinx (vertigo) 27, 232
independence 47
individual sessions 92, 95–6
individualism 42–3

individuation, adolescent
    separation and 137–9
inner critic drawing 144
inscribed body 59–60
isolation of therapists 200–1,
    206
institutional issues 199–203
  anxiety 179–82
  defences 180–1, 200, 201,
    202–3, 240
  identity 38, 39, 41–2
    contradictions 42–3
  values 7

Jaspers, K. 27, 66
Jung, C.G. 26, 65, 119, 164, 227,
    236–7

kairos (opportunity) 19–20
Kavuri, S. 25
Klein, M. 67, 68, 181, 236
Kleinman, A. 15, 16, 52
Klement, V. 69

Lakoff, G. and Johnson, M. 17
Langellier, K.M. 63
Lawton, J. 57–8, 69, 236
Learmouth, M. 133, 134, 221
limbo 15, 16–18, 222, 224–30
liminal(ity)
  cancer experience 14, 30–1
  characteristics 15
  communitas 15, 28–30, 232–3
  constructive 69
  definition 13
  limbo 15, 16–18, 222, 224–30
  managing acute and sustained
    235–6
  metaphors 17–18, 18–19, 82–3,
    220–1, 240
  personal 224–41
  playing 15, 22–8, 69, 231–2
  power/powerlessness 15, 21–2,
    24–7, 230–1
  professional 236–40
  rites of passage 14, 26, 67–8
  secondary 239–40
  space 18–19

time   19–21
see also embodied liminality
literature review   85–91, 128–30,
     185–7, 199–208
Little, M. *et al.*   13, 14, 16, 19, 21,
     25, 27, 30, 55–6, 65, 68, 70,
     71, 224, 230, 235, 236, 240
loved ones
     death of (images)   168–70
     see also family; friends/peers;
         specific family relationships
lumbar puncture (LP)   120, 121–2,
     124
Luzzatto, P.   104, 124, 186–7,
     187–8, 195, 217
     and Gabriel, B.   128, 129
Lyth, I.M.   180

McNiff, S.   25, 26, 27, 29, 146
Macquarrie, J.   51, 66
Malchiodi, C.A.   21, 138–9, 226
mandalas   139, 141, 142
Marie Curie Hospice, London
     91–7
Marx, K.   8–9, 39, 41, 46
masculinity   62–3
media/advertising   43–4, 46
medical/nursing staff   200–2, 239,
     241
     anger towards   215–16, 217
Meeks, J.E. and Bernet, W.   137–8
metaphors   216, 229
     liminality   17–18, 18–19, 82–3,
         220–1, 240
methodology, autoethnographic
     study   13
Miller, B.   18, 53, 66
mimicry   24, 231
Minar, V.M.   143–4
mind–body relationship   102, 159
mirror metaphor   18–19
missed diagnosis   225–6, 230–1
mobile graffiti board   92, 93–4
Montgomery, C.   29
mother–daughter relationships
     169
     case studies
         Felicia   122–3

Mary   139–40, 141–2, 145,
     148
Mrs Verdier   105–6, 107, 113,
     115–16
Rita   123
see also parent–child
     relationships
motivations of therapists   211
multi-sensory experience   54–5
multiple sessions   215–21
Muuss, R.E.   138
Muzzin, L.J. *et al.*   15–16, 55, 229,
     241
Myerhoff, B.   29
     et al.   55, 56, 64

Nathanson, D.   66, 67
National Institute for Clinical
     Excellence (NICE)   86–90,
     205
Navon, L. and Morag, A.   62–3
'negative behaviours'   123–4
NHS Care Plan   86
NHS settings
     multiple sessions   215–21
     therapist's perspective
         211–13
     see also single sessions
Nitsun, M.   173–4, 177, 178
nursing staff *see* medical/nursing
     staff

object relations theory   138–9
     cancer experience   67–8, 69
     transitional objects   27–8, 65,
         124
objectification of body   8–9,
     43–7
open art therapy studio   92, 94–5
'ordeals'   53–4
organizational issues *see*
     institutional issues
Owoc, M.A.   26

pain   52–3
     supporting children in   121–4
     therapeutic effects of clay
         modelling   53, 104

paintings
case studies 214–15
James 219–21
Mrs Verdier 106, 107,
108–10, 111, 112–13
images from dreams 166–7
paper tree 125
paranoid-schizoid position 67,
181, 236
parent–child relationships
in adolescence 137–9
case studies 125–6, 130–1,
158–9
see also father–daughter
relationship, case study;
mother–daughter relationships
peers see friends/peers
performance art 146
permission
to exhibit art 85
to play 23–4
personal liminality 224–41
photography 140–1, 147
collage 141, 145–6
physical perspective, group work
152
physicality 51, 52–5
playing 15, 22–8, 69, 231–2
post-treatment outcomes
147
power
father–daughter relationship,
case study 110–11
and powerlessness 15, 21–2,
24–7, 230–1
structural inferiority and 52,
55–62
Pratt, M. 175
and Wood, M.J.M. 187
prodromal symbols 226–8
professional liminality 236–40
projective identification 67–8, 69,
181, 237
psychodynamic psychotherapy
brief 129
theories of self 40
see also object relations theory;
therapeutic relationship;

transference; transference-
countertransference
psychological perspective, group
work 153
puppet, use of 122

rebellion see resistance
referral 206, 207
self-referral 207, 215
research see evaluation and research
resistance 39, 42, 48
in therapy group 175–7
restimulating 238–9
revelatory expression 65–7
'reverie' 28
rewards of therapists 203–4,
207–8, 211
Riskó, A. 237
et al. 17, 67, 229, 237
rites of passage 14, 26, 67–8
see also liminal(ity)
ritual(s) 14–15, 20
redefinitional 29, 68
'ritual powers' 231
threshold art symbols 25
Rogers C.R. 23, 237
Rogers, N. 53, 54

sacred circle dance 155
sacred space 153–4
sand pictures 213
visual impairment 214
scapegoat, artwork as 27–8
scars 59–60
Schaverien, J. 22, 25, 27, 56, 65,
96, 129, 188, 190, 192,
199–200, 203, 204, 231, 233,
237, 238
Schechner, R. 14, 20
Schore, A.N. 60, 237
scientific perspectives 8, 9, 10,
40–1, 48
Searles, H. 190, 191, 195
secondary liminality
239–40
Segal, J. 69
self 40, 41–2
'false self' 200

see also identity; independence; individualism
self image *see* body image
Self, M.   17, 229
'self-collage'   227, 231
self-referral   207, 215
'self-supervision'   216
separation, adolescent   137–9
settings   204–5
  group work   153–4, 165, 173, 179–80
  see also NHS settings
sexual embodiment   52, 62–4
shame   66, 67
Shoreline (group work project)   82–101
silence, group   165
silencing the therapist   178, 182
silk paints   214
Simon, R.M.   18, 19, 26, 28
single sessions   128–30, 134–5
  art materials   213–15
  case studies   130–4
Skaife, S.   188–9, 190, 195, 202
  and Huet, V.   15, 174
social act of dying   5
social construction of identity   39–42
social and institutional values   7
social support *see* communitas
sociological theories of identity   40
soul   41, 48–9
space
  liminal   18–19
  sacred   153–4
  time space (chronotope)   20–1, 55
Speck, P.   181, 200, 201, 202
spiritual perspective, group work   153
splitting   67, 69, 181
Stacey, J.   96
staff *see* institutional issues; medical/nursing staff
Stanley, L.   13, 50, 223, 224
stigma, body image and   55–7
Stokes, A.   65, 178, 179, 181

stress
  art therapists   200–1, 207
  medical staff   200–1
  see also anxiety
superstition   25
supervision of therapists   196, 207, 236, 237, 238–9
  'self-supervision'   216
symbolic component of art   185–6
symbolic objects   27–8
symbols   26, 65
  prodromal   226–8
Symington, N.   181
Synnott, A.   50, 51, 55

talismans   25, 231
teamwork   206
therapeutic methods   91–7
therapeutic process   67–8
therapeutic relationship   139, 191–2
  case study   215–18
  beginnings   212–13
  endings   97
  see also transference
therapists
  collusion in defence mechanisms   182–3, 190–1
  NHS settings   211–13
  role in group work   182–3
  silencing of   178, 182
  supervision of   196, 207, 236, 237, 238–9
  'self-supervision'   216
  see also art therapists
'third way' approach   164
time, liminal   19–21
time space (chronotope)   20–1, 55
touch   54–5
traditional societies   9–10, 25, 26
transference   187–9
  case studies   192–6, 219–20
  countertransference   189–91, 237–9
transference–countertransference   64, 135, 202, 203
  single sessions   129–30
  case studies   130–4

transitional objects   27–8, 65, 124
transitional states *see* embodied
    liminality; liminality
tree(s)   145, 160
  paper   125
  'self-collage'   227, 231
Turner, V.W.   14–30 *passim*,
    50–71 *passim*, 223–41 *passim*

'unboundedness'   57–9, 69,
    236
uncertainty   212, 221–2
'unthought known'   226, 228,
    237–8

Van Gennep, A.   14, 50, 55, 58,
    223
'verbal feedback'   166
'verbal sharing'   166
visible bodies   43–4
'visual feedback'   166
'visual sharing'   165

vulnerability and mortality
    (images)   170

Walter, T.   175, 176, 183
Weber, M.   5, 8, 41
White, E.C.   19–20
White, M.   29
  and Epston, D.   18, 70
Wilson, B.   22
Wilson, L.   143
Winnicott, D.   23, 27, 28, 29, 56,
    120, 124, 139, 200, 241
Wood, M.   51, 56, 63–4, 85, 96,
    102, 128, 129, 186, 188, 200,
    201, 204, 205, 206
wounded storyteller   224

Yalom, I.D.   173–4, 178–9, 188,
    190–1, 191–2, 195, 201
Young, R.M.   27, 190, 191, 195

Zammit, C.   174

LOSS, CHANGE AND BEREAVEMENT IN PALLIATIVE CARE

Pam Firth, Gill Luff and David Oliviere

- How do professionals meet the needs of bereaved people?
- How do professionals undertake best practice with individuals, groups, families and communities?
- What are the implications for employing research to influence practice?

This book provides a resource for working with a complex range of loss situations and includes chapters on childhood bereavement, and individual and family responses to loss and change. It contains the most up-to-date work in the field presented by experienced practitioners and researchers and is relevant not only for those working in specialist palliative care settings, but for professionals in general health and social care sectors.

Strong links are maintained between research and good practice throughout the book. These are reinforced by the coherent integration of international research material and the latest thinking about loss and bereavement. Experts and clinicians draw upon their knowledge and practice, whilst the essential perspective of the service user is central to this book.

Loss, Change and Bereavement in Palliative Care provides essential reading for a range of professional health and social care disciplines practising at postgraduate or post-registration/qualification level. It challenges readers, at an advanced level, on issues of loss, change and bereavement.

Contributors
Lesley Adshead, Jenny Altschuler, Peter Beresford, Grace H. Christ, Suzy Croft, Pam Firth, Shirley Firth, Richard Harding, Felicity Hearn, Jennie Lester, Gill Luff, Linda Machin, Jan McLaren, David Oliviere, Ann Quinn, Phyllis R. Silverman, Jean Walker, Karen Wilman.

Contents
Notes on the contributors – Series editor's preface – Acknowledgements – Foreword – Introduction – The context of loss, change and bereavement in palliative care – Mourning: a changing view – Research in practice – Illness and loss within the family – Life review with the terminally ill – Narrative therapies – The death of a child – Interventions with bereaved children – Involving service users in palliative care: from theory to practice – Excluded and vulnerable groups of service users – Carers: current research and developments – Groupwork in palliative care – Cultural perspectives on loss and bereavement – Conclusions – Index.

240pp   0 335 21323 5 (Paperback)   0 335 21324 3 (Hardback)

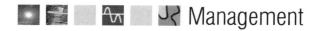
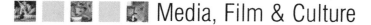
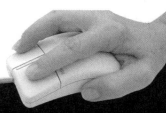